CULTURES OF PLAGUE

Cultures of Plague

Medical Thinking at the End of the Renaissance

SAMUEL K. COHN, Jr

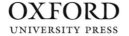

OXFORD
UNIVERSITY PRESS

OXFORD

UNIVERSITY PRESS

Great Clarendon Street, Oxford OX2 6DP

Oxford University Press is a department of the University of Oxford.
It furthers the University's objective of excellence in research, scholarship,
and education by publishing worldwide in

Oxford New York

Auckland Cape Town Dar es Salaam Hong Kong Karachi
Kuala Lumpur Madrid Melbourne Mexico City Nairobi
New Delhi Shanghai Taipei Toronto

With offices in

Argentina Austria Brazil Chile Czech Republic France Greece
Guatemala Hungary Italy Japan Poland Portugal Singapore
South Korea Switzerland Thailand Turkey Ukraine Vietnam

Oxford is a registered trade mark of Oxford University Press
in the UK and in certain other countries

Published in the United States
by Oxford University Press Inc., New York

© Samuel K. Cohn, Jr 2010

The moral rights of the authors have been asserted
Database right Oxford University Press (maker)

First published 2010
First published in paperback 2011

British Library Cataloguing in Publication Data

Data available

Library of Congress Cataloging in Publication Data

Cohn, Samuel Kline.
Cultures of plague : medical thinking at the end of the Renaissance / Samuel K. Cohn Jr.
p. ; cm.
Includes bibliographical references and index.
ISBN 978–0–19–957402–5 (hardback : alk. paper) 1. Epidemics—Italy—History. 2. Plague—Italy—History.
3. Medicine, Medieval—Italy. 4. Public health—Italy. I. Title.
[DNLM: 1. Disease Outbreaks—history—Italy. 2. Plague—history—Italy. 3. History, Early Modern
1451–1600—Italy. 4. History, Medieval—Italy. 5. Public Health—history—Italy. WC 11 GI8 C678c 2009]
RA650.6.I8C64 2009
614.5′732—dc22   2009026994

Typeset by Laserwords Private Limited, Chennai, India
Digitally printed and bound in Great Britain by
CPI Antony Rowe, Chippenham and Eastbourne

ISBN 978–0–19–957402–5 (Hbk)
ISBN 978–0–19–960509–5 (Pbk)

Dedicated to the Librarians of Edit 16

Contents

Acknowledgements

Made possible through a project grant from the Wellcome Trust (Grant no. 079190), this book benefited from the kindness and professionalism of librarians in fifty rare book rooms and archives from Palermo to Berkeley. The most intense period of research was conducted in Rome, when I was a visiting professor in March 2007. I wish to thank the director of the American Academy in Rome, Camilla Franklin, the head librarian, Christina Huemer, and others among the staff and fellows, who made my stay productive and pleasant. Professor Guido Alfani helped with photographing documents in Milan and Turin and with his detailed information of early modern Italy. In addition, I wish to thank Alexandra Bamji for sharing her knowledge of seventeenth-century plague in Italy and for reading drafts of Chapter 9 and the conclusion, to Colin Miller, FRCA, who read Chapter 2, criticizing it from a medical perspective, to Debra Strickland for reading the preface and other sections that I found stylistically problematic, to Tom Laqueur, who read and discussed sections from his broad knowledge of nineteenth- and twentieth-century medicine, and to Jane Stevens Crawshaw and Aaron Shakow for corrections for the paperback version. I thank Professors Rudolph Binion, Bryan Dick, Paula Findlen, Vivian Nutton, and the anonymous readers of Oxford University Press, who read critically the entire manuscript. In addition to correcting errors, they forced me to rethink my positions at every turn. I thank Rupert Cousens and Seth Cayley at Oxford University Press for their patience and encouragement. Finally, this book is dedicated to the efforts of Italy's research librarians over the past several decades and their ongoing census of imprints, 'Edit 16'. Without their work this and many other scholarly works based on sixteenth-century imprints would be much more difficult, timely, and expensive to complete.

RARE BOOK ROOMS CONSULTED

France

Bibliothèque nationale de France (Paris)
Bibliothèque Sainte-Geneviève (Paris)

UK

British Library
Cambridge University Library

National Library of Scotland, Edinburgh
Special Collections, Hunterian, University of Glasgow
Wellcome Library, London

USA

Bancroft Library, Berkeley, California
Countway Library, Harvard Medical School
Houghton, Harvard University
National Library of Medicine, Bethesda, Maryland (microfilm collection)
Robins Collection, Berkeley, California

Vatican City

Biblioteca Apostolica Vaticana

Italy
Bergamo

Biblioteca civica e archivi storici 'Angelo Mai'

Bologna

Biblioteca comunale dell'Archiginnasio
Biblioteca universitaria

Borgomanero

Biblioteca pubblica e Casa della cultura. Fondazione Achille Marazza

Chiavari

Biblioteca della Società economica

Florence

Archivio di Stato
Biblioteca Berenson (Villa I Tatti)
Biblioteca Biomedica (Careggi)
Biblioteca nazionale centrale
Biblioteca umanistica, Sede di Lettere
Laboratorio di ristauro e libri alluvionati di Sant'Ambrogio (BNCF)

Genoa

Biblioteca civica Berio

Jesi

Biblioteca comunale Planettiana

Lucca

Biblioteca statale

Milan

Archivio di Stato
Biblioteca nazionale Braidense

Naples

Biblioteca nazionale Vittorio Emanuele III

Palermo

Biblioteca comunale

Pavia

Biblioteca Universitaria

Perugia

Biblioteca comunale Augusta

Pisa

Biblioteca Universitaria

Rome

Biblioteca Angelica
Biblioteca Casanatense
Biblioteca dell'Academia nazionale dei Lincei e Corsiniana
Biblioteca della Pontificia Facoltà teologica Marianum
Biblioteca nazionale centrale
Biblioteca romana Antonio Sarti
Biblioteca universitaria Alessandrina
Biblioteca Vallicelliana

Trent

Biblioteca Comunale

Turin

Biblioteca civica centrale
Biblioteca dell'Archivio di Stato di Torino
Biblioteca nazionale universitaria
Biblioteca Reale

Urbania

Biblioteca Comunale

Venice

Biblioteca nazionale Marciana

Verona

Archivio di Stato
Biblioteca civica

List of Maps, Figures, Tables, and Illustrations

Map

Figures

Tables

Illustrations

Introduction

The Black Death of 1348 ushered in a new form of medical writing, the plague tract,[1] which, according to the medical historian Arturo Castiglioni, became by the fifteenth century the first form of popular literature in the West.[2] Until the plague crisis of 1575–8 (often called the plague of San Carlo), these were written in Italy almost exclusively by academically trained physicians and only rarely by surgeons or clerics (usually bishops). In the fourteenth and fifteenth centuries they could either concentrate on preventative measures, on remedies, or both.[3] These ranged from highly philosophical tracts based on theology or astrology, aimed at explaining the 'superior causes' of human history and disasters, to straightforward lists of plague recipes to protect or cure the individual from plague.[4] Though not the earliest, the *Compendium* or *Report of the Medical Faculty of Paris*, commissioned by King Philip VI of France in October 1348, remains the best known plague tract across five hundred years of this medical genre.[5] While it offered some remedies, the emphasis of the Paris doctors was placed on the astrological and remote causes of plague, its origins in the celestial conjunction of Saturn, Jupiter, and Mars that occurred on 20 March 1345. Various historians have maintained that this literature remained more or

---

[1] Plague tracts antedated 1348: one is known for the plague 1340 and at least two from earlier in the century; see Thorndike, 'A pest tractate before the black death'. However, the number takes off in 1348, with between sixteen and twenty known survivals between 1347 and 1351. To date, the historiography has concentrated on these, giving little attention to broader trends over the late Middle Ages or the early modern period; see Cohn, *The Black Death Transformed*, 67.

[2] Castiglioni, 'Ugo Benzi da Siena', 75.

[3] By the sixteenth century, tracts concentrating either on the curative or the preservative alone had become extremely rare. An exception is one by the Roman citizen and personal doctor of Pope Clement VII, Emanuele, *Opus utilissimum contra pestilentiam*.

[4] Our knowledge of plague tracts from 1348 to 1500 still derives from Karl Sudhoff's collecting, editing, and abbreviation of 288 of them in 'Pestschriften aus den ersten 150 Jahren' [hereafter, Sudhoff], vols VI–XVII from 1910 to 1925. This selection was highly biased by the libraries Sudhoff could investigate during the turbulent years of the First World War and shortly thereafter. Tracts from France are poorly represented, while those from German-speaking regions are over-represented.

[5] 'The Report of the Paris Medical Faculty, October 1348', in *The Black Death*, ed. Horrox (hereafter, Horrox), 159; and for the full text, 'Compendium'. On its manuscript tradition and diffusion, see Coville, 'Écrits contemporains sur la peste', 336–58; and more recently, Bazin-Tacchella, 'Rupture et continuité du discours médical'.

less fixed until the end of the sixteenth century, if not later,[6] and that from its first appearances in 1348, writing on plague was caged within intellectual systems devised in antiquity (principally by Aristotle and Galen) and modified by Arabic physicians, philosophers, and commentators of the early and central Middle Ages. These ideas and models, so it is alleged, blinded late medieval and early modern doctors from observing the pathological and epidemiological realities of plague, of seeing the disease's obvious mechanisms of transmission (supposedly rats and fleas). In several books on plague concentrating on seventeenth-century Italy, the prominent economic and medical historian Carlo Cipolla concluded that doctors would not begin to tear themselves from the 'scientia' of ancient authorities until the seventeenth century. Even then practising physicians on health boards,[7] and not academics, were the ones who supposedly began to focus on the realities before them, and they too continued to place the facts they gathered into the constructs of ancient dogma.[8]

More recently, other historians who have read far more plague tracts than Cipolla, especially for the sixteenth and seventeenth centuries, have come to similar conclusions: this genre of medical literature remained much the same over the long term.[9] Thus Andrew Wear begins his chapter on medical literature principally in England:

This chapter comes close to providing an example of *l'histoire immobile*. There was a great deal of consensus about health advice, with no controversies or significant new arguments across the sixteenth and seventeenth centuries, with the exception of some Helmontian

---

[6] Recently, La Croix, 'Vergelijkende studie', 361, draws a line from the 1348 report of the Paris Medical Faculty to Dutch medical tracts in the second half of the seventeenth century to argue that little changed in attitudes towards or knowledge of the plague over these centuries.

[7] The earliest health boards or special magistracies to confront epidemic disease appear with the Black Death itself in 1348 in cities such as Pistoia, Florence, and Venice. These were, however, temporary emergency councils that were disbanded as soon as the threat of plague subsided. The first permanent health offices do not appear in Italy until shortly before the mid-fifteenth century: Milan was the leader, and other city-states were slow to follow. Turin and Palermo, for instance, did not have a permanent board until 1576. Yet northern Italy was the model for cities and kingdoms north of the Alps, where these institutions did not take root until the sixteenth century or later. Moreover, even during the sixteenth century these boards were comprised principally of those outside the medical profession. On health boards and health legislation, see Chapter 6, n. 208.

[8] See Cipolla, *Public Health and the Medical Profession*, 2–3. For a similar view of late medieval and early modern physicians and science, see Cantor, *In the Wake of the Plague*, 17 and 196: 'Essentially it [pre-modern Europe] had only non-biomedical responses to devastation of a breakdown in societal health—pray very hard, quarantine the sick, run away, or find a scapegoat to blame for the terror' (196).

[9] In the words of Cosmacini, *Storia della medicina*, 94: 'I medici del '500 sono edotti dei nuovi fatti, ma prigionieri delle vecchie idee . . . ' On the supposed unchanging character of these tracts into the sixteenth century in Italy also see Henderson, 'Epidemics in Renaissance Florence': 'Each of three Florentine *Consigli* mentioned—those by del Garbo, Ficino and Buonagrazia—demonstrate the extraordinary continuity of ideas about the origin and spread of epidemics over these 170 years' (168). Also see Naso, 'Les hommes et les épidémies' on the Parisian compendium of 1348: 'Elaborées à l'échelon universitaire, les théories astrologiques étaient considérées encore comme tout à fait valables au XVIIe siècle' (308). On the early modern plague tract as neglected and disdained in present historical studies, see Jones, 'Plague and Its Metaphors', esp. 100–1.

attacks on the whole enterprise of giving health advice . . . [there was] a continuity in the health advice literature.[10]

Lawrence Brockliss and Colin Jones go further:

From the account of the 'Plague of Justinian' in 588 given by Gregory of Tours in his *History of the Franks* right up to the accounts of the last outbreak of plague on French soil, which was to take place at Marseilles in 1720, there is a remarkable family likeness in the story-telling. The *History of the Franks* constitutes a kind of ur-text for plague writing, a script for a plague outbreak which brooked little alteration.[11]

As with attitudes of fear, pessimism, and apocalyptic doom, historians such as Jean Delumeau have viewed Europe as transfixed on the same plane until the Enlightenment.[12] Few historians have even considered that attitudes and ideas about the plague, or indeed the plague itself, may have evolved over nearly five hundred years with numerous strikes from 1347 to the nineteenth century.[13]

This book will not examine the entire course of this disease's evolution or of ideas and attitudes about it but will concentrate on the sixteenth century, principally in Italy. After an examination of sources, it will analyse the remarkable 'Necrologies' of Milan at the end of one of the worst plagues of the fifteenth century—that of 1449–1452—until the plague of 1523–4, when these records cease to be complete in plague years. They reported deaths across Milanese urban society in plague and normal years and are distinguished from earlier city-wide burial records—those at Arezzo, which begin in 1373, and those at Florence at the end of the fourteenth century as well as many later ones in Europe.[14] In contrast to the earlier single-line records, in which diagnoses of grave-diggers or clerics only occasionally distinguished plague deaths

---

[10] Wear, *Knowledge and Practice in English Medicine*, 155.

[11] Brockliss and Jones, *The Medical World of Early Modern France*, 67. More broadly, Maclean, *Logic, Signs and Nature*, treats medical thinking c.1500 to 1630 as a historical block without significant changes, characterizing it as 'a static discourse in which certain lines of thought did not evolve, and intellectual change was slow to occur' (333). Calvi, 'L'oro, il fuoco, le forche', goes further, seeing the thinking and defences against plague as without significant change until 1894 (esp. 406–7). More recently, other historians have shown the vitality, innovation, and challenges to antique authorities in the medical literature more generally during the fifteenth and sixteenth centuries; see for instance, Park, 'Natural Particulars', esp. 360–1; and Nutton, 'Medicine in Medieval Western Europe'.

[12] Most prominently, see the work of Delumeau, *La peur en Occident*; *Le péché et la peur*; and *Rassurer et protéger*. Also, see Calvi, 'L'oro, il fuoco, le forche', esp. 405, 409, 424, who sees 'the myths' of plague, resulting in 'the persecution of witches, plague spreaders, Jews, heretics, and revolutionaries' as a constant over the long history of plagues in Europe, which they were not. On the sudden and long-term disappearance of Jews and other outsiders as scapegoats of plague after the Black Death, see Cohn, *The Black Death Transformed*, ch. 9; and idem, 'The Black Death and the Burning of the Jews', 10–11.

[13] Moote and Moote, *The Great Plague*, 279–80, boldly assert: 'not only do the symptoms described in the past fit a present-day diagnosis . . . the disease's pathology has not fundamentally changed during a long history'.

[14] On the Florentine burial records, see Herlihy and Klapisch-Zuber, *Les Toscans et leurs familles*; and Carmichael, *Plague and the Poor*. The earlier Aretine records kept by the Fraternità dei Laici have yet to be systematically studied; see del Panta, *Le epidemie nella storia demografica italiana*, 23–5; and Cohn, *The Black Death Transformed*, 171–2.

from others by a marginal 'P', the Milanese physicians gave the causes of death. These descriptions of corpses, discussions of causes of death, and indications of the duration and course of illnesses that led to death could fill long paragraphs.

Plague clearly prompted the collection of these detailed records. For the most part the doctors' diagnoses were dichotomous, aimed at establishing whether a death had been caused by plague or not, regardless of the names used for plague ('sine contagio', 'sine aliquali contagione', 'absque signo pestifero'). When plague was not suspected, the entry was usually short, listing little more than the victim's name, parish, and occasionally the duration of illness or a generic characteristic such as continual or tertian fever. By contrast, the reports of plague victims were longer, especially when the accidents did not include the normal telltale signs of buboes, pustules, or continuous fever, headaches, and vomiting, but when death was quick, within a week. In such questionable cases ('casi dubiosi') the descriptions reflect discussions and debates among the examining doctors of Milan's health board as they searched for further details from relatives and neighbours of the victim as to the first signs of illness and whether the patient had died in a household where others had been afflicted.[15]

From this source, chapter 2 will investigate the range of signs and symptoms of the late medieval and early modern plague, not only to see whether they matched 'so unquestionably' with *Yersinia pestis*, but to explore a new question: did the signs, symptoms, or epidemiological traits of plague, whatever its agent, change after its initial outbreak in 1348 with successive strikes of plague during the late fourteenth to the end of the sixteenth century? In this evaluation of the disease the archival records from Milan will be interpreted and compared with descriptions from the plague tracts across Italy. The clinical reports will provide a check on academic physicians and other authors of plague tracts to examine whether they were trapped so indefensibly in paradigms of antiquity, unable to observe the physiological facts they confronted.

The bulk of this book will concentrate on plague writing in Italy during the sixteenth century, authored principally by university-trained doctors but which during the plague of 1575–8 suddenly engaged a wide spectrum of authors from cardinals to cobblers, in prose and verse. This book will argue that such writing was hardly static over the five hundred years of the plague or over the sixteenth century; rather, it evolved as did the plague itself. Almost a century before Thomas Sydenham (1624–89), physicians and others, across the Italian peninsula, struggled to understand their biggest killer in new ways. They did so by tracking the disease's contagion person to person and defining it essentially by its clinical traits. The fillip of change was the 1575–8 plague that invaded

---

15 On these Milanese records, see Albini, *Guerra, fame, peste*; Carmichael, 'Contagion Theory'; 'Epidemics and state medicine'; 'Universal and Particular'; Zanetti, 'La morte a Milano'; Nicoud, 'Médecine et prévention de la santé'; and Cohn and Alfani, 'Households and Plague'.

the Italian peninsula simultaneously from its extreme north across the Alps into the Trentino to its far south, afflicting major ports and small towns and villages of Sicily. This epidemiological crisis, I will argue, formed the creative crucible of a new outpouring of plague literature and medical analysis. No plague had so threatened Italy as a whole since 1400 or probably even as far back as 1348.[16] This crisis reshaped the plague genre, doctors' ideas about plague, and how to combat it.

Chapter 1 shows the effect of this late sixteenth-century plague threat quantitatively. In two years alone, 1576 and 1577, almost half the century's published writings on plague appeared. This pattern was unique to Italy not only for these years but across the history of plague in Europe from the Black Death to at least the seventeenth century and probably beyond.[17] In addition, the language of plague writing, whether composed by academic physicians or others, shifted abruptly from a majority in Latin (fuelled by the revival in classical medical writing over the previous century) to an overwhelming preponderance in the vernacular. The subsequent chapters explore the qualitative significance of this change.

Chapter 3 concentrates on one of the longest and most influential plague treatises of the century, that of the Sicilian *Protomedico* Giovanni Filippo Ingrassia, written mainly in 1575 and published the following year. Despite his Counter-Reformation piety and classical erudition, his treatise was the first to break the physician's mould of plague writing. Instead of proposed preventative measures and cures directed to the individual patient, it concentrated on the duties of the prince and local magistrates for public health policy and the best strategies to be pursued. Moreover, unlike other tracts even during the plague crisis of 1575–8 or afterwards, Ingrassia's opinions and advice took immediate effect through the financial force of city magistrates of Palermo and the Spanish viceroy in Sicily. These measures included the creation of new plague hospitals, places for the quarantine of suspected goods, the locking of afflicted houses and procedures for ensuring the separation of the ill, the suspected, and the healthy, new organizations for reporting and controlling the disease, clearing of filth, improvements in sewage, issuing plague passports, and more. In addition, by utilizing his international contacts and public health statistics, which his recommendations had in fact implemented, Ingrassia was the first physician to pay serious attention to tracking a disease—the possible paths of its arrival to a region and its detailed spread within neighbourhoods once it had entered a city.

---

[16] See Corradi, *Annali*, vol. I.

[17] No 'Edit 17' as yet exists to make systematic comparisons with the sixteenth-century; however, Corradi, *Annali*, II, 71–4, and 186–93, made lists of medical plague tracts published during the pestilence of 1629–33 and 1656–7. For 1630–1, he listed 46; some of these, however (Luca Boerio, Cesare Mocca, Giovanni Castagno, Ascanio Oliveri), were reprints of late-sixteenth-century works. For the plague of 1656–7, sixty-nine appear but these include also secondary works published into the nineteenth century; only sixteen were published during the plague years 1656–7 or the year afterward. According to Conforti, 'Peste e stampa', p. 136, the production of plague tracts in Genoa during this plague was 'piuttosto limitata'; in Rome only two were published.

Chapter 4 turns to northern Italy, where the majority of 1575–8 plague publications were written. These suddenly broke physicians' near monopoly over these manuals since the Black Death. Now bishops, parish priests, gentlemen, government administrators, gate guards, notaries, and even artisans suddenly felt compelled to describe and explain the plague in a new genre of plague writing often called the *Successo della peste*. These began not with erudite definitions or 'superior' or 'remote' causes of pestilential fevers in a variety of languages or with notions of the mutation of air but with detailed chronicling of the paths by which this highly contagious disease had spread via persons and goods from one region to another and then within an author's own town. Once the disease had arrived within the city, these authors (like Ingrassia) used local health office records to trace precisely the plague's spread and 'progress'. Then, against the ebb and flow of mortality figures, they plotted human reactions to it—administrative decrees and health control measures, new and old forms of ecclesiastical organization, processions and other forms of spiritual solace, and modes to placate God's ire. In addition, these authors narrated changes in the landscape and collective psychology of the city along with their own mental anguish as the plague brought civil life to its weakest and darkest moments.

Chapter 5 reveals other forms of plague writing spurred on by the peninsula-wide threat of 1575–8—new forms of thanksgiving and liberation literature that detailed the celebrations offered for their heavenly and secular deliverance and especially an explosion of plague poetry that parted with plague verse of the past going back to Lucretius. Instead of grim pictures of corpse-strewn horrors, plague poetry of 1575–8 sung the praises of local heroes from heads of health boards to bell-ringers, celebrating their epic deeds that buttressed communities against imminent destruction and that defeated the 'hydra-headed' plague. Chapter 6 shows another side of the intellectual vitality stimulated by the 1575–8 crisis. An unprecedented denial of 'true plague' suddenly swept through medical circles. Best known are the arguments voiced by Padua's academics Girolamo Mercuriale and Girolamo Capodivacca, invited by the Venetian government to diagnose the disease in the summer of 1576. Similar arguments, however, were voiced across the peninsula from Trent to Sicily in these years, some appearing a year or more before as in Palermo and Verona. An impassioned rebuttal from those within and outside the medical profession met head-on these theoretical arguments used to rescind public health measures such as quarantine. Now notaries and others outside the ranks of physicians challenged the definitions and theories of plague propounded by those from the highest chairs of academic medicine. In so doing, administrators and even artisans questioned long-held models of medieval and Renaissance medicine with their admixtures of Galen, Avicenna, and God. In their place, they focused on that which could be observed, from particular plague signs and symptoms and epidemiological patterns such as the quickness of death and the clustering of deaths in households to tracing the paths of the disease's rapid contagion. These debates did not, however, neatly split plague-denying physicians from hard-nosed empirical bureaucrats of health boards or others. Instead, the 1575–8 plague deeply divided the medical profession, leading many to challenge head on the old universals of medical theory.

On this empirical and pragmatic level, Chapter 7 argues that plague writers across Italy in 1575–8 paid new attention to the social causes of plague. In seeing the plague as one principally afflicting the poor, they went beyond previous explanations grounded in Galen and other texts of classical, Arabic or Renaissance medicine—differences in complexion, humours, diet, and spoilt food. The new authors of 1575–8 pointed to class differences in the availability of medical care, treatment of the poor by political authorities, social characteristics of neighbourhoods, inadequate and overcrowded housing, poor plumbing, and contaminated water to explain the plague's clear class divisions and transmission. Chapter 8 shows how these pragmatic and social concerns created a new approach to plague and medicine among academically trained physicians. With the plague crisis of 1575–8 new sections often called 'on governing the plague' suddenly appeared, transforming the traditional plague tract. These shifted and expanded the physician's remit and frame of reference from the patient's bedside to society as a whole. Just as the causes of plague were now seen as essentially social, the remedies had to become political. As a consequence, doctors addressed city magistrates and princes directly with 'recipes' that went beyond drugs and particular surgical procedures and pertained instead to street cleaning, the organization of plague controls at city gates and mountain passes, punishments for the theft of contaminated property, treatment of the poor, new forms of charity, the construction of hospitals, directives for ensuring safe water and effective means for removing excrement and other sources of contamination. Physicians now stressed political organization and public health as the best 'remedies' for combating epidemic disease.

Chapter 9 explores the psychological ramifications of plague that provoked social conflict and mass fear, which doctors and others in 1575–8 now saw as adding significantly to plague mortalities. This turn to the psychological and moral ramifications of plague did not mean that the crisis of 1575–8 was fought under the dark cloud of Counter-Reformation piety and authority, a return to apocalyptic notions of plague and a rejection of the 'realism' of physicians and health boards seen earlier in the sixteenth century as some historians have asserted. Against the general picture of a Church–State conflict in plague time with two fundamentally different views of the plague's cause, this chapter shows the mutual respect and cooperation between these two forces in combating the pan-Italian plague of 1575–8: both passed ordinances steeped in the realization that plague spread because of human contagion and the contamination of goods. Of the manifold divisions wrought by this plague, that between Church and State does not appear among them. The book concludes by stressing that major mortalities and epidemics do not necessarily lead to transcendental religiosity and the weakening of state formations as is commonly generalized across the world history of epidemics. Italy's most important plague of the sixteenth century had the opposite effect. The mobilization of massive resources to combat the plague in 1575–8 and the successful encouragement and coercion of clergy and health workers to remain at their posts, risking their lives for their communities, fuelled the growth of the new Counter-Reformation Church and secular states alike across Italy. This success proclaimed in plague poetry and prose led to the glorification of individual rulers and instructed on the need and value of subjects to obey, thereby boosting absolutist authority at the end of the sixteenth century and into the next.

Far from being unchanging documents from the Black Death to the seventeenth century, physicians' plague tracts and other plague writing by those outside the profession shifted fundamentally over time. The plague crisis of 1575–8 was the crucible of one such caesura in these medical and literary works and engendered two heretofore unnoticed developments in medical history: the first attempts seriously to track diseases through detailed health-board statistics and doctors' newly perceived mandate to engage in politics and instruct princes on public health. With new health-board records plague writers of 1575–8 created new forms of plague writing, which wove stories of dark comedy, pathos, and personal trauma into narratives of the plague's relentless 'progress' as measured by its death counts. Similar journals of plague, unknowingly indebted to these sixteenth-century works, would later develop into masterpieces of plague literature, from Defoe to Camus.[18]

---

[18] Recent literary historians remain unaware of these sixteenth-century antecedents; see for instance Gordon, 'The City and the Plague', esp. 67–8, who makes numerous assumptions about innovations in post-1720 plague writing, which in fact were well embedded in plague tracts, 1575–8, such as concerns with the collapse of commerce (82) or that these authors began their descriptions with rhetorical claims that plague's ravages were indescribable (86–7).

1

Sources and Perspectives: A Quantitative Reckoning

Authors of plague tracts from at least the 1360s to the first half of the fifteenth century were far from slavish followers of abstract ancient theories.[1] Instead, like physicians in antiquity, they relied on their experience and experimentation, and occasionally referred to cases from their own practices. For instance, from observation and not ancient doctrine ('sicut nos vidimus ad experienciam') they concluded that their plague was highly contagious through observing its mortalities clustering in households. As a professor of medicine and rector of the University of Prague at the end of the fourteenth century concluded, if one case arose in a home, the rest of the household would probably catch the disease, because it was so extraordinarily contagious.[2] Many other doctors of the late fourteenth and fifteenth centuries stressed the remarkable, even unique contagion of this disease through touching, breathing, or supposedly by sight, almost two centuries before Girolamo Fracastoro in 1546 categorized contagion into the three principal forms—by direct contact, *ad fomites* (through contamination of goods by a disease's venomous atoms), and by distance.[3] Although Galen had a notion of 'seeds of contagion', as Vivian Nutton has shown, transmission of epidemic disease by goods and persons was not a principal plank of his or any other ancient physician's notion of the spread of disease,[4] none of whom had witnessed an illness similar to the Black Death or its successive waves through the early modern period in Europe. Later, the Milanese necrologies and parish

---

[1] In addition to the remarks of Cipolla, see Carmichael, 'The Last Past Plague': 'This kind of medical commentary, characteristic of late medieval plague treatises, was formulated with good Galenic universalism. It is difficult to deduce physicians' first-hand experience from the information included' (158). Also, see idem, 'Universal and Particular', 21; and for others who hold that these tracts remained much the same from 1348 to the seventeenth century, see ibid., 21.

[2] 'Causae, signa et remedia . . . per Magistrum Henricum', 85.

[3] On these doctors, see Cohn, *The Black Death Transformed*, 235. On Fracastoro and contagion, see Fracastoro, *De contagione*, ch. 1–5; and Nutton, 'The Reception of Fracastoro's Theory of Contagion'. Fracastoro, however, went beyond these late medieval physicians by inventing 'another order of living things, the seeds of disease' (*seminaria contagionis*); ibid., 211. On the philosophical underpinnings of Fracastoro's theory of contagion, see Fracastoro, *De sympathia et antipathia*; and Pennuto, *Simpatia, fantasia e contagio*, for a different notion of Fracastoro's *seminaria*, ch. 8, esp. 381–5.

[4] Nutton, 'Seeds of Disease'; 'The Reception of Fracastoro's Theory of Contagion'; and 'Roman Medicine', 54.

burial records attest to the truth of these late medieval observations. These records allow a comparison of the extent of the clustering of deaths in households for various diseases, which were in fact contagious—*pondi*, *lenticulae* (which modern historians have assumed was typhus), dysentery, or even influenza. None of these came close to approximating the degree of household clustering seen in numerous plagues of Milan from the mid-fifteenth to the seventeenth century.[5]

Furthermore, as testimony to such direct experience, most late medieval plague tracts were written in the midst of a plague, or just afterwards, and their opening sections gave evidence of these plagues in the author's town or region. Others of the late fourteenth and fifteenth centuries confirmed their cures and theories with phrases such as that used by the famous doctor of the Milanese Visconti, Pietro da Tossignano, 'and this I have seen by experience'.[6] This pattern continued through the sixteenth century in Italy, as can be seen in numerous introductory dedications that justified publishing a new plague treatise.

Others, such as John of Burgundy in the 1360s, went further: not only did he claim that his advice came from 'long experience', which gave credence to his recipes and cures; experience of two or three plagues bequeathed him and his generation of practitioners a new seal of authority. His subsequent references to ancient authority hardly bore the stamp of obsequious devotion to any ancient thinker. Beginning with Galen, John listed a number of Hellenistic, Arabic, and Jewish compilers, doctors, and natural philosophers as authorities who had never witnessed a plague of the duration and magnitude of the plagues in his day. Because of their lack of experience, he alleged, 'the knowledge found from Hippocrates on had now become obsolete'. Just as these masters had to rely on experience for treating the diseases of their day, John held that experience ought to become the key for healing once again (*quod experientia facit artem*): from this 'long experience, modern practitioners everywhere' ('magistri moderni ubicunque terrarium'), he claimed, are now more expert in curing pestilence and epidemic diseases than all the doctors of medicine and authors from Hippocrates onwards.[7]

John was not alone in this new medical confidence infused by plague experience. With the third strike, Johannes Jacobi of Montpellier said much the same: since the plague had invaded us so frequently, we have much to say from

---

[5] See Cohn and Alfani, 'Households and Plague'. Already by 1348, doctors were struck by plague deaths clustering in households. Examples are also found for the sixteenth century; Mignoto, *Mignotydea de peste*, raises the question: 'why if one in a family dies [of plague], do almost all the rest die of it, and in other households, none die from it?'

[6] 'Der Pesttraktat des Pietro di Tussignano (1398)', 395; also, see 'Prophylaxe und Kur pestilentialischer Fieber', 341: 'et sic etiam experientia demonstavit maxime'.

[7] 'Die Pestschriften des Johann von Burgund', 68. Of course, these late medieval doctors knew only a small portion of the ancient corpus of medicine and mostly through Arabic intermediaries, but often (and more often than doctors of the early modern period) they sensed that neither Hippocrates nor Galen had witnessed a disease that was the same as the Black Death. On the variety of ancient medicine and the small portion of it that remains, see Nutton, *Ancient Medicine*: 'By 600 at least', the proper interpretation of Galen had supplanted 'the lively and wide-ranging medical debates of the Early Roman Empire'; and Nutton, 'The Fortunes of Galen', 363.

experience, while 'the ancients could say little'.[8] By the next plague in 1382, the papal doctor Raymundus Chalmelli de Vinario granted the ancients even less respect. They neither understood the causes of plagues nor knew how to deal with them: 'plainly, they could not cure' such victims and had 'left everything in confusion'.[9] In 1406 the physician of the king of Aragon added Hippocrates, Galen, Alexander, Serapion, Rhases, Averröes, Avicenna, and Haly to the list of ancient authorities who were of no use with the current plague. In place of this 'scientia', he trumpeted his own credentials—forty years of plague diagnosis in Toulouse, Montpellier, and Sicily.[10]

This emboldened view of their science spelled a new confidence in their powers to heal, especially in cases of plague.[11] Guy de Chauliac's about-face from the first plague to the third one in 1361, from few possible cures, if any, to a long list of specific recipes, was hardly unique. Other doctors cured themselves (or so they believed) and wished to make their experiences and remedies known to fellow doctors, their 'own citizens, and to the world'.[12] At the end of the fourteenth century, a Dr Stephen of Padua turned to personal experience, describing his own and his wife's affliction with plague—four days 'of horrendous fevers and the detestable signs' with himself 'at the head of the bed and she at the foot'. Ultimately, with his regime of remedies he proclaimed to have 'triumphed over the plague', curing himself, his wife, and 'many other citizens of Padua'. He now wrote them down to benefit his fellow citizens—to whom he dedicated his tract.[13]

With confidence, others pointed occasionally to specific clinical histories of patients as proof of the remedies' success. At the time of the third (1372) or fourth plague (1382) John of Tornamira, a professor and practising physician at Montpellier, supported one of his procedures for bloodletting and another for surgery on a boil by referring to treatments of named patients.[14] While others did not name their patients, they were no less confident about their procedures based on experience. In a tract from 1371–2, doctor Heinrich Rybinitz of Bratislava recommended rubbing plague boils with his own concocted recipe for a *tyriaca*. He maintained that this was a cautious method of healing 'as I along with many

---

[8] Cited in 'Die Identität des Regimen contra pestilentiam', 58.

[9] 'Das Pestwerkchen des Raymundus Chalin de Vinario', 38–9.

[10] 'Die Pestschrift des "Blasius Brascinensis" ', 104.

[11] In *The Medical World of Early Modern France*, Brockliss and Jones describe traditional histories of medicine as a 'grand narrative', which sees the history of Europe from the ancient Greeks to the Industrial Revolution 'as marking a two-thousand-year period of stasis' (3). However, when it comes to plague, their narrative fits well with this traditional one. Only with the Enlightenment was '[t]he diseased body . . . no longer a plague-wracked site of lethal trauma, a living death . . . .' Only then: 'The mood of medicine was shifting from an erudite scepticism to a "can-do" functionalist meliorism' (23). They further contend that '[t]he plague script did not leave much room for positive action' from doctors, and as proof they cite one case of a doctor at Saint-Lô who was thrown into prison for witchcraft because of his success in curing plague victims (69).

[12] 'Ex libro Dionysii Secundi Colle', 169.   [13] 'Ein Paduaner Pestkonsilium', 356.

[14] Johanns de Tornamira, 'Praeservatio et cura apostematum', 53.

others have seen and experienced'.[15] A late fourteenth-century doctor in Venice claimed to have cured a hundred patients with his plague recipes.[16] The doctor of the Portuguese Cardinal Philip of Alenzolo boasted that none had died under his care during the last big plague (at the beginning of the fifteenth century); 'his methods' had cured 'an infinite number'.[17] At about the same time, a doctor from Danzig claimed that his concoction of *luto armenico* mixed with weak wine had cured many plague victims.[18] At the end of the fifteenth century, a doctor from Cologne began his tract by saying that his 'little work' had already proven itself successful for the treatment of plague cases in Rome and other places throughout Italy. For him and others north of the Alps, as evinced by their training and earlier practice in Italian towns, the Italian experience was the model: as the Cologne physician pointed out, 'through their industry and medical procedures many plague victims had been sagaciously liberated from the illness'.[19]

The doctors also assured themselves, their colleagues, and their patients that certain preventative measures were effective in warding off plague. They described fires to be burnt from exotic woods, the use of scents in homes, and special diets and herbal recipes, the best directions for houses to face and the opening and closing of windows and doors depending on the seasons, the stars, and the winds. Others recommended simple sanitary measures—washing hands with warm water after coughing and defecating, covering mouths and noses with bread or sponges soaked in vinegar and rose water when near the infected, and simply avoiding public places and especially enclosed ones, such as churches, in times of plague. At least one modern commentator on these texts with a professional competence in pharmacology and herbal medicine has remarked that these fires, scents, and herbs would have served as effective disinfectants and would have had value, not against modern bubonic plague, but in protecting against a number of airborne diseases.[20] Further, these doctors' stress on cleanliness and elementary sanitation (seen in these texts as well as in post-plague sanitary manuals, which also soar in number)[21] may not have been without beneficial consequences, especially if the disease was highly contagious, as they maintained and the quantification of plague mortalities underline. The proof of their methods, at least as far as they and their patients were concerned, was their own survival. No doubt it had less to do with their recipes than their bodies' immune systems

---

[15] 'Tractatus de praeservationibus . . . Hinricum Rybbinis', 222.

[16] Varanini, 'La peste del 1347–50', 305. Unfortunately, he neither names the doctor nor cites the source.

[17] 'Eine Pestbeulenkur', 342.   [18] 'Ein Compendium epidemiae', 174.

[19] 'Ein Kölner Pestinkunabel kurz vor 1500', 152. Although less praising of the Italians, the fifteenth-century doctor from Besançon began his tract by bragging that he had previously practised in Bologna; 'Der Tractatus pestilentialis eines Theobaldus Loneti', 53–4.

[20] Trillat, 'Etude historique'; and Panebianco, ' "De preservatione a pestilencia" ', 352.

[21] On these see Castiglioni, 'I libri italiani della pestilenza', 140–52, and more recently Rawcliffe, 'The Concept of Health', and Nicoud, *Les régimes de santé*.

adapting to the new toxic germ, which, as the death data from a wide variety of sources—last wills and testaments, confraternal and religious necrologies, and burial records—have shown,[22] was rapidly becoming domesticated over its first hundred years of invasion.

Later in the fifteenth century, Johannes Cleyn of Lübeck continued to believe that he and his generation of doctors 'because of their great experience' had surpassed the ancients.[23] This evolving confidence over the first hundred years of the Black Death paralleled the plague's evolution: although it remained the late medieval 'big killer', its mortality and morbidity declined more or less progressively. The confidence of the physicians of the late fourteenth and early fifteenth centuries was a far cry from the desperation of doctors' tracts seen with the Black Death and the years that immediately followed, when physicians such as the Montpellier-trained Simon de Couvin (*c.*1350) viewed the plague as unprecedented, completely confounding all medical knowledge. Doctors' principal recourse then was to turn to God and pray.

***

The confidence of doctors such as Raymundus was not, however, to endure through the fifteenth century. By mid-century such examples from the sources edited and extracted usually in highly abbreviated form by Karl Sudhoff become rare: confidence and sweeping indictments against ancient authority waned. Again, physicians' tone and recommendations followed the contours of their plague experience: in contrast to the plague's rapid downturn during its first fifty or hundred years, by the mid-fifteenth century doctors had to recognize that their plague was here to stay and would remain a fixture of Renaissance demography. With the widespread epidemics in 1449–52 and 1478–80, plague mortalities climbed and reversed the fourteenth-century trend towards plague becoming increasingly one that affected children. These plagues also marked a change in medical consciousness. With Marsilio Ficino's tract of around 1481 and more so during the early sixteenth century, such emboldened criticism of the ancients and hyper-confidence in their own curative powers disappeared from doctors' plague manuals.

More than at any time since the Black Death, references to Greek and Latin authorities filled plague manuals of the last decades of the fifteenth and the early sixteenth century. Most significantly, this Renaissance return to the sources produced numerous published editions of Galen and Hippocrates in Latin translations from 1490 and Greek editions by 1525.[24] It also saw a revival of Aristotle (who had almost completely disappeared from plague tracts from the

---

[22] See Cohn, *The Black Death Transformed*, ch. 8.

[23] Cited in Johannes Jacobi, 'Tractatus de peste', 21.

[24] On the Renaissance in medicine and changes in language see Nutton, 'The Changing Language of Medicine'; 'Humanist surgery'; and 'The Fortunes of Galen', 368–71; and below, Chapter 6, n. 120.

late fourteenth to the mid-fifteenth centuries)[25] as a principal authority on plague along with the inclusion of other ancient authors rarely cited, if known at all, in the late medieval tracts, such as Thucydides, Homer, Lucretius, Pliny, and Plato. But with plague mortalities on the rise, did this Renaissance drive to uncover ancient sources of medicine lead to a slavish adulation of antique authority? While the boldness, even arrogance of a Raymundus, may have disappeared, these later texts did not abandon observation and experience. Many sixteenth-century tracts, such as Ingrassia's *Informatione*, which listed fifty-two signs and symptoms of the plague as he observed it in Palermo during the epidemic of 1575–6, or that of the Genovese surgeon Luchino Boerio, show an acute awareness of the 'accidents', signs, and symptoms of plague; they drew sharp distinctions in the positions and colours of various skin disorders, the course of the disease, and remedies according to the formation of buboes and carbuncles. Their detail of clinical description in fact goes far beyond anything seen in fourteenth- or fifteenth-century tracts.[26]

As the Black Death disease had not been known in antiquity, none of these signs and symptoms had been so catalogued. In the sixteenth century, doctors added new sections to their tracts aimed at teaching practical lessons on how to recognize the plague, its various signs on the living as well as on plague corpses, and to distinguish them from the accidents of other diseases.[27] Some,

[25] Cohn, *The Black Death Transformed*, 69–71.

[26] Considerable discrepancy in notions about differences in the status of early modern Italian surgeons and physicians persists. One view puts surgeons' status a little above that of barbers, claiming that they were mostly illiterate (in Latin), their knowledge came from *ars* not *scientia*, and their status worsened during the late fifteenth and sixteenth centuries; see for instance Cartwright, *A Social History of Medicine*; and Cipolla, 'A Plague Doctor', 69, and *Public Health*, 3, 74, and 91. These authors, however, have little evidence to support their claims for early modern Italy. Cipolla even presents evidence against this picture by showing the power and responsibilities entrusted to the surgeon Michelangiolo Coveri in upholding the dictates of the Florentine health board within the walled town of Montelupo during the plague of 1630–1; *Faith, Reason, and the Plague*, 46. By contrast, with detailed textual and archival evidence Bylebyl, 'The School of Padua', offers a different picture of the surgeon, his relations with physicians, and his change in status during the sixteenth century in Italy. First, against the stereotypes above, physicians were not bookish scholars who rarely saw or touched patients. Instead, during the sixteenth century, they became increasingly involved in treating patients (and not only the rich) and employed surgical practices. One reason for the attraction of the University of Padua for training doctors outside Italy during the late Renaissance was its focus on clinical practice and use of the hospital for training. By the mid-sixteenth century, hospitals such as Santa Maria Novella in Florence were also used for bedside teaching and practical demonstrations for medical students (see Henderson, *The Renaissance Hospital*, 242 and 250). Furthermore, chairs in surgery were not rarities at Italian universities and, with the growing importance of anatomy in the sixteenth century, these became the most important chairs when combined with anatomy. The careers of surgeons such as Gasparre Tagliacozzi (1545–99) and Ambroise Paré confound generalizations such as Cipolla's that surgeons were like porters in nineteenth-century hospitals (*Public Health*, 74). See Gnudi and Webster, *The Life and Times of Gaspare Tagliacozzi*; and Castiglioni, *A History of Medicine*, 473–7. For a trenchant critique of the traditional view of physicians as the villains and surgeons as the heroes, see Nutton, 'Humanist surgery'.

[27] One of the earliest to include a substantial section on how to recognize the signs and symptoms of the plague was Corvi, *De febribus tractatus optimus*. In addition to Boerio, *Trattato delli buboni*, 8 and 50, see Daciano, *Trattato della peste*, 37–40; [Eustachio], *Regimento mirabile et verissimo*, 7r and 12r; Lini da Correggio, *Trattato contra peste*, part 2 of the tract, divided into five parts; Napolitano, *Trattato di mirabili secreti* [1576], ch. 9; Bellicochi, *Avvertimenti*, 413r, 415r, 420v–3v; Massa, *Ragionamento,*

such as the Veronese druggist Bellicocchi, declared that these sections were their most important contributions. In cases such as Boerio's tract, one written by a Mantuan doctor in 1576, and another written by a doctor of Turin during the plague of 1584, the entire tract was devoted to the problem of observation and plague recognition.[28] These were addressed to citizens and doctors alike.

By the sixteenth century city magistrates and health boards depended on such knowledge, first from doctors, then from elected guards and parish officials, and finally from household heads, who predominantly were the poor: they were responsible for calling plague cases to the attention of clerics and health board officials as soon as possible. During the plague of 1575–6 the magistrates of Palermo passed legislation demanding that all the doctors of its city and territory be instructed in recognizing plague signs ('questo pestifero contagio') to isolate and sequester the plague-inflicted.[29] Furthermore, various Italian cities passed new and stringent decrees, obliging householders on pain of death to report to their parish doctors, guards, or priests any appearance of suspected signs of plague among family members and other co-residents, from the initial rise of pestilential fevers to the emergence of buboes, carbuncles, and pustules.[30] In Palermo, new city plague ordinances of 1575 instructed the public on the four signs of the 'morbo contagioso' that they should recognize.[31] As we shall see, physicians' instructions in academic plague tracts, moreover, correspond closely with the descriptions and decisions seen in the death records of the Milanese health board drawn up by physicians in their daily evaluations of corpses throughout the city in plague and non-plague years.

Sixteenth-century Italian plague tracts show other more subtle changes from those of the later Middle Ages. A prominent feature of many plague tracts from

---

9v–11v; Ajello, *Breue discorso*, 29v–30r; Parisi, *Auuertimenti*, 20–1; Argenterio, *Porta tecum rimedii piu veri*, 41–3. I have not spotted a single tract within Sudhoff's collections from 1348 to 1500 with a section on 'how to recognize the plague'. The closest example comes in fact from the end of his period and from Italy, a tract written by Antonius de Salomonibus, a physician and canon at the cathedral of Bologna ('Notizen zur Pestkur'). In one short paragraph, it lists 'four or five *certa noticia de peste*, to recognize when a person is ill with the said affliction' (124).

[28] Susio, *Libro del conoscere la pestilenza*; Bucci, *Modo di conoscere*; Ingrassia, *Informatione*, 52, 106, and 172. Compare these to Marsilio Ficino's ch. 4, 'Signs of the Plague', in the most famous plague tract of the previous century (*Il consiglio*, 6r–7r). This section discusses fevers and urine but does not even mention swellings—buboes or *carbunculi*. In later discussions of treatments, he mentions apostemes dwelling on their colours but shows none of the clinical clarity that becomes common in sixteenth-century tracts especially after 1575. At least one example can also be found of an early sixteenth-century tract that dwelled on pestilential signs both as predictors (such as the multiplication of toads) and as symptoms but which showed no precise awareness of the disease. With nine small-print columns on pestilential signs Rustico's *Qui atrocem horres pestem* . . . points to fevers, angst, stinky breath, spiky tongue, vomiting, aspects of the heart, pulse, breathing, and urine, but fails to mention swellings of any sort in its ch. 5, 'Signs of Pestilential Fevers', 8v–10v. A second part raises questions about the first part, with one query regarding the colours of spots (*macule*) but, as with the first part, neither carbuncles nor buboes are mentioned (21v–2r).

[29] Ingrassia, *Parte quinta*, 12–13.

[30] See for instance *Bando et ordinationi fatte per . . . città di Palermo*, 3v–4r.   [31] Ibid., 4r.

1348 to 1500 was bloodletting, instructing doctors, surgeons, and barbers on which veins to tap given the positions of pestilential swellings, whether they were buboes, carbuncles, or pustules, occasionally based on age, sex, and complexion of the patient and even the time of year.[32] By contrast, sixteenth-century plague tracts rarely mentioned bloodletting or else did so with caution. Moreover, those tracts that did advise bloodletting appeared almost exclusively in the earlier part of the century and were mainly manuals of surgeons. The surgeon Giovanni Bassino in the earliest tract found in this study (1501) supplies the fullest discussion of bloodletting, giving instructions similar to what had been commonplace during the previous hundred and fifty years, with details of the veins to be opened corresponding to the swellings' positions. His advice, however, was more cautious than that of most fifteenth-century doctors: bloodletting was not to be considered in all cases and in its place syrups, powders, and treatments for 'sucking out the poison' should be employed.[33] The tract of the surgeon and physician of Pope Julius II, Giovanni da Vigo, also advised letting blood with caution: it was to be done only on the first day of plague illness; by the second, the poison had circulated through the blood, and thus bloodletting would weaken the patient, making matters worse ('& faria più pericolo assai').[34] Giovanni Pietro Arluni in a plague tract first published on 18 April 1515 discussed bloodletting but was not wholly convinced of it as a cure for plague patients and was more sceptical of it as a preventative measure.[35] The Augustinian and head of Naples' public health board, Giovanni Battista Napolitano, recommended it but only for strong and ruddy men with the right complexion ('homo robusto & sanguigno').[36]

An unpublished compilation of plague remedies by various French druggists, surgeons, and physicians composed between 1562 and 1566 and translated into Italian paid greater attention to bloodletting as a therapy for plague patients than any sixteenth-century Italian tract I have found. These tracts, however, also indicate that the practice was by then being hotly contested in France. The Parisian druggist Maestro Nicolas Novel in the first of these cites Ambroise Paré, the famous surgeon of the king of France. While travelling with the king

---

[32] See Cohn, *The Black Death Transformed*, 69, 71, 226, and 234; and the tracts edited by Sudhoff.

[33] Bassino, *Modo e ordine securo*, esp. 7–8 (not in Edit 16 as of January 2009). Another exception is the early, short tract of Torella, *Qui cupit a peste*.

[34] Da Vigo, *Secreti mirabilissimi* (the title does not appear in Edit 16). Castiglioni, *A History of Medicine*, 470, rated Da Vigo (Rapallo, 1460–1525) 'among the better-known Italian surgeons'.

[35] [Arluni], *La peste*, 25–31. The modern editor mistakenly dates the first publication to 1517. (See Edit 16 for the correct date.)

[36] Napolitano, *Opera et trattato che insegna* [1527], 7v; and idem, *Opera et trattato che insegna* [1556], 13v. Other exceptions were Cittadoni da Cassia, *Regole per conseruar l'huomo*, n.p., but he only mentions in passing that if a pain or tumour appears on the neck, the vein to be taped is in the head called the *Cephalica*; Carcano, *Trattato di peste*, 7v–8v, stressed that it was a risky and dangerous procedure of which he was dubious, that it had caused great controversy, and was not to be used with the weak, young, or old. Finally, an undated anonymous short tract that survives in one copy alone, *Del regimento della vita*, 2v, comes closest of the sixteenth-century tracts to fifteenth-century ones edited by Sudhoff that specified the vein to tap depending on the place of the pestilential swelling.

in the plague-stricken region of Bagiona in 1565, Paré questioned doctors, surgeons, and barbers of the region about their success in bloodletting plague patients. They unanimously affirmed that all those from whom blood had been taken or who had taken strong purgatives ('che si erano grandemente purgati') had died, while those spared the treatments had survived.[37] At about the same time, the Venetian Niccolò Massa claimed much the same about such treatments for all cases of 'putrid fevers', which included plague, *petecchie*, and other diseases.[38] Fracastoro reported doctors making these observations as early as 1505 and 1528, and in his treatise of 1546 denounced the practice as well as strong drugs to evacuate the germs in most cases of pestilential fevers.[39] In Italy by the 1570s bloodletting appears to have sunk further into abeyance. Girolamo Donzellini said doctors were no longer recommending it to cure fevers because of the side effects.[40] In 1576 the Sicilian physician Ingrassia discussed at length opinions on bloodletting of doctors from antiquity to the sixteenth century. After listing those who had earlier recommended it, he concluded his survey by citing two doctors who 'worked from experience', Fracastoro and Jean Fernel [Fervelio]: both had argued against it.[41] In other places, Ingrassia supported his own suspicions, approaching this treatment with extreme caution: barbers could not be entrusted with such decisions alone; doctors had to be present to take the patient's pulse, examine the complexion to make sure that the operation should proceed, and determine the quantity of blood to be taken.[42]

Finally, he cited the famous anatomist and professor at Padua, Gabriele Falloppio, and the Aragonese doctor Jaun Tomás Porcell, both of whom had condemned the practice outright.[43] Similarly, during the 1570s plague doctors

---

[37] *Consigli contro la peste (da un manoscritto della Braidense)*, 37. For other places in these tracts where bloodletting is discussed, see 26, 31–2, 35–9, 45–6, and 68. Emanuele's *Opus utilissimum contra pestilentiam* is another tract to recommend phlebotomy but concentrated on cases when it was not to be employed (15r–16v). Also, see Prezati, *Tractatus flagellum*, 15r. In addition, distrust of bloodletting may have been growing in France by the middle of the sixteenth century; at least one of France's most prominent physicians, Jean Fernel (1497–1558), denied its efficacy with plague treatment; see Brockliss and Jones, *The Medical World of Early Modern France*, 156. Similarly, at Leipzig, the Paduan-trained physician Simone Simoni took a cautious view of it along with the use of strong purgatives, recommending instead gentle cathartic drugs; see Nutton, 'With Benefit of Hindsight', 16.

[38] Palmer, 'Nicolò Massa', 402.

[39] Fracastoro, *De contagione*, 210–21, 226–9, and 242–3: 'In these fevers I do not approve of phlebotomy' (243).

[40] Donzellini, *De natura*, 6r.

[41] Ibid., 91. One exception is the short tract of the Bolognese druggist Pastarino, known by no other name, who appears in Venice during the 1576–7 plague (*Preparamento*, 8v). Unlike authors of fourteenth- and early fifteenth-century tracts, however, he spent no time explaining the procedures. His advice in fact was more moral than surgical: during plague he urged his co-citizens of Bologna to purge themselves of all superfluities from the body and the soul—bad blood, evil thoughts, and dirty words (*i pensieri cattivi, le parole immonde*).

[42] Ingrassia, *Informatione*, Parte Quarta, 28 and 90.

[43] Ibid., 105–14. Nonetheless, these authors conclude: 'approval of phlebotomy, it must be stressed, was ubiquitous' (157). On Porcell, see Carreras Panchón, *La peste y los medicos* 109–16.

such as Calzaveglia and the College of Physicians of Brescia[44] became cautious and critical of another practice, which along with bloodletting is usually assumed to have been an unchanging fixture of doctors' practices and pharmacology before the Enlightenment—strong purgatives, theriacs, and poisons for attacking the venomous disease with venomous antidotes.[45]

The most significant change in the writing about plague, however, came with the plague of 1575–8. This threat of plague ignited an explosion in plague publications in Italy, marking the most significant increase in plague writing during the 500-year period of European plague including the Black Death of 1348 or France's finale in 1720 and has escaped notice by subsequent historians.[46] The 1575–8 plague also created a more significant caesura in mentality and plague literature than any future plague including that of 1629 to 1633 dramatized later in Alessandro Manzoni's *The Betrothed* and *The Column of Infamy*. This now more famous early modern plague in fact occasioned the republication of several key tracts written a half century earlier, which now served as the models for plague writing in the 1630s—tracts by the Florentine Francesco Rondinelli, the Milanese Giuseppe Ripamonti, Alessandro Tadino, Agostino Lampugnani, and Federigo Borromei.

PLAGUE AND DEMOGRAPHY
IN SIXTEENTH-CENTURY ITALY

The demographic data now available do not allow us to say that the plague of 1575–8 was without doubt the most devastating one of the sixteenth century or of any since 1478–80, 1449–52, or 1399–1400. But it was the most extensive as far as the geographical coverage of the Italian peninsula goes, more so than

---

[44] See Redmond, 'Girolamo Donzellino', 59–150; Calzaveglia, *De theriacae abusu*; and Donzellini, *De natura*. Also, see Findlen, *Possessing Nature*, 272–85, who argues convincingly that these disputes intensified with the plague of 1575–7 (esp. 285).

[45] On the theriac, see Watson, *Theriac and Mithridatium*; and more recently, Fabbri, 'Treating Medieval Plague': 'There was little evolution in the antipestilential regimen as regarded diet, hygiene, medicines, or surgical procedures. On the contrary, late medieval physicians—in the face of what was by all accounts a terrible disease—retained their long-established practices and remedies . . . Throughout the period . . . 1348 to the close of the sixteenth century—the treatment of plague . . . was strikingly continuous, attesting to an overarching conservatism of medical practice' (248). 'Until the nineteenth century, the drugs used were remarkably consistent, and change was resisted' (280). Also, see Siraisi, *Medieval and Early Renaissance Medicine*: 'Certain basic physiological concepts and associated therapeutic methods—notably humoral theory and the practice of bloodletting to get rid of bad humors—had a continuous life extending from Greek antiquity into the nineteenth century' (97); Lindemann, *Medicine and Society*, cites this passage as an astute observation (68). For early modern theriacs, see Gentilcore, *Healers and Healing*, 113; and idem, *Medical Charlatanism*, 213. For an overview of Galen's methods, theory, and pharmacology, see Nutton, *Ancient Medicine*, 230–47. On public control and ceremonious rituals of the theriac, see Pomata, *Contracting a Cure*, 89–92.

[46] For the French numbers, see Jones, 'Plague and Its Metaphors', 103; this plague produced the highest number of plague tracts in French history—around sixty of them.

the plague of 1478–80, which stimulated one of the most famous plague tracts of the medieval or early modern period, the humanist tract of Marsilio Ficino. According to the sixteenth-century doctor Jean Fernel, the late fifteenth-century plague spread through 'Italiam per Germaniam, vero Galliae et in Hispaniae'.[47] But at least for Italy, no evidence points to any place afflicted south of Rome or that it even reached Milan and Lombardy.[48] By contrast, plague between 1575 and 1578 had two near simultaneous starting points at the peninsula's opposite ends: in the extreme north it spread over the Alps of the Swiss cantons to Trent, then southward to Mantua, Verona, Venice, Brescia, and through villages and small towns in Lombardy, such as Monza, before striking Milan. To the west, it afflicted villages and small towns on the eastern borders of Piedmont and eventually struck Genoa in 1579. This plague's southern trajectory appears to have had the same origins as the northern one—the Levant—but arrived from northern Africa, probably from ships from Tunisia or Alexandria that docked in Sicily. It struck first Messina and then Sciacca, Giuliano, and Palazzo d'Adriano in the south-west, and then Palermo, Agrigento, Naro, and Trapani.[49] From one direction or the other, the 1575–8 plague threatened Naples, the Marche, Umbria, and Tuscany. However, despite expectations, it seems never to have built momentum in central Italy, perhaps as a result of the controls health boards in these regions vigorously put in place. While this plague was most devastating in Sicily and the cities of Lombardy and the Veneto, plague tracts also sprung up in towns where it appears never to have reached. Threatened by a north–south pincer movement, doctors, local governments, and health boards in the centre prepared for the worst. In dedicatory prefaces, physicians and other writers at Pieve Santo Stefano,[50] Monte Sano, near Fermo,[51] Lucca,[52] Perugia,[53] Bologna,[54] Bagnoregio (Lazio),[55] Salerno,[56] Naples,[57] Lanciano (Abruzzi),[58] and the pope in Rome[59] explicitly remarked on this threat, seeing it as a pan-Italian phenomenon.

---

[47] Corradi, *Annali*, I, 289.

[48] Ibid., I, 282–9; and IV, 154–61, has uncovered pestilence at Venice, Lugano, Como, Cremona, Mantua, Perugia, Rome, Florence, and other places in Tuscany, Romagna, and the Marche for this plague. No evidence of it appears in the Milanese *Libri di morti*, Archivio di Stato, Milano (hereafter ASM), Fondo popolazione, parte antica (hereafter Popolazione).

[49] Corradi, *Annali*, I, 581 and 589.

[50] Tronconi, *De peste*, 1: 'Dum dira pestilentiae lues iam per Italiam publice grassari ceperit, nonnullasque urbes iam saeviter angat, ut Tridentina Urbs, Venetiae, Mediolanum quoque magna cum strage suorum modo experiuntur.'

[51] Augenio, *Del modo di preservarsi*, n.p.

[52] Puccinelli, *Dialoghi sopra le cause della peste*, n.p.; and Minutoli, *Avvertimenti*, n.p.

[53] Tranquilli, *Pestilenze che sono state in Italia*, 21–2.

[54] *Lettera pastorale di Monsig. Ill Card. Paleotti*, 371v (Biblioteca Apostolica Vaticana pagination, hereafter BAV).

[55] Locati, *Italia trauagliata*.   [56] Alfani, *Opus, de peste*.

[57] Ajello, *Breue discorso*, n.p.   [58] Tranzi, *Trattato di peste*.

[59] *Gregorii PP. XIII Iubileum ad avertenda pestis pericula Venetiis*, n.p.; and *Gregorii PP. XIII [S.D.N.D.] Iubileum ad avertenda pestis pericula*, n.p.

The plague that struck Italian regions before 1575–8—one in 1555–6—was far more localized: restricted to parts of Friuli, and the Veneto, it was principally a plague of two cities, Padua and Venice.[60] In geographic coverage, if not in total devastation, the 1575–8 plague was even more extensive than the more famous and last major Italian plagues of the seventeenth century, those of 1629–33 or 1656–7. The one of 1629–33 was restricted to northern and central Italy (but failed to strike Genoa), while that of 1656–7 spread through the south but struck only Genoa in the north and spared all other major Italian cities except Naples and Rome.[61] The second most important plague of the sixteenth century, that of 1522–4, also swept with a wider arc than the two more deadly seventeenth-century plagues, hitting places in Piedmont (Saluzzo, Oncino, and other neighbouring localities), Siena and Foligno in central Italy, and at least touching Sicily (Castrogiovanni [Enna] and the province of Caltanissetta).[62] It had a presence at Rome and in Sardinia,[63] and various Italian authors[64] as well as the French doctor Jacques Dubois commented that it spread 'almost through all of Italy'.[65] However, as far as evidence from chroniclers and plague tracts go, the 1522–4 plague was concentrated largely in central and northern Italy—Rome, Florence, Perugia, Parma, Mantua, Vercelli, Novara, Alessandria, Pavia, Piacenza, and especially Milan and its territory. Moreover, its spread through the north was not universal: it failed to reach (or at least afflict seriously) two of Italy's most important centres of population and commerce, Genoa and Venice.[66]

Estimating the severity of these plagues, even in places for which numerous narrative and archival sources survive, is more difficult. For Milan, where health-board officials meticulously recorded plague deaths in the city, in locked houses of the plague-stricken, and in lazaretti, the plague of 1576–7 killed 17,239.[67] This was the city's worst annual mortality, whether absolutely or in relation to its population, by plague or any other malady since at least 1449–52, for which no statistics or contemporary estimates of mortality survive.[68] The next worst plague in Milan had been that of 1483 to 1485. Unfortunately, the health board's 'necrologies' do not survive for 1484, but in 1483 only 534 died of plague and

---

[60] Corradi, *Annali*, I, 532–5; and IV, 452–6.

[61] Corradi, *Annali*, II, 183–4; Del Panta and Livi Bacci, 'Chronologie', 411–13. This plague was also virulent in Sardinia, lasting from 1652 to 1657, and devastated towns and villages in southern Lazio; see Sonnino, 'Cronache della peste a Roma', 35–6.

[62] Corradi, *Annali*, IV, 333.   [63] Ibid., I, 392.

[64] Previdelli, *Tractatus legalis de peste*, n.p.; Tranquilli, *Pestilenze che sono state in Italia*, 19–20.

[65] Dubois, *De febribus commentarius*, 71r–v.

[66] Corradi, *Annali*, I, 391–8; and IV, 332–53. The plague of 1527–8 reached Venice, but Corradi describes the mortality as 'non poca, ma non tanta' (398). From the archival sources, however, Palmer, 'The Control of Plague', 355, also finds cases of plague in Venice in 1523 and 1524.

[67] Besozzi, *Le magistrature cittadine milanesi*, 11.

[68] In a contemporary chronicle cited by Albini, *Guerra, fame, peste*, 27, 60,000 died in this plague; by another chronicle, 30,000; in neither case does the rounded estimate make clear whether it pertained to the city alone, the diocese, or the territory.

in 1485, the worst plague year recorded in the surviving necrologies, 4,829 died, including those sent to the pest-house of San Gregorio.[69] By contrast, the plague of 1523 loomed much larger in the historical imagination than that of 1483–5, at least among some Milanese chroniclers, and was part of a larger plague sweeping across northern Italy. According to Milan's death records, however, it killed far fewer, only 1,457.[70] This figure contrasts dramatically with the historical memory of the Dominican chronicler Gasparo Bugati, who was born in that plague year but wrote about it just after the 1575–8 plague. He claimed that 100,000 died in 1523 alone from plague, which would have been almost Milan's total population. In fact Bugati described the city as having been left 'dishabitata, incolta, & selvaggia' ('emptied of people, grass had taken over the city').[71] Yet, according to the health board's detailed statistics, somehow the city continued to possess a sizeable enough population to lose as many the following year as recorded in 1523. By these records the aggregate mortalities of the 1520s do not even show these plague years as ones of abnormal crises: the total mortality in 1523 and 1524 was about the annual average of the early sixteenth century.[72] Bugati's childhood memories may have been influenced by his experiences in 1576–7, magnifying his recollections of Milan's previous plague.[73]

On the other hand, Milan's plague mortality in 1576–7 was relatively light in comparison with that of Venice, which lost 51,000 in this plague (some have estimated 60,000),[74] accounting for between a quarter to a third of its population. In absolute terms this was probably Venice's worst plague since the Black Death, taking an even heavier toll (in raw numbers) than the plague of 1629–30. Venice was the only major city in Italy for which this was the case.[75] Palermo's experience was different. The fear and appearance of

[69] These figures come from my analysis of the death records in 1483 and 1485, Popolazione, no. 77. In 1485, the records were divided into 'new cases' (4,357), cases of recidivism (210), and those who died in the Lazaretto of S. Gregorio (262).

[70] My tallies derive from the registers of Popolazione, no. 87. In that year the health officials set aside a separate *filza* for plague victims. It continued until early September. However, other plague victims can be found in the general register for all deaths during that year.

[71] Bugati, *Historia universale*, 770–1.

[72] Ferrario, *Statistica medico-economica*, 374. For a discussion of these statistics, see Cohn and Alfani, 'Households and Plague'.

[73] I have calculated the annual averages of mortality from Ferrario, *Statistica medico-economica*, 374. Ferrario copied his numbers directly from summaries made in 1791. According to Albini, *Guerra, fame, peste*, 158, these contain errors when compared to figures computed from the surviving volumes of the *Libri dei morti*; she does not, however, indicate or correct the tallies. On the other hand, Saba, 'Una parrocchia milanese', 414–15, finds a close correspondence between the 1791 summaries and his counts from the surviving *libri*, 1607 to 1640, except where the *libri* are damaged or parts are missing.

[74] Biraben, *Les hommes et la peste en France*, II, 92.

[75] Preto, 'La società veneta'; and idem, 'Le grandi pesti', 123–6. Brescia (then under Venetian control) also experienced high mortalities during this plague, as much as 16,396 within the city and 20,677 in its territory by one account. (The figures, however, do not derive directly from death lists or other official archival documents.) Brescian chroniclers also point to the paucity of health controls in the city, the mixing and the social exuberance at Carnival time, and the over-confidence of its *popolo*; see Corradi, *Annali*, I, 593.

plague gave rise to one of the most important and most cited plague tracts of the sixteenth century, which called for and successfully implemented the city's first permanent health board and building of its first lazaretto, called Cubba, along with two other plague hospitals and numerous plague decrees enforced with draconian efficiency.[76] The plague mortality both in the city and its plague hospitals was only 3,100 of a population of nearly 100,000.[77] These smaller plague-infected death rates may well attest to the vigilance and methods of Ingrassia and his health board, its militant policies of quarantine and sequestering plague victims and suspects in the city's new plague hospitals, and its daily provisioning and charity to the poor. This was certainly Ingrassia's opinion: he pointed to much higher percentages of plague cases and deaths in the smaller towns to the south—Palazzo Adriano, Sciacca, and Giuliana—as well as in the city of Messina, where governments had been less vigilant in implementing new plague controls.[78]

As the experience of Palermo shows, sheer mortality figures were not necessarily the only factors that might spur an individual's or community's consciousness into implementing new and concrete changes in health policy and preventative measures against the plague. Across Italy, between 1575 and 1578, a new urgency and mentality can be charted, even in regions where no evidence of this plague survives.[79] The measure of this change can be seen in creative shifts and innovations within a genre of writing that was to all extents and purposes born with the Black Death of 1348—the plague treatise or tract.

EDIT 16

The Italian census (*censimento*) of all known sixteenth-century publications compiled from over 1,500 Italian libraries both public and private, called Edit 16, allows us to investigate quantitatively the importance of the 1575–8 crisis on the literary production of plague works.[80] This census of printed materials,

[76] Il Borgo detto di Santa Lucia, o ver di Fornaia fuor della porta di San Giorgio, and Borgo di Sant'Anna for convalescents.

[77] Preti, 'Giovanni Filippo Ingrassia', 398, citing Ingrassia, claims that it was around 3,000. However, Ingrassia's figure at least until 21 November puts it at 2,100. Further, his arithmetic is mistaken: by his tallying 150 died between 1 June and 18 July, another 150 between 18 July and 3 August, 750 between 3 August and 28 September, and from then 900 to 21 November, giving a total of 1,950 deaths for both the city and the hospitals in the surrounding *borghi* (Ingrassia, *Informatione*, 70, 71, and 77–8). According to Aymard, 'Epidémies et médecins en Sicile', 10, the population of Palermo around 1570 was 80,000 but had risen to 99,000 by 1591.

[78] Ingrassia, *Parte quinta*.

[79] See Chapter 6 on the sharp rise of plague and sanitary decrees issued in 1575–8 and thereafter in Bologna.

[80] *Edit 16: Censimento nazionale delle edizioni italiane del XVI secolo*, Ministero per i beni e l'activitá culturali. Istituto Centrale per il Catalogo Unico delle biblioteche italiane e per le informzioni bibliografiche-ICCU, <http://edit16.iccu.sbn.it>. When I began research on this topic, Edit 16 had surveyed 1,200 libraries; by January 2009 it had reached 1,500.

ranging from broadsheets to scholarly tomes almost 1,000 pages long, also includes printed works known from typographical sources alone and for which the Edit 16 team of librarians has yet to find surviving copies. At present the only other country to have assembled a comparable electronic resource for the sixteenth century is Germany. By using various forms of pest* (*peste, pestis, pestilentia, pestilentium, pestifero*, etc.) as keyword title searches in Edit 16, 356 titles appear.[81] Some words for plague such as *lue* or *lues* produce no further titles.[82] Other names for plague or pestilential fever that appear in these plague writings and which became especially important during the plagues of 1575–8—variations of 'contag*', *mal contagioso, contagioso morbo, de contagione*, and the like—yield further works.[83] Probably the most important theoretical work on plague and disease of the sixteenth century, Fracastoro's *De sympathia et antipathia rerum liber vnus* and *De contagione et contagiosis morbis et curatione libri III* (published together in 1546), would not appear in the plague list had pest* been the only keyword search. Other key words produce less impressive harvests such as variations of *epidemia*. Thirteen titles appear in Edit 16, but of those that relate to plague all but one is captured also by variations of *peste*.[84] No doubt, other writings on plague will have escaped this net, and no matter what or how many keyword searches are tried, some titles centred on plague may not appear.[85] Nonetheless, I feel that my net of keywords along with cross-references from other plague works has succeeded in finding the vast majority of plague titles published in sixteenth-century Italy.

Still other works might be counted in this survey such as Bugati's *L'aggiunta dell'Historia universale, et delle cose di Milano* (Milan, 1587). Fifteen pages of this chronicle are in effect a *Successo della peste* for the Milanese plague of 1576–7. Other chronicles and diaries could be added such as Andrea Morosini's *Historia veneta ab anno M.D.XXI usque ad annum M.DC.XV*, of which fewer than 12 of

---

[81] This number is continually rising (last searched in January 2008). When I first compiled a list from Edit 16 in 2005, 295 titles appeared.

[82] In one case the title refers to venereal diseases, and for the other one, *pestifera* also appears in the title.

[83] Thirty-eight appear, sixteen of which, however, are captured also by the pest* searches, such as Ingrassia's *Informatione*. Two others pertain to other diseases and have been subtracted.

[84] However, no copy of this exception—Capra's *De morbo epidemico*—has yet to be located in any Italian library.

[85] For instance, I discovered within the multi-book 'miscellanea' volume of the Biblioteca Apostolica Vaticana, R.I.IV.1551, Sebastiano Montecchio's poem on the plague of Padua, *Carmen epicum* (no. 96), and *Ricordi di m. Paolo Clarante da Terni medico in Roma* that describes plague there in 1576 (no. 99). Furthermore, the title of another tract, *Due discorsi volgari in materia di Medicina*, by Leveroni, a doctor from Fossano in Piedmont, gives no hint that it is a plague tract: his first 'discourse' on healthy living (*Del reggimento della sanità*) 'teaches principally how to protect oneself when plague threatens', and the second recommends cures for plague swellings and pestilential fevers. Donzellini's attack against Calzaveglia's definitions and treatment of plague written under a pseudonym, *Eudoxi Philalethis Adversus calumnias*, is another title not captured by any obvious keyword designating plague.

its 1,846 pages pertain to the plague of 1576–7[86] or the diary of the Milanese carpenter who devotes about 16 of 127 pages to this plague.[87] These three sources will be used in this book for illustrative purposes but have not been counted as plague imprints, that is, as works devoted principally to the medical analysis of plague or the description of a single plague.

On the other hand, not all titles containing pest* concerned plague, the disease. One such title was a tract published between 1502 and 1550 on the immortal sins described in the Bible; another six were invectives against heresy, mostly diatribes against Martin Luther and one against Bernardino Ochino.[88] As might be expected, these works clustered in the years immediately after Luther posted his Ninety-five theses, and all of them were published before mid-century. Another was a tract on the immortality of the soul, which used *pestifero* in its paragraph-long title to refer to the arguments of the sophists and Epicureans.[89] A tract published in 1556 used *peste* in reference to the invasions of the Turks.[90]

To view the Italian production of plague writing, still other tracts might be subtracted from the keywords' lists. The humanistic tradition of the sixteenth century was rich in the revival, translation, and reprinting of classical medical texts from Greek, Roman, and Arabic doctors containing variations of pest* in their titles—works by the ninth-century philosopher and doctor Al-Razi (two tracts), the sixth-century AD Greek physician Alexander Trallianus (three tracts), and most importantly new editions of the second-century Roman physician Galen (nine editions listed in Edit 16), which survive in libraries across Italy. Furthermore, modern pre-sixteenth-century Italian tracts on plague written since the Black Death were printed for the first time or reprinted in the sixteenth century. Most prominent of these was Ficino's *Consiglio contro la pestilentia*, written during the 1478–80 plague. Seven new editions of this work were printed in sixteenth-century Italy, and several of these included tracts by other fourteenth- and fifteenth-century doctors, such as the fourteenth-century Florentine Tommaso Del Garbo, the late fifteenth-century Mengo Bianchelli, and the fifteenth-century doctor and professor at Padua Niccolò Rainaldi. The survival in libraries across Italy in over fifty collections illustrates the remarkable success and influence of Ficino in the sixteenth century, and is corroborated by copious references to his *Consiglio* in numerous tracts by sixteenth-century physicians. Finally, I have read but subtracted from the tallies of Italian Cinquecento production the few works of non-Italians: those of the French doctor Jacques Houllier, who died in 1562 (one edition), the

---

[86] Morosini, *Degl'istorici delle cose veneziane*, VI, 617–35 (and not all these pages concern the plague).

[87] *Il diario di Giambattista Casale*, for the plague: 289–304. On Casale, see Amelang, *A Journal of the Plague Year*, 21.

[88] Some, such as Politi's *Rimedio a la pestilente dottrina de frate Bernardino Ochino*, used forms of *peste* in adjectival form.

[89] Flandino, *De animorum immortalitate*.   [90] Darezia, *Auisi Dongaria del'assedio de Strigonia*.

French nobleman and Cavaliere of Malta Nicolas Durand de Villegagnon (one edition), the late sixteenth-century physician at the Sorbonne and court librarian Lorenzo Condivi, and the mid-fifteenth-century physician Johannes Ketham from Würtemberg (three editions).

Physically, the Italian publications ranged in cost and quality from the plague poems dedicated to Cosimo I de' Medici in 1549 trimmed in gold leaf to cheap octavo prints in vernacular consisting of only several leaves or even a single sheet with antiquated Gothic type and without covers, publication dates, or the names of the press.[91] The preponderance of the cheaper varieties of print along with authors' stated intentions of appealing to and instructing populations at large strongly suggests that the readership of these tracts was often a lay one and certainly more vast than that of any other form of medical writing (which had indeed been the case since at least the early fifteenth century in Italy).[92] In addition, with the mass publication of ephemeral single-sheet plague broadsheets plastered in prominent places throughout cities, especially during and after the 1575–8 plague, the scope of medical instructions in print expanded further down the social ladder. Now beggars, scroungers, scoundrels, and other forms of low life, no doubt mostly illiterate, were nonetheless required to take notice of these broadsheets and act immediately on draconian decisions taken by health boards and princes or face punitive measures, including execution.[93]

THE PLAGUE OF 1575–8: A QUANTITATIVE RECKONING

Without making any adjustments, the importance of the plague 1575–8 for the production of plague publication is overwhelming. Of 378 printed publications with plague or variations of *contagioso morbo*, and so forth, 68 were printed before 1550 (18 per cent), 66 (17.5 per cent) between 1550 and 1575, and 69 (18.3 per cent) after 1578, leaving the lion's share, 170 (45 per cent),

---

[91] The secondary literature on the variety of Cinquecento printing and its readers is large. See Hirsch, *Printing, Selling and Reading*, and, more recently, Grendler, 'Form and Function in Italian Popular Books'; Bell, *How to Do It*, 1–16; de Vivo, *Information and Communication in Venice*; and Fenlon, *The Ceremonial City*, 233–71.

[92] See Introduction, n. 2. A possible contender may have been *Regimen sanitatis*, from which plague tracts had derived. For the *Regimen*'s tradition principally in England and during the later Middle Ages, see Rawcliffe, 'The Concept of Health'. The production of new works of the *Regimen* (or *Reggimento*) in sixteenth-century Italy was, however, far less impressive than that of plague tracts. From a quick search through Edit 16, I find only twenty new *Regimen* in Latin (9) or Italian (11) published during the sixteenth century in Italy. (On the other hand, there were many translations and reprints of the famous thirteenth-century *Regimen sanitatis Salernitanum* and works of healthy living from antiquity, especially by Aristotle, Galen, and Avicenna.) A study of the *Regimen* in early modern Italy is badly needed.

[93] For a discussion of these broadsheets, see Chapter 6, 'Government Reactions'.

to four years alone. Most of these (115) were published in the peak two years of this plague, 1576 and 1577, giving an annual production of plague publications at 57.5, compared with 1.4 during the first half of the century, 2.6 from mid-century to the beginning of the plague wave, and three per annum for the last twenty-three years of the century. Subtracting texts where *peste* refers to heresy rather than disease, translations and republications of Arabic, Greek, and Roman classics, tracts written before the sixteenth century, works by foreign authors, and tracts on contagion which did not concern plague puts the 1577–8 production in bolder relief. By this reckoning, the total number of plague publications decreases by 41 to 337.[94] Of those subtracted, only two (a new edition of Ficino's *Consiglio* and a translation of a plague prayer by Saint Cyprian) were published 1575 to 1578. With these adjustments, half the plague writings of the entire century (49.9 per cent) were printed in two years alone. The other two principal transregional plagues in Italy of the Cinquecento show no comparable influence on plague writing. For the plague of 1522–4, only eight tracts appear plus two new editions of Ficino's *Consiglio*.[95] The plague of 1556 produced slightly more—eleven new Italian works and four reprints of classics, Ficino, or of foreigners, amounting to less than 7 per cent of the 1575–8 production. The 1575–8 plague did more: it broke the virtual monopoly of university-trained physicians in Italy in composing these published pamphlets and ushered new professions and social groups into giving advice on plague. Before 1575, almost 90 per cent of the authors were physicians (106 of 119); after 1578 to the end of the century, the dominance of physicians as the authors returned—92 per cent (56 of 61). By contrast, non-physicians during the four years of the Italian-wide threat of 1575–8 scripted 44 per cent of the plague publications (not including the massive increase in broadsheets issued by city oligarchies, princes, and health boards).[96]

Further scrutiny, moreover, shows the preponderance of plague writing in 1575–8 as even more remarkable than that seen from keyword searches in Edit 16 alone. First, Edit 16 has yet to find or list a number of published works of plague verse and to a lesser extent, plague prose. Numerous examples of free-standing

---

[94] This figure is considerably larger than that calculated by Brockliss and Jones, *The Medical World of Early Modern France*, 41, for France over two and a half centuries, from 1500 to 1750: it amounted to less than 300. Also, see Jones, 'Plague and Its Metaphors in Early Modern France', 102, where the number is 263 from 1550 to 1770.

[95] According to Henderson, 'Epidemics in Renaissance Florence': 'The news that "pestilenza" was spreading throughout Italy in the early 1520s led to a flurry of printing activity; many earlier treatises, which had by now become standard texts, made their re-appearance and new ones were written especially for the advice of the reading public' (166). But he shows no evidence for it, and Edit 16 does not substantiate it.

[96] The percentage becomes even higher if the collection of poems on Verona's 1576 struggle against plague is counted by author (*Raccolta delli componimenti*). Of thirty-five poems, eight authors can be identified by occupation (some wrote more than one poem). They were local literati or bureaucrats; none was a physician.

as well as collections of poems on plague can be found in miscellanea volumes in the Vatican Library that have yet to be thoroughly catalogued.[97] These pertain almost entirely to 1575–8. In addition, large numbers of decrees and regulations (called *gride* in Milan, *bandi*, *proclami*, or *provvisioni* elsewhere)—broadsheets posted on street corners and in other public places—were published by the Church, lieutenants of the Spanish throne, city magistrates, and health boards in plague years to govern against the spread of plague and to instruct residents on matters as simple as boiling water and washing hands. These also listed plague recipes and gave instructions on the preparation and use of purgatives for cleaning various types of contaminated goods. Some appear from the keyword searches, but most do not. From my searches through Edit 16 for imprints on plague, subtracting those that pertained to heresy but adding many other titles found from my own research in fifty libraries in France, the United States, Britain, and Italy with chance encounters in libraries such as the Vatican and the Braidense of Milan, I have amassed a total of 609 imprints on plague during the sixteenth century published in Italy or housed in Italian libraries. Without doubt, more examples could be accumulated through further assiduous research in Italian and foreign libraries or just by waiting for the indefatigable investigation of Italy's librarians to add new titles to Edit 16.

While this figure represents a large and representative picture of sixteenth-century Italian plague publications, it must nonetheless be considered a sample; yet from it the importance of the 1575–8 plague becomes extraordinary. While the average per annum production of these texts across the century was six a year, the plague years 1575–8 produced 301 plague texts, 75.3 per annum. If only 1576 and 1577 are considered, the annual count soars to over 140. With this larger sample of 609, these two plague years alone constitute almost half the entire century's production of printed plague works. Furthermore, other writings such as Asciano Centorio Degli Ortensi's lengthy treatise on the Milanese plague of 1576–7 published in 1579, Sebastiano Tranzi's work on Lanciano in 1576, published in 1586, or Carlo Borromeo's statutes and advice for the plague in Milan in 1576, but not published until 1593, could be added to the 1576–7 list. If published plague decrees, *gride*, and broadsheets, which may not be considered plague tracts proper (even though they did concentrate on preventative measures and occasionally included medical recipes) are subtracted, the peaks for 1576 and 1577 are not quite as sharp, but the quantitative significance of this plague remains much the same: overwhelmingly, 47 per cent of the publications come from these four plague years and 42 per cent from 1576 and 1577 alone when the plague peaked in most places.

This spike in production did not ride a steady wave or sudden increase in printing activity in Italy during the 1570s. In fact, the opposite was the story: as

---

[97] Since I began this work, Edit 16 has made considerable progress in including previously uncatalogued plague tracts and verse.

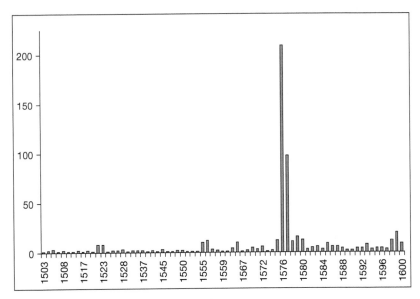

Figure 1.1. Sixteenth-century Italian Plague Imprints.

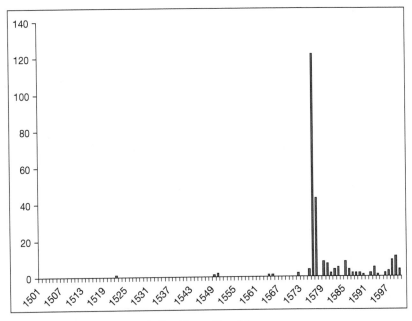

Figure 1.2. Sixteenth-century Italian Plague Broadsheets.

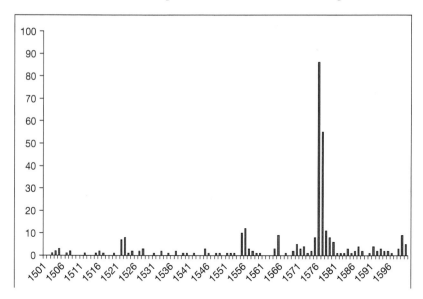

Figure 1.3. Italian Plague Tracts, 1501–1600 (Not including Broadsheets).

plague depressed commerce and other productive activities, especially. in cities, the same happened in printing. According to Edit 16, 8,629 new titles and re-editions appeared during the decade 1570–79. For the critical years 1576 and 1577, the numbers, however, fell to 718 and 550 respectively, the latter constituting the lowest number of the decade, the lowest in fact since 1561 (549 titles).[98] In Venice, the capital of sixteenth-century publishing, where this plague hit hardest, the decline may have been the most dramatic. For instance, production of the Giolito press, which produced between thirty-five and forty editions in a good year in the sixteenth century, suddenly collapsed to seven in 1576.[99] Moreover, the 1575–8 peak in plague publications was not accompanied by any signs of a boom in the production of other medical texts. Instead, new titles and re-editions of the principal medical textbook, the *Practica*,[100] remained at a low ebb until the mid-1580s.[101]

---

[98] For the 'paralysis' of the printing industry in Venice during these plague years, see Fenlon, *The Ceremonial City*, 253 and 375. The Venice industry did not recover until the late 1580s.

[99] Robin, *Publishing Women*, 199 and 327. For the problems suffered by the printing industry in Rome during the plague of 1656–7, see San Juan, 'The Contamination of the Modern City', 205–6.

[100] For the increasing importance of these texts in fifteenth- and sixteenth-century medical training, see Park, 'Natural Particulars', 351.

[101] Plague could (and probably did) often lead to the temporary closure of presses as in Leipzig during its plague in 1575, when printers refused to come to their workshops, delaying the publication, among other works, of Simone Simoni's plague treatise; Nutton, 'With Benefit of Hindsight', 8. Another supposedly popular medical manual may have been the *Regimen sanitatis*. Nicoud, *Les régimes de santé au*

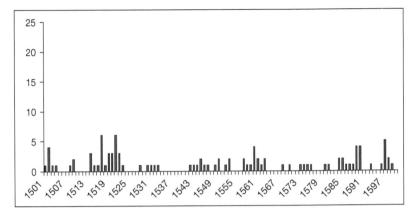

Figure 1.4. Medical 'Practicae'.

Was Italy part of a larger, general European trend? To find plague writings during the sixteenth century for other areas of Europe I have turned to other sources: the library catalogues of the University of Leiden; the National Library of Medicine in Bethesda, Maryland (the largest single collection of sixteenth-century medical literature); the Wellcome Library, London; and J.-N. Biraben's bibliography of plague writing compiled largely through a search in French libraries and the Wellcome catalogues. From these, not only did the plague years of 1575–8 fail to produce a sudden rise in the production of plague manuals and other imprints outside Italy, but no plague of the sixteenth century had such an impact on plague writing and publication in any other area of Europe (see Fig. 1.3). Use of the German database of sixteenth-century imprints (*Verzeichnis der im deutschen Sprachbereich erschienenen Drucke des 16. Jahrhunderts* [VD 16]) traces a slightly different trend from that seen in various medical library catalogues: keyword searches with variations of *peste, pestelentz, contagium, lues, plag* from VD 16 produces many more religious titles than those gathered from searches in medical catalogues, even after titles concerned with biblical plagues, pestilential heresies of the Turks, Martin Luther, or Protestant condemnations of Roman Catholics and anti-popes have been subtracted. Nonetheless, the pattern for German-speaking regions differs from the Italian. The imprints increase over the century especially with the plague years of the first half of the 1560s, the mid-1580s, and in the last years of the century, but no two-year period constitutes more than 10 per cent of these imprints (72 for the years 1564 and

Moyen Age, I, ch. IX, has recently shown, however, that it was a genre that remained limited largely to an elite scholarly community and that the number of new works fell precipitously in the second half of the fifteenth century and with extremely few new productions in the sixteenth century. A search for new titles in Edit 16 confirms her conclusions.

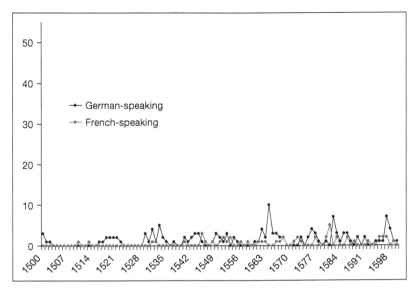

Figure 1.5. Plague Imprints: French- and German-speaking Regions.

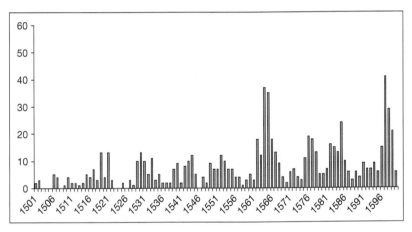

Figure 1.6. Plague Imprints: German-speaking Regions (VD).

1565 of 778 titles), compared with at least 42 per cent for the years 1576 and 1577 in Italy.[102]

[102] When the online *Universal Short Title Catalogue* of all books published in Europe before 1601 has been completed (scheduled for 2012) such comparisons across countries will be easier and more complete; on this enterprise, see Pettegree, 'Centre and Periphery', 108.

The significance of 1575–8 in Italy highlights other changes. Overall 461 of these plague works were written in Italian and 142 (just under a quarter) in Latin.[103] These were not, however, distributed equally over time; nor did the trend move progressively towards the vernacular. Before mid-century, the majority were in the vernacular (34 of 63, or 59 per cent) in marked contrast with other medical books such as the *Practica*, which were almost exclusively in Latin. From mid-century to just before the plague of 1575–8, however, Latin dominated with over 57 per cent (39 of 68)—a reversal indicative of the 'Renaissance in Medicine of the sixteenth century': the recovery of classical texts of Hippocrates, Galen, and others in Greek and Latin had influenced medical writing throughout, down to its most popular manual, the plague tract.[104] But this trend came to an abrupt end with the plague years 1575 to 1578: the language of plague reverted dramatically to the vernacular at levels previously unseen: 288 of these texts were written in Italian (87 per cent), only 42 in Latin. Even the decrees and advice on plague issued by the papacy and local bishops in these years were principally in Italian. Afterwards to the end of the century, Italian continued to predominate, with slightly over 80 per cent of the imprints in the vernacular (120 of 147). A substantial proportion of the plague imprints for 1575–8 were published broadsheets, decrees, and advice by religious leaders and more predominantly by health boards and secular states. These account for almost half these publications (169 of 330 or 48 per cent) and were overwhelmingly written in Italian (157 of 169 or 93 per cent). Yet excluding these does not change the picture substantially: instead of 87 per cent drafted in Italian, the proportion falls only to 81 per cent, more than doubling the proportion in the vernacular before this plague.

A CONCEPT OF ITALY

Did 'Italy' exist in the sixteenth century? Is it justifiable to study ideas and attitudes or medical knowledge that was 'Italian' as opposed to Florentine or Sicilian on the one hand or as European on the other, especially given that large areas of Italy were then part of the Spanish Empire, that areas such as the Alpine zones of the Trentino were linguistically as much German as Italian, and that Piedmont formed part of French-speaking Savoy? Recent texts on early modern Italy begin by stressing the peninsula's regional variety as though by necessity.[105] The distinctiveness of regional zones—the Veneto, Lombardy, the

---

[103] Four works contain substantial parts in both languages.   [104] See n. 24 above.

[105] See for instance Di Scala, *Italy: From Revolution to Republic*; Hanlon, *Early Modern Italy*, ch. 1: 'Italy circa 1700: a Geographical Expression'; Black, *Early Modern Italy*, ch. 1: 'Disunited Italy'; Lyttelton (ed.), *Liberal and Fascist Italy*, 3. Hanlon, *Early Modern Italy*, 1 and 5–6, argues for the exclusion of Piedmont from a consideration of Early Modern Italy until the eighteenth century.

Papal States, the kingdom of Naples, and Tuscany—may have even increased with the consolidation of a myriad of city-states into territorial states after the Black Death and especially with the collapse of 'Italian independence' during the sixteenth century. Even after unification (1861–70), Italy hardly presents cultural or linguistic unity: only between 2.5 and 12 per cent of the peninsula's population spoke Italian.[106] With political unification and industrialization during the late nineteenth and twentieth centuries, the division between north and south, in fact, continued to grow. Many scholars now stress the legacy of Italy's disunited past in the present-day weakness of the Italian central state and the importance of its regions.[107] How can we then justify a book on plague in sixteenth-century Italy?

The plague tracts give a strong voice to an intellectual unity of Italy in the sixteenth century, at least as concerns this branch of medicine and the fear of plague. The references of sixteenth-century doctors to modern doctors and other sources on plague are overwhelmingly to Italians, that is, to those who inhabited *grosso modo* the present borders of the peninsula: the fourteenth-century author-ities were Gentile da Foligno, Tommaso del Garbo, Giovanni Boccaccio, and Matteo Villani;[108] for the fifteenth, Marsilio Ficino, and Saladino Ferro; and for the sixteenth the list of Italian physicians, surgeons, and pharmacists cited in plague tracts runs into the hundreds. Moreover, these Italian works are the ones that Italian presses reprinted or printed for the first time from manuscripts. By contrast, few foreign doctors or their works are mentioned—whether in Latin or the vernacular, and according to the resources of Edit 16, few foreign works were translated, published, or republished in Italy, and few can currently be found in rare book rooms across the peninsula.[109] Even citations within the published Italian tracts to two tracts of the most-read medical authors of the sixteenth century—those of Ambroise Paré (none) or Paracelsus (two cita-tions)—were extremely rare. The transfer of information and theories about plague appears to have flowed in one direction. Unlike foreigners who readily translated and plagiarized Italian plague tracts,[110] the Italians did not recip-rocate. One exception was a northern Italian translation of several tracts by doctors, surgeons, and druggists from Poitiers and Paris who offered remedies based on their experiences during the French plagues from 1562 to 1566. This compilation, however, which also included extracts from the Florentines Tommaso Del Garbo and Marsilio Ficino, remained in manuscript, published only in 1966.[111] As Ian Maclean has noted more generally, the learned medical book may have become international by 1600, but 'little direct presence of

106 Black, *Early Modern Italy*, 1.   107 See for instance Putnam, *Making Democracy Work*.
108 The one exception is a reference to the popes' doctor at Avignon in 1348 and 1362, Guy de Chauliac; see for instance Ingrassia, *Informatione*, 102 and 188.
109 In addition to Edit 16, see Maclean, *Logic, Signs and Nature*, 66.
110 See Slack, *The Impact of Plague*, 45.
111 *Consigli contro la peste (da un manoscritto della Braidense)*.

books produced in the north of Europe' appeared in Italian libraries at this time.[112]

On the other hand, references within these tracts sketch a lively intellectual network among sixteenth-century Italian doctors that was neither parochial nor regional as might have been expected. For the Black Death of 1348 the two most cited works in these sixteenth-century tracts were by Florentines: Giovanni Boccaccio's *Decameron* (despite Counter-Reformation condemnations of it)[113] and Matteo Villani's continuation of his brother's chronicle from 1348 to 1363. These were hardly the intellectual property of Florence or Tuscans; instead, they were cited by doctors across the peninsula—the Torinesi Francesco Alessandri,[114] Agostino Bucci,[115] and Filippo Maria Roffredi,[116] professor of medicine at Padua Girolamo Mercuriale,[117] the Mantuan Giovanni Battista Susio,[118] the Sicilian physicians Pietro Parisi[119] and Ingrassia,[120] and the Vicentine, Vittorio Bonagente.[121] Curiously, I do not find sixteenth-century Tuscan doctors in their own plague tracts citing them.

The Sicilian Ingrassia, appointed *Protomedico* for the kingdom of Sicily by the king of Spain, illustrates this peninsula-wide intellectual network and consciousness in one of the longest of plague works of the sixteenth century. He reflects on examples of epidemic disease in Sicily, central Italy, and northern Italy from the Black Death to the present plague of 1575–6.[122] Citations to numerous works, experiments, drugs, and plague experiences, historical and contemporary, fill his treatise and come almost exclusively from Italian doctors even though Sicily was then a part of the Spanish Empire. Ingrassia dedicated his tract of 1576 to Philip II king of Spain and his second one of 1577 (*Parte quinta*) to Philip's Spanish lieutenant, Don Carlo of Aragon, Duke of Terranova, to whom Ingrassia periodically reported and on whom he depended for funds to build Palermo's new lazaretti and to support the poor. Nonetheless, of the hundreds of doctors Ingrassia cited, I find only one doctor from the Iberian peninsula, Juan Tomás Porcell, concerning his experiences during epidemics in Zaragoza of 1558 and 1564.[123]

Most prominent among the myriad of contemporary sources cited by Ingrassia were physicians currently holding chairs at the University of Padua or who had taught there. This is perhaps not surprising given that Padua was the powerhouse of medical teaching, not only for Italy, but for all of Europe in

---

[112] Maclean, *Logic, Signs and Nature*, 66.

[113] Boccaccio's works were placed on the index of forbidden books in 1559.

[114] Alessandri, *Trattato della peste*, 44r.   [115] Bucci, *Reggimento*, n.p.

[116] Roffredi, *Pestis, et calamitatum Taurini*, 26 and 42.   [117] Mercuriale, *De pestilentia*, 70.

[118] Susio, *Libro del conoscere la pestilenza*, 51.   [119] Parisi, *Auuertimenti*, 45.

[120] Ingrassia, *Informatione*, 14, 84, 187, and 196.

[121] Bonagente, *Decem problemata de peste*, 5v.

[122] On Ingrassia and the office of the *Protomedicato*, see Chapter 3, n. 4.

[123] Ingrassia, *Informatione*, 101, 147; Parte quarta, 71 and 105. The title of Ingrassia's 1577 tract may have in fact derived from Porcell's *Informaciòn y curacion de la peste de Çaragoça* . . . (Zaragoza, 1565).

the sixteenth century.[124] Moreover, Ingrassia had been a student and taught there for a few years after graduating. His tract refers to his Paduan training and to an experience with infectious disease there when he was a student in 1537.[125] He cited frequently colleagues with whom he must have kept a lively exchange with the circulation of books and letters—Oddo degli Oddi and his son Marco, Francesco Frigimelica, Bassiano Landi, Bernardo Tomitano, Vittorio Bonagente, Prospero Borgarucci, the anatomist Falloppio.[126] But he relied even more heavily on the Venetian physician Niccolò Massa (1489–1569), who never held a chair at Padua.[127] He also cited doctors from northern Italy, who were prominent in the first half of the century—the surgeon and professor at Padua Alessandro Benedetti (who died sometime shortly after 1511), Pietro Mainardi, who also taught surgery at Padua and died in 1529, the Ferrarese doctor and astrologer Giovanni Mainardi (1462–1536), who taught at the University of Ferrara,[128] and most prominently the Veronese Girolamo Fracastoro.[129]

Ingrassia read and cited recent publications on plague by others in northern Italy such as Girolamo Cardano, then practising in Rome,[130] and those outside university centres entirely, such as the Tridentine physician Andrea Gallo, and the communal doctor of Udine, Gioseffo Daciano.[131] Of fifteenth-century doctors, he relied on the Florentine Marsilio Ficino,[132] the Ferrarese chronicler Giovanni Herculano,[133] and the early fifteenth-century doctor of Pavia, Antonio Guainerio.[134] Furthermore, his detailed recommendations for the separation of the infected from the healthy, with separate rooms in lazaretti for the sick, the suspected, and those convalescing, relied on models from Milan and Venice, from which he added his own original variations.

Was this referencing a one-way street: Sicilian doctors citing those from the north but not the reverse? Before Ingrassia, it appears to have been the case, but by the end of the century, doctors in Piedmont including Alessandri,[135] Bucci,[136] and Roffredi,[137] from Turin and Cesare Mocca, the communal doctor of Poirino in the region of Turin,[138] and the professor of medicine at Padua, Ercole Sassonia,[139] were among northerners who cited Ingrassia along with other

---

[124] Bylebyl, 'The School of Padua'.   [125] Ingrassia, *Informatione*, 16.

[126] Ibid., 20, 28, 47–8, 107; Parte quarta, 89–90, 93, and 142.

[127] On Massa's life and work, see Palmer, 'Nicolò Massa'.

[128] Ibid., 75 and Parte quarta, 70 and 115. On Mainardi's Hippocratic astrology and critique of the heavens' occult influences and determination of health and disease, see Pennuto, *Simpatia, fantasia e contagio*, 390–2.

[129] Ingrassia, *Parte quinta*, 20 and 75.   [130] Ingrassia, *Informatione*, 169.

[131] Ingrassia, *Parte quinta*, 10 and 13.

[132] Ibid., 20 and 75; and Ingrassia, *Informatione*, 19, 70, and 102.

[133] Ingrassia, *Informatione*, 19.

[134] Ingrassia, *Parte quinta*, 20 and 75; *Informatione*, Parte quarta, 70.

[135] Alessandri, *Trattato della peste*, 4r.   [136] Bucci, *Modo di conoscere*, 5v.

[137] Roffredi, *Pestis, et calamitatum Taurini*, 14, 17, 34, and 38.

[138] Mocca, *Trattrato della peste*, 22   [139] Sassonia, *Disputatio de Phoenigmorum*, 4r.

Sicilian doctors such as Pietro Parisi from Trapani.[140] Moreover, physicians in Piedmont cited doctors, chroniclers, and poets, and described plagues and other afflictions across the length and breath of Italy: in Pavia,[141] Bologna,[142] Milan,[143] Genoa,[144] Udine,[145] Florence,[146] Venice,[147] Siena,[148] Padua,[149] Palermo,[150] Trent,[151] Mantua,[152] and Macerata.[153] They also argued for models that had been instituted and developed in other regions of Italy, such as citing Ingrassia's three-pronged approach to plague during the 1575–6 plague and public health in Palermo—'Oro, Fuoco & Forca'.[154] In addition, the Piedmontese Bucci had a detailed knowledge of the organization of the Milanese lazaretto of San Gregorio, including its number of beds and division into three sections. He also cited Milanese plague decrees and recommended several for implementation in Turin in his 1586 plague tract.[155]

Not only was Piedmont a part of the duchy of Savoy, a separate political entity in the sixteenth century and perhaps politically more integrated into the Realm of France than with any territorial state of Italy; ecologically the region can be argued to have been more a part of eastern France or southern Germany than of Italy. On the one hand the region escaped unscathed the great plagues that swept Italy in the sixteenth century, in 1523–4 and most importantly 1575–8; on the other, it was afflicted by plagues that swept through eastern France and Germany but remained largely without incident in Italy, principally the plague of 1564 that, according to the contemporary Torinese doctor Bucci, 'began in Lyon and spread through France, Spain, and Germany';[156] and those of 1585 and 1598–1600, which again were confined to parts of France and

---

[140] Parisi, *Auuertimenti*, 33 and 46.

[141] Roffredi, *Pestis, et calamitatum Taurini*, 8 (cites the doctor of Pavia, Guainerius); and Bucci, *Modo di conoscere*, 54v.

[142] Roffredi, *Pestis, et calamitatum Taurini*, 14 (Fioravanti).

[143] Ibid., 14 (Bugati); Alessandri, *Trattato della peste*, 21r, 25r, 27r, and 48v; Bucci, *Modo di conoscere*, 12v.

[144] Roffredi, *Pestis, et calamitatum Taurini*, 14.   [145] Ibid., 17, 35, and 43 (Daciano).

[146] Ibid., 42 (Boccaccio, Archbishop Antoninus, and Ficino); Alessandri, *Trattato della peste*, 44r (Boccaccio); Bucci, *Reggimento*, n.p. (Boccaccio); Alessandri, *Trattato della peste*, 5v (Ficino).

[147] Alessandri, *Trattato della peste*, 4r; Bucci, *Modo di conoscere*, 7v, 12v.

[148] Alessandri, *Trattato della peste*, 5r.   [149] Ibid., 44v; Bucci, *Modo di conoscere*, 7v.

[150] Ibid., 5v, 7r.   [151] Ibid., 12v.   [152] Ibid., 12v.   [153] Ibid., 54v.

[154] Ibid., 18r. This was the principal organization of a highly abridged version of Ingrassia, *Avertimenti contra la peste*. It is not clear whether Ingrassia or someone else brought together these strands of Ingrassia's two publications of 1575–7. Despite its highly abbreviated form, some of its directives seem new at least in his plague tracts. For instance, he warns that 'no one should trouble, taunt, or make derisive gestures towards gravediggers or those who clean infested houses and belongings' (4r). These strictures can be found, however, in the plague laws of Palermo (1575) which Ingrassia inspired, *Bando et ordinationi fatte per . . . città di Palermo*, 3r–v.

[155] Bucci, *Modo di conoscere*, 22v–23r.

[156] Bucci, *Reggimento*, n.p. Also, see the *bando* issued by the Florentine health board on 28 September 1564 (*Bando dell'ill. . . . Duca di Firenze . . . sopra la tere, e provincie infette dalla peste*), which blocked the passage of goods and persons from fifty-four enumerated cities and regions in Spain, France, Switzerland, the lands of the Grigioni of southern Germany and western Austria, Carintia (Slovenia), and all of Piedmont, except Vercelli, Asti, and Santra.

Germany but failed to cross into Lombardy or spread through northern Italy into Liguria and beyond. Yet, intellectually, the references in these doctors' plague tracts show them as practitioners within an Italian world that stretched south to Sicily and east to Udine. Despite the importance of foreign lands and especially of France to Piedmont's plague experience, its sixteenth-century plague writers (Bucci, Alessandri, Mocca, and Roffredi) did not cite a single Spanish, French, or German author;[157] their modern sources were entirely Italian.[158]

The clearest notion of 'Italy' in these tracts, however, comes with the plague of 1575–8, when doctors, surgeons, notaries, judges, noblemen, and churchmen across much of Italy in Sicily, Naples, the Abruzzi, Rome, Florence, Lucca, Perugia, Genoa, Milan, Venice, Verona, and other places wrote plague manuals, reports, poems, and songs in record numbers because of a plague that they then perceived as threatening all of Italy from Trent in the north to Sciacca on the southern shores of Sicily. Along with forcing those in places where the 1575–8 plague had yet to strike and in fact would not strike—Florence, Lucca, Perugia, Naples, and the Abruzzi—to envision this plague as an 'Italian' catastrophe, it created the first plague tracts with an expressed Italian focus with Italy in their titles as opposed to ones centred on a doctor's own city or region. In 1576 Umberto Locati published his *Italia trauagliata*, which pictured all the present troubles then besieging Italy.[159] In the same year the Perugian humanist, historian, and member of the Academy of the Insenati Vincenzo Tranquilli attempted to write a history of Italian plagues over 2,311 years to discover if various sorts of natural occurrences or 'prodigies' could be correlated with pestilence through Italian history.[160] In 1591, Antonio Carrarino wrote a similar work in its longitudinal survey and subject matter, *Delle pestilenze et prodigii che sono stati in Italia avanti N.S. e doppo*. Here again, Italy was the frame.[161]

From the plague tracts, this Italian unity appears well entrenched before the Counter-Reformation clampdown and decline of Italian medical students seeking degrees in Protestant countries and the restraints placed on northerners attending Italian medical schools.[162] As Jerome Bylebyl has argued, Padua remained the medical school of Europe throughout the sixteenth century.[163] And as Richard

---

[157] This is particularly puzzling given the importance of Lyon as a perceived starting point of plagues, such as the 1564 outbreak, and its rich tradition of plague writing (see Biraben's bibliography of sixteenth-century plague writings and Durling, *A Catalogue of Sixteenth Century Printed Books*). At least one of the Lyonnais tracts was written in Italian: Condivi [Condio], *Medicina filosofica contra la peste*.

[158] Findlen, 'The Formation of a Scientific Community', esp. 380–94, shows Pietro Andrea Mattioli's 'botanical republic' as chauvinistically 'an Italian republic, created to restore glory to Italy in the spirit of Petrarch's and Machiavelli's famous statements to the same effect' (380).

[159] Locati, *Italia trauagliata*.   [160] Tranquilli, *Pestilenze che sono state in Italia*.

[161] Published in Orvieto by Antonio Coaldi. I have not read this work. According to Edit 16 only one copy survives; that one supposedly in the Biblioteca Nazionale Centrale, Firenze is, however, missing. Moreover, Palmer, 'The Control of Plague', 179–80, has suggested that the increasing sophistication of plague measures during the sixteenth century fostered a new 'sense of Italianità' that was strengthened by the negligence for health controls across the Alps.

[162] See Israel, 'Counter-reformation'.   [163] Bylebyl, 'The School of Padua'.

Palmer has shown, sixteenth-century Italian doctors could and did make contacts with doctors from Protestant countries and could collect northern medical tracts so long as they did not push their luck, as did the brazen late sixteenth-century Veronese Donzellini, who collected Protestant religious tracts at the same time.[164] Yet, despite this freedom and Italy as the European melting-pot of medical studies, the plague tracts reflect a remarkably strong Italian intellectual identity in the sixteenth century.

Before turning to the focus of this book—the medical and cultural consequences of the 1575–8 crisis on plague writing—we will consider the character of the disease in the sixteenth century, how it may have changed since the Black Death, and to what extent academic physicians and other writers on plague were aware of its physiological trends and realities. For this we will investigate another source—an archival one—the daily examinations of deaths in Milan from its earliest records in 1452 to the last plague that appears in these detailed reports of practising doctors, that of 1523–4.

[164] Palmer, 'Physicians and the Inquisition'.

2

Signs and Symptoms

Scientists and historians have insisted that the Black Death and its successive outbreaks through Europe up to the early nineteenth century were the same disease as the bubonic plague that spread worldwide at the end of the nineteenth century. The reason for such assurance has rested largely on the supposed similarity of the signs and symptoms of the Black Death disease and the rodent-based bubonic plague first cultured at the end of the nineteenth century, *Yersinia pestis*. Some, such as Ann Carmichael, have pointed out epidemiological differences between the two but have insisted: 'Boccaccio leaves no doubt that bubonic *Y. pestis* was the disease that ravaged Florence in 1348'. For the medieval and early modern bubonic disease, the perception has relied largely on a few statements from a handful of contemporary commentators and mainly from the first outbreak of the Black Death—Giovanni Boccaccio, the pope's doctor Guy de Chauliac, Petrarch's friend the Avignon musician Louis Heiligen de Beeringen, and a few others.[1]

The clinical presentation of many diseases when first introduced to newly discovered lands such as the Americas or previously isolated regions such as the Faroe islands and Greenland differed strikingly from those well-known characteristics of a disease after a pathogen has established some symbiosis with its host. When tuberculosis, for instance, afflicted the Indians of western Canada, it manifested extensive glandular involvement; only by the third generation did it settle in the lungs, becoming the pulmonary disease we recognize today.[2] In the sixteenth century, contemporaries also observed the rapid change in the symptoms and character of syphilis from the last years of the fifteenth to the mid-sixteenth century.[3]

No one to date, however, has attempted to chart possible changes in the most commented upon disease of European history, the one for which we possess the greatest number of historical sources—statistical and narrative, medical and lay—before the twentieth century, the Black Death and its recurrences over nearly five centuries. Historians and scientists have not attempted to investigate

---

[1] Walløe has gone through the narrative sources more thoroughly in *Plague and Population* and 'Medieval and Modern Bubonic Plague'.

[2] Kiple, 'Scrofula', 48.

[3] Among other places, see Fracastoro, *De contagione*, 138–41 and 154–7.

a wide range of narrative and especially medical descriptions of the plague over time to detect change in the disease. Few have analysed case records of symptoms and signs of plague to enquire where the buboes appeared, their number, what other skin disorders, if any, accompanied the larger swellings, the course of the disease, how long patients survived from the onset of illness to death, and more.[4] For the late Middle Ages to 1450, these questions are difficult to pursue. In my examination of the Black Death, I found few sources that described individual cases, especially case histories examined by the medically trained. Before 1450, the largest number of individually described cases are found in saints' lives, and here I was able to gather only thirty-six, where the observers, sometimes with notarized testimony, attested to the number of buboes, their specific locations, other skin disorders, symptoms, and indications of the disease's course.[5]

In contrast to the Black Death's first hundred years, records from the early modern period, beginning with the remarkable sources from Milan, permit far greater scrutiny of the plague's clinical traits with abundant case histories as opposed to generalized statements by chroniclers or physicians in their plague treatises. From 1452 to 1523 in city-wide necrologies or *Libri dei morti*, university-trained doctors diagnosed the causes of death of all (or at least most)[6] of the urban population to ascertain whether the dead had been victims of plague.

Before turning to these documents, we need to consider another problem: the great variability of symptoms and skin disorders displayed by *Yersinia pestis* since its discovery in 1894. Doctors and health workers in the twentieth century divided *Yersinia pestis* into various groups according to its supposed origins or biovars, its DNA, and, most useful for historians, its clinical manifestations. For these, four or five groups were proposed early on: *Pestis Minor*, the cellulocutaneous type, bubonic, septicaemic, and pneumonic plague. By far the most important in terms of mortality and global spread over the twentieth and twenty-first centuries has been the bubonic form, but even this category has hardly shown consistently the same signs since Alexandre Yersin's discovery over a century ago.

Clinicians have observed that bubonic plague manifests painful swellings in lymphatic glands on the second or third day of illness, that usually only one such swelling forms, and that the usual places for it are in the groin, axilla (armpits), or side of the neck. Those in the groin are the most common, with as many as 75 per cent (and most recently in Madagascar, 80 per cent) of the swellings; those in the axillary glands come next with 20 per cent, and those in the cervical glands third with 10 per cent.[7]

---

[4] Ann Carmichael in various studies of the Milanese necrologies has investigated several of these questions but to date has not endeavoured to show any evolution in the plagues' clinical characteristics. See most recently her 'Universal and Particular'.

[5] See Cohn, *The Black Death Transformed*, 71–81, and appendix I.

[6] Deaths of infants are in some years under-recorded.

[7] Chun, 'Clinical Features', 314, states that as many as 70% of swellings were in the groin. At Hong Kong in 1894, Yersin reported 75% in that area. In the recent epidemic of *Yersinia pestis* in

Yet bubonic plague can show widely divergent patterns, with swellings forming (even if rarely) outside the lymph nodes and in almost any part of the body—the feet, face, head, back, abdomen, and arms. In addition, rare forms of plague have appeared since Yersin's discovery: for instance, in Chile (1903), Ecuador (1909),[8] and Mauritius. Sore throat followed by greyish matter exuding from the neck and then multiple swellings forming in the cervical region were the clinical manifestations of a plague in 1925 in Mauritius.[9] In Chile and Ecuador, sufferers discovered spots similar to smallpox or measles forming in different parts of the body, accompanied by black vomit. Few of the general texts on infectious diseases have pointed to these rare forms of plague, and none has given much sense of their frequency.[10]

However, clinical reports for the first half of the twentieth century, now perhaps of more interest to the historian than to present-day physicians, provide more specific characteristics of these unusual forms of *Yersinia pestis* and their variability. In 1909, the Indian plague doctor K. H. Choksy found pustules (which he labelled 'Cellulocutaneous plague') developing in 3.7 per cent of 13,600 cases of bubonic plague collected at two hospitals in Bombay over the course of twelve epidemics, between 1897 and 1908.[11] From cases in Brazil, Peru, Ecuador, and Chile at the beginning of the twentieth century, Atilio Macchiavello observed in the 1930s and 1940s that carbuncles could form on the wrists and ankles of plague victims a day or two before the bubo or simultaneously with it. Further, he concluded: 'cutaneous lesions—petecchiae, ecchymoses, pustules, and gangrene, generally called "carbuncles" of variable sizes may appear over the buboes or independent of them, especially on the abdomen or extremities'. He also observed 'pustular plague eruptions' that at times resembled smallpox and could occur 'on any part of the body' but most often appeared in the gluteal and scapular regions.[12] Unfortunately, neither Macchiavello nor J. W. H. Chun quantified the numbers or proportions of such cases. They must have been extremely rare: not

Madagascar, that proportion has been 80% in adults but lower for children; Sallares, 'Ecology, Evolution, and Epidemiology of Plague', 233. Chun also groups those in the maxillary glands (under the breasts) with those in the cervical region (on the neck and behind the ears). However, his results and others show those under the breasts to have been extremely rare.

   8 Martinez Vinueza, 'Peste eruptiva'.

   9 Chun, 'Clinical Features', 321–2. These physicians did not speculate on the reasons for the appearance of these rare forms: did they emerge because of a strain of the pathogen or were they related to the genetic conditions of a previously isolated population?

   10 See for instance Craven, 'Plague', 1,306: 'pyogenic, necrotic, infarctive, inflammatory, hemorrhagic, and edematous lesions have formed on those afflicted with *Yersinia pestis*.'

   11 Choksy, 'The Various Types of Plague'. This statistic combined cases of pustules forming on the bubo as well as across other parts of the body. Chun, 'Clinical Features', 311 and 313, also reports that haemorrhages in different parts of the body and 'pustules may coalesce and form areas of necrosis, the so-called carbuncles' or 'blains' as they were called in the Plague of London in 1665, but he does not quantify their frequency. In his tables plague pustules do not even appear (314–5) or are later classified cases with vesicles and pustules as 'atypical cases' (321–4).

   12 Macchiavello, 'Plague', summarizes his earlier clinical work on plague.

only do none of them appear in the published hospital reports from the Presidency of Bombay during the plagues of 1896–7 (only two cases of over 3,000 hospital patients report even skin rashes or blisters covering parts of the body);[13] numerous authors of standard texts such as the various editions of *Manson's Tropical Diseases* from 1898 to the twenty-first century, either were unaware of these rare forms of *Yersinia pestis*, thought them of such insignificance as not worthy of mention, or stated explicitly that they were rare.[14] Furthermore, from thousands of plague cases in India over two decades, Chun could only point to 'two cases which showed vesicles and pustules on the trunk and legs', and in one of these, the disease was mistaken for chickenpox.[15] In the Mauritius plague of the 1920s, only one case of a papular rash was found. It changed to vesicles that appeared on the face and neck, and Chun points to only one or two other 'atypical cases'.[16]

For cases of bubonic plague where human fleas as opposed to rat fleas were suspected as the plague's vector, swellings in the groin were rare,[17] and with primary pneumonic and septicaemic forms of plague, skin disorders have no time to form. Given this great variability, how can scientists and historians then be so sure that the signs of the medieval and early modern plagues matched so unmistakably those manifested in the subtropical disease whose agent was discovered by Yersin?[18] As doctors working in the field warned throughout the twentieth century, without proper biological tests it is often easy to mistake plague (*Yersinia pestis*) for any number of other diseases—chickenpox, smallpox, pneumonia, influenza, typhoid, and most often typhus. In the 1920s and 1930s Chun had gathered specific examples of such misinformed clinical diagnoses and confusions with these and other diseases in areas of the subtropics where plague was prevalent. Closer to our own time, costly confusion of misdiagnoses accompanied the outbreak of plague in Surat, western India, in September 1994.[19] Thus, even today trained health workers and doctors can misdiagnose plague when dependent on clinical evidence alone.[20]

---

[13] Gatacre, *Report on the Bubonic Plague*; and Cohn, *The Black Death Transformed*, 77–9.

[14] On the various editions of *Manson's Tropical Diseases*, see Cohn, *The Black Death Transformed*. None of its editions cites examples of bumps covering entire bodies; it turns instead to historic plague, such as the plague of London in 1603. See Smith, 'Plague' in the latest edition (22nd, 2009), 1,121.

[15] Cited in Chun, 'Clinical Features', 322.   [16] Ibid., 321–2.

[17] Laforce et al., 'Clinical and Epidemiological Observations'. Of twenty-six cases, only three (12%) had buboes in the groin or 24% if only those with buboes are considered.

[18] Most recently, see Little, 'Life and Afterlife of the First Plague Pandemic', 3–4, who asserts: 'Plague, however, is a major exception [to other illnesses] because of the unmistakable appearance of buboes on most its victims . . . .' He fails to heed the advice of health workers throughout the twentieth and twenty-first centuries citing a wide variety of diseases that manifest such swellings and can easily be misdiagnosed without laboratory tests; see for instance *Manson's Tropical Diseases*, 7th edn, 270; *Manson's Tropical Diseases*, 19th edn, 594–5; Smith and Thanh, 'Plague', 920; and Chun, 'Clinical Features', 327–33. For others who claim that the swellings in lymph nodes 'leaves no doubt that bubonic *Y. pestis* ravaged' Europe in 1348 or during the early modern period, see examples in Cohn, *The Black Death Transformed*, ch. 3.

[19] See for instance Mavalankar, 'Indian "Plague" Epidemic'.

[20] On other diseases confused with plague by health workers, see editions of Manson cited above and for other cases of misdiagnosis, also see Moseng, 'Climate, Ecology and Plague', 25.

As double Noble Prize-winner Macfarlane Burnett cautioned, reliance on signs and symptoms for the identification of diseases in past time is risky, and it is better to turn to epidemiological features and trends.[21] Nonetheless, let us make an attempt to describe systematically the symptoms and signs with actual cases from the European past and not just from doctors' and chroniclers' generalizations about them. The records of Milan offer the historian a rare opportunity.

LANGUAGE

Any attempt at cross-temporal comparison of clinical traits that runs from 1348 to the twenty-first century must confront the difficulties of language, especially given such broad differences of clinical practice and classification that have developed since the Enlightenment and, more fundamentally, after the late nineteenth-century 'laboratory revolution'.[22] Modern terms that are cognates of those of the Middle Ages or early modern period may not denote exactly the same bodily parts. Most significant and problematic is the Italian and Latin word for the hip. After swellings in the groin—*in inquine* or *inquinibus*—those in the *coxa* took pride of place with almost a quarter of all swellings (23.1 per cent) or 1,405 of 6,088 buboes, *carboncelli, tumori, pustuli* and other such swellings located by physicians of the Milanese health board with cases of plague.[23] For the plague year 1483, the number of swellings in the *coxa* exceeded ones in the groin: 27.1 per cent (118) as against 24.1 per cent (105). Clearly, the Milanese doctors did not use *in coxa* as interchangeable with *in inguine*. Often they distinguished swellings on the same victim as forming in both places, as with a forty-year-old man who died of plague with a bleeding nose and flux, *morbili* or spots all over the body, and two buboes: one in his groin (the side was unspecified); the other on his right *coxa*.[24] Or, as in the plague of 1523: after four days, a sixteen-year-old girl died with a bubo on the right side of her groin and a *carbunucullo* on her left *coxa*.[25]

Were swellings in the *coxa* within the glandular region of the inguinal? Occasionally the Milanese reports suggest that they may not have been, as with a twenty-eight-year-old plague-victim, Caternia de Ferrariis, resident of the parish

---

[21] Burnet, *Natural History of Infectious Disease*, 296.

[22] For a recent appraisal of these philological problems with ancient medical texts, see Leven, ' "At Times these Ancient Facts" '.

[23] Rondinelli, *Relazione del contagio*, 192, distinguished between buboes in the groin and the thigh or hip (*nell'inguine, e nella coscia*) during the Florentine plague of 1630–3 and held that those in the latter were the most numerous and deadly.

[24] Popolazione, no. 73, 23.x.1452. In the time of the Black Death, doctors such as Guy de Chauliac distinguished between swellings in the groin and the hip. His chapters grouped those around the hip with ones on the shins and the foot (*de apostematibus coxarum et tybiarum sive pedem; Inventarium sive chirurgia magna*, I, ch. 8, 130) and not with swellings in the three principal glandular nodes (ch. 5, 117–22).

[25] Popolazione, no. 87, 4.i.1523.

of San Lorenzo outside the walls, who died on 13 July 1485. She was afflicted with one swelling—a *carbone pestifero*. According to her death report this formed in the right 'coxa' and wrapped around to her back ('et parte posteriori').[26] Either this was one gigantic swelling (although *carbone* as opposed to bubo usually indicated a smaller bump, rash, or even a pustule) or the *coxa* meant, in fact, the hip. Moreover, of 3,068 cases of swellings in either the groin or the *coxa*, only one case of a swelling in the *coxa* is explicitly linked to the groin: on 12 August 1485 a woman died of plague with a single *glandula* that was 'partially in her groin and partially on her *coxa*' (which also suggests a physiological separation of the two).[27]

In a further nine swellings in the *coxa*, the doctors may have indicated that they were near the groin as opposed to the hip bone. But here, too, the language is ambiguous. The doctors described the buboes, glandules, or antraces as 'in the domestic part' ('in domestice parte') of the *coxa*, as on 3 May 1483 when a twenty-two-year-old woman died of plague in four days with purple spots (*morbilli*) and an 'antrace in her left *coxa in domestyce*'.[28] In anatomical terminology of the Renaissance, *parte domestice* was contrasted with the *parte silvestris*; the domestic being the inner or underside[29] and the silvestran, the outer side. Here, the swelling was on the inner side of the hip, perhaps towards the groin and perhaps within its glandular duct.[30] However, in the vast majority of cases, the Milanese doctors' clinical descriptions suggest no association between the *coxa* and the groin.

As fundamental as the now lost precision of places on the body that anatomical words from the late Middle Ages and early modern periods may denote, the terms physicians used to describe the swellings, rashes, bumps, and other skin disorders show still greater perplexities for anatomical translation. No drawings accompanied the Milanese death records or the more academic plague tracts (that I know of) to illustrate precisely what a *carbone* as opposed to a bubo, anthrax, *tumore*, or other type of swelling might have resembled and their differences; nor did the Milanese necrologies employ quantitative means to distinguish these various bumps or swellings as medical researchers provide today, indicating in inches the diameters of various swellings.[31] Other than the number of swellings, the only quantitative measures used by the Milanese doctors were occasional

---

26 Popolazione, no. 77, 16r.

27 Ibid., 26v. It was not, however, unusual to find in these records swellings and rashes that spread from one identified region of the body to another, especially between the neck and ear and the neck and shoulder. Perhaps *coxa* could also mean *coscia* or thigh. In Italian, however, there is a similar ambiguity: *coscia* can mean thigh, side, or hip; *Grande dizionario*, III, 879.

28 Popolazione, no. 76, n.p.   29 *Grande dizionario*, IV, 932.

30 The 'domestic part' is also used with other parts of the body such as arms, knees, shins, and even ears; see for instance two cases in 1468, ASM, Miscellanea Storica, no. 1, 1.vi.1468 (no. 156 and 366); and Popolazione, no. 77, 20.v.1485. In a case during the plague of 1485, a sixty-year-old woman died with an unspecified number of carbuncles (*carbonibus*) on her right shin (*tibia*) in both the domestic and silvestran parts, along with an unspecified but plural number of buboes in her armpits; Popolazione, no. 77, n.p. [45r].

31 See for instance Choksy, 'The Various Types of Plague', 357–8; Chun, 'Clinical Features', 313.

descriptions of the position of a swelling. For instance, a twelve-year-old daughter of a cobbler died of plague with a carbuncle on her stomach, that was four inches from her navel in a place commonly called the *bastardela* ('in ventre per 4 digitos infra umbilicum que vulgus bastardelam vocant').[32] In general the reports suggest two broad categories of skin disorders: swellings or rashes in specific places on the body, which in most cases the doctors reported in number ranging from one to seven; and smaller bumps (*morbilli*), stripes (*vergulentum*), or the general blackening (*denigrato*) of entire bodies. Almost invariably these bumps, spots, and rashes were not counted or linked to specific parts of the body. Instead, they were reported as 'many' (*copia, plures*), 'notable', 'horrible' and to have covered entire bodies. Let us begin with the larger swellings.

THE SWELLINGS AND THEIR NOMENCLATURE

At least twenty-two terms are employed to name the pestilential swellings in the Milanese death records. Several such as *cunetia, barutiara, herispilla* occur only once. *Petracia* and ulcer, often used for descriptions of skin disorders not associated with plague in these death reports, occur only twice to describe a plague swelling. Other terms are not used consistently through the seventy years charted by the six Milanese plagues (1452 to 1523). In the earliest records, relating to the plague of 1452, *dragonzellus* is the third most commonly used term for a plague swelling but declines thereafter, disappearing altogether by the sixteenth century. On the other hand, except for the plague year of 1503, when nearly three-quarters of the cases were not diagnosed with the larger individuated swellings at all, four terms predominated—*apostema* or *apostemata, bubonus, carbone* (and its various spellings, such as *carboncellus*), and *glandula*. These four constituted over 90 per cent of the terms doctors gave for pestilential swellings, with bubo used the most often (2,254 times, 41.2 per cent), followed by *carbone* and its variants (1,046, 19.1 per cent).

While judgements on whether a swelling was a tumour, an aposteme, or a bubo certainly may have varied from one doctor to another, these were not words used interchangeably or at whim. Often these physicians used different terms with the same plague victim to distinguish swellings in different parts of the body. For example, on 6 June 1523 a thirty-six-year-old woman died after three days with a bubo (*bubone*) in her armpit, another bubo on the left side of her groin, and two carbuncles (*carboncellis*) on her right thigh.[33]In the same plague, a servant girl died with three carbuncles (*carbonculis*), two on her chest (*in pectore*), another on her back (*in dorso*), and a bubo (*bubone*) on her right hip (*in cossa destra*).[34] The same region in the same victim could also host more

[32] Miscellanea Storica, no. 1, fasc. 1, slip no. 164, 13.vi.1468.
[33] Popolazione, no. 87, n.p.   [34] Ibid., n.p, 4.v.1523.

than one variety of swelling, as with a forty-year-old plague victim with three *carbonchulis* and a bubo all in the right groin.[35]

What was the significance of these terms? Unlike the smaller and more numerous *morbilli*, *signis malis*, *nigris*, or *rubeis*, for which the colour of the swelling or inflammation was often stated, almost none of the thousands of pustules, tumours, *carbonicelli*, *apostemate*, *anthraces*, or *buboni* was described by colour and most of these could be either large (*magnus*) or small (*parvus*). Perhaps the *carbonicelli* were distinguished by their blackness. When colours are given, the *carboni* were often black. But other swellings could also be black, as with the death on 27 June 1503 of a nine-year-old girl with two black tumours (*tumore dinigrato*) in her right groin along with black *morbilli*, presumably all over the body.[36] Nor do the academic plague tracts give precise guidance with these terms, even though sixteenth-century authors paid much greater attention to pestilential signs and symptoms than their predecessors had done over the first 150 years of this medical genre.[37]

If the Milanese doctors used *carbonicello* and its various derivatives similarly to doctors of the twentieth and twenty-first centuries, then, the two diseases—historic plague and *Yersinia pestis*—appear more different than has heretofore been suggested. The terms used by twentieth-century plague doctors for pestilential swellings have been mostly 'buboes', sometimes ulcers, sometimes 'glandular swellings'. Carbuncles and its derivatives have been used infrequently. Such swellings refer to the unusual spread of necrosis of the tissues that leads to dark eschars or rashes in cases of 'cellulocutaneous plague' found at most in only 3 per cent of plague cases.[38] If the 'carbone' of the early modern period had the same meaning as the carbuncle of the twentieth century, then by these terms alone plague in early modern Milan was not 'typical plague', even before we begin to examine the prevalence of spots, pustules, and the like, which covered entire plague bodies in such numbers that early modern plague doctors did not count them. For the early modern plagues in Milan, carbuncles constituted just under a fifth of swellings and inflammations, a far greater proportion of such swellings than seen with any recorded modern plague. Still, by the early nineteenth-century a thoroughgoing physician's report of Italy's last plague, which struck Noja (Noicattaro) in the region of Bari in 1815, distinguished *carboniche*, along with antrace, from the *gandole* by size and position: the *gandole* appeared principally in the armpits and groin, while antrace and *carboniche*

---

[35] Popolazione, n.p, 9.viii.1523.   [36] Ibid., no. 80, n.p.

[37] Instead of drawing distinctions, earlier tracts often defined various types of swellings in terms of one another as with Guy de Chauliac, *Inventarium sive chirurgia magna*, I, 72: 'De antrace. Antrax secundum Guillelmum de Saliceto nichil aliud est quam carbunculus malignatus.'

[38] Choksy, 'The Various Types of Plague', 356. Also, see Smith, 'Plague', 1,121, who comments that pestilential skin lesions rarely form a carbuncle.

were grouped with the small lentil-sized typhus-type bumps and could appear anywhere on the body, that is, close to our sense of the terms today.[39]

In the early modern Milanese reports, *magnus* was used principally with tumours, then buboes, but also (though much less frequently) with *carboncelli*, while *magnus* never modified an anthrax, *pustula*, or *morbillo*. If distinguished at all by size, these bumps were called small (*parves*). As with tumours and buboes, *carbonicelli* were almost invariably numbered and their positions specified. Only occasionally were they described as 'many', a 'notable' number, or left vague but in the plural as with a plague victim of 28 June 1523 with 'multis carbonculis et mobilis nigris' and no particular part of the body specified. Notable numbers of these swellings or ones left vaguely in the plural as 'cum bubonibus' also were described for *dragonzellis*,[40] buboes,[41] *glandulae*,[42] anthraces,[43] tumours,[44] aposteme,[45] and *eminentiae*.[46] These, however, were rare, constituting only 2.4 per cent of all the swellings that were not *morbilli*, *signi nigri*, and the like. On the other hand, *carbonicelli* appeared in multiple numbers, were modified by 'many' (*plures* and *multitudine*), and were described as covering plague victims' bodies more often than was the case for buboes, tumours, and apostemes. From the quantitative evidence, I speculate that while 'carbonicelli' may not have been exactly equivalent to our modern usage of carbuncular, they were larger than the spots (*morbili*) but smaller than buboes or tumours, and of a different shape: they should not be understood as just another term for the larger bubo.

If we consider the multiple swellings that the doctors counted in their death reports, the distinctiveness of the *carbonicelli* becomes more pronounced. More than any of the other large swellings, even the perhaps smaller *pustula* and anthrax, the *carboncello* predominated as the one doctors specified in multiple sites on plague corpses, appearing more than four times more often in multiples than buboes or tumours, and this ratio held through the plague years at Milan, 1452, 1468, 1483, 1485, 1503, and 1523.[47]

---

[39] Morea, *Storia della peste di Noja*, 5: 'i cui sintomi erano . . . Febbre con delirio, diarrea, abbattimento di forze, accompagnata nel principio da ingorgo indolente e inerte delle gandole inguinali e ascellari, nella maggior parte; nel rimanente da carboniche o antraci, e da petecchie lenticolari e rare'.

[40] Popolazione, no. 73, n.p.; two cases from 28.vii.1452 and one from 29.vii.1452.

[41] Ibid., 17.ix.1452; no. 87, 3.xi.1483; no. 77, 27.vii.1485; 30.viii.1485; 4.ix.1485; 9.ix.1485; 12.ix.1485; 25.ix.1485; 28.ix.1485; 30.ix.1485; 4.x.1485; 8.x.1485; 2.v.1523; 13.xii.1523.

[42] Ibid., no. 76, n.p., 9.ix.1485; 15.ix.1485; 22.ix.1485; 4.x.1485; no. 80, n.p., 3.iii.1503; 18.vii.1503; 7.x.1503; 17.x.1503.

[43] Ibid., no. 80, n.p., 13.vii.1503.

[44] Ibid., no. 76, 11.ix.1483; no. 77, n.p., 8.i.1485; 8.iv.1485.

[45] Ibid., no. 76, 12.ix.1485; 19.ix.1485; 25.ix.1485; 29.ix.1485; no. 80, n.p., 17.x.1503.

[46] Ibid., no. 76, 6.ix.1483; no. 77, n.p., 13.ii.1485; 24.ii.1485; 27.vii.1485; 30.viii.1485; 12.ix.1485; 22.x.1485; no. 80, n.p., 29.iii.1503; 28.xi.1503.

[47] When three swellings occurred on victims with two different types (say buboes and *carboncelli*) doctors did not often indicate which type was the multiple one.

Table 2.1 Multiple Pestilential Swellings that were not Counted

Name of swelling	Number, not counted but in plural	Total	Percentage
Aposteme	8	742	1.08%
Eminenita	12	79	15.2%
Carbone	48	1046	4.6%
Bubone	38	2254	1.7%
Tumour	4	267	1.5%
Pustule	3	61	4.9%
Glandula	15	899	1.7%
Antrace	1	37	2.7%
Dragonzello	3	26	11.5%
Other	4	65	6.2%
Total	136	5476	2.5%

Table 2.2 Multiple Pestilential Swellings that were Counted

Name of swelling	No. >1	Percentage of multiple swellings	Total no.	Percentage of type
Aposteme	48	12.9%	742	6.5%
Eminenita	2	0.5%	79	2.5%
Carbone	177	47.6%	1046	16.9%
Bubone	86	23.1%	2254	3.8%
Tumour	10	2.7%	267	3.8%
Pustule	5	1.3%	61	8.2%
Glandula	39	10.5%	899	4.3%
Antrace	4	1.1%	37	10.8%
Dragonzello	1	0.3%	26	3.9%
Other	3	0.8%	65	4.6%
Total	372	100%	5476	6.8%

SWELLINGS IN SIXTEENTH-CENTURY PLAGUE TRACTS

Like the death books, physicians' plague tracts in the sixteenth century also possessed a wide vocabulary for pestilential swellings—*giandussa, aposteme, carbone, bubone, antrace*, and more. A few tracts appear to have used the terms more or less interchangeably[48] or, like the death reports, without clear definitions of the differences.[49] Some even claimed that all the symptoms came about

---

[48] See for instance De Forte, *Il trattato de la peste*, where the positions more than the type of swelling—*gonfiando l'anguinaglia, carbone*, or anthrax—made the critical difference in his tripartite division of plague signs and symptoms; and Venusti, *Consilium de peste*, 12v and 21r.

[49] See for instance Bucci, *Reggimento*, n.p.: 'se li scoprono nella persona anguinaie, antrace, carboni, macchie livide o' nere, che in queste bande si dicono cenespioni.' See also Centorio Degli Ortensi, *I cinque*

together[50] or were basically the same.[51] Other plague commentators made no distinctions at all, among them the Milanese historian and theologian Gaspare Bugati describing Milan's plague in 1576–7. He grouped *carboni* with other terms, such as *gonfiamenti* and *bugnoni*, to designate the larger swellings, which he called 'the black pestilential signs'. These were apparent, he claimed, everywhere the disease spread, from Zurich to Bellinzona to Venice and then to the outskirts of Milan, and formed indiscriminately 'on breasts, the neck, in the armpits, on the back, arms, legs, groin, and elsewhere'.[52] For some, the word *carbone* was the only term used for the larger pestilential swellings.[53] Moreover, the physician Prospero Borgarucci advised similar treatments for both *carbone* and buboes: the site of the swelling, not its size, determined the procedure.[54]

More often, however, doctors reflected on differences between the two types of swellings. The Torinese physician Alessandri said that treatment of the two was similar; however, with buboes the physician had to dig deeper with the scalpel. Perhaps, similar to present-day notions of carbuncles, the *carboni* of early modern Italy appear here to have been a flatter rash, while the bubo, tumour, and *glandula* were the more bulbous growths that could swell as large as a pigeon's egg.[55] Still others, such as a doctor of the commune of Udine during the plague of 1576, divided the pestilential skin disorders into three classes: *petecchie*, *posteme*, and *carboni*. The *petecchie* were either spots or bumps the size of lentils and resembled flea bites and appeared all over the body. The pestilential *postemes* or as Avicenna named them, the *buboni*, appeared 'in the lymph nodes (*emontorij*), that is, in the glands' ('nelli luoghi giandulosi'), behind ears, under arms, and in the groin, and hence their name, *giandussa*. The third category was the *carboni*, also called *antraci*, which were distinguished by their presence anywhere on the body and gave birth to malignant fevers. The *carboni* were also more variable ('di più qualitadi') in shape and colour: some were flat and black, while others were raised and white, more like *vesche* or pustules.[56] Later, his section 'on the signs or accidents of the plague', emphasized a division into

libri degl'avvertimenti, 12, who tried to trace the networks and means by which the 1576–7 plague arrived in Milan—'si scoperse la peste, di che in due & in tre giorni ne morirno molti con segni de carboncelli, di buboni, d'Anguinaglie, e d'altri pestiferi segni': he must have assumed that his audience would have known the precise meaning of these various words for clearly different forms of pestilential swellings. Also, see Cavagnino, *Compilatione delli veri et fideli rimedii*, ch. 5: 'Segni di peste'.

50 *Informatione*, ch. 15: 'al bubone, sudore, carbone, petecchie o ver macchie, . . . quanto a tutti gli altri syntomi insieme'.

51 Frigimelega, *Consiglio sopra la pestilentia*, n.p.: 'Succede poi la inquietudine & altri accidenti detti sopra, gli apostemi, carboncoli, pruni & altre esiture che si veggono in alcuni sono causati per la ebullitione delli humori fatta dalla gran putredine . . . seguitano tumori, piu o meno velenosi.'

52 Bugati, *I fatti di Milano*, 3.

53 See for instance Susio, *Libro del conoscere la pestilenza*, 51, who referred to 'un vero Carbone'.

54 Prospero Borgarucci, *De peste perbrevis tractatus*, 57. On Prospero and his brothers, see Firpo, 'Borgarucci'.

55 See for example Alessandri, *Trattato della peste*, 86v.   56 Daciano, *Trattato della peste*, 3.

two categories, seen in other plague tracts as late as the 1816 report on Noja. The critical divide now was whether the spots were in the glands or outside them. Here, as in the nineteenth century, the *carboni* were categorized along with the smaller black spots (*petecchie nere*).[57]

Again writing during the plague of 1575–8, the Genoese surgeon Luchino Boerio devoted his treatise entirely to the 'accidents' or signs of plague, drawing a still sharper divide between bubo and *carbone*.[58] He provides one of the most detailed descriptions of pestilential skin disorders found in these texts before the nineteenth century, beginning by defining the bubo: '[it] is a tumour which at first is elongated and mobile but becomes round and pointed and fixed to "the emunctories" '.[59] For the brain, they form behind the ears and are called *parotide*; for the heart, in the armpits, and for the liver, in the groin and thus called *inguinaglie*.[60] They were of various colours—yellowish, purple, or black (*citrini, lividi, e negricanti*).[61] Starting with Avicenna but following with recent experience—the plague of 1528—Boerio argued that if these swellings were black, patients had little chance of survival.[62]

In Boerio's descriptions, the *carboni* were small, round, and pointed. Initially, they could be as big as a grain of millet or a chick-pea. They were 'immobile', so that the skin did not rise or become separate from the skin underneath it. They could spread to some parts of the body quickly and to other parts later and could form a crust of dried blood.[63] They could appear below the chin where they might grow into large tumours down to the Adam's apple (*alle calvicole*) even strangling the patient, or they could form 'where the foot separates from the leg' or on the shoulders (*brazzo dalla spalla*). They could also be tiny spots 'as if made by points of needles' or they might appear as thousands of herpes blisters.[64] These *carboni* (at least at certain stages in their development), thus may have been more similar to the *morbilli* and *signi nigri* in the Milanese reports and appear close to present-day descriptions of carbuncles. Unlike what might be implied by their name—*carbone*—these could be of various colours (which Boerio describes in detail). Furthermore, pestilential *carboni* were always accompanied by continuous fever and 'other very cruel symptoms, often followed by a heart attack'.[65] As with the pustules and spots described by chroniclers and diarists from the Black Death to the early fifteenth century—the Sicilian Michele da Piazza, Geoffrey le Baker, the Florentine Giovanni Morelli, and others[66]—these

---

[57] Daciano, 38.   [58] Boerio, *Trattato delli buboni*.
[59] The three springs of life found in Galenic texts.   [60] Boerio, *Trattato delli buboni*, 7.
[61] Ibid., 11.
[62] Ibid., 11: 'che quando il color è negro pochi campano, come dice Avic, e nell'anno 1528 accadeva . . . .'
[63] Ibid., 48–9.
[64] Ibid., 55: 'il piede separarsi dalla gamba, il brazzo dalla spalla . . . si fanno certe picicle vesiche, come se fussero stati ponti da ortiche, o come quelle, che si veggono alli herpeti miliari . . . '.
[65] Boerio, *Trattato delli buboni*, 50.   [66] Cohn, *The Black Death Transformed*, 62–3.

smaller spots were for Boerio the most deadly signs, from which patients could die within twenty-four hours.[67]

Perhaps the most famous doctor of the last quarter of the sixteenth century, Girolamo Mercuriale, at first drew a similar schema of these plague signs. The larger buboes were confined to the lymph nodes—in the groin, under the arms, and behind the ears—while *carbunculi* formed in all parts of the body and were often numerous.[68] Mercuriale, however, distinguished the carbuncles from a third category of pestilential skin disorders: scabs, blotches, and spots that were black, purple, or red. These formed on the back, sometimes in small numbers, sometimes in great numbers, and sometimes spread over the entire body. For Mercuriale these were the most deadly signs and the most contagious: few recovered from them or could survive for more than five days.[69]

A Lucchese physician of the same period, Alessandro Puccinelli, adopted much the same tripartite division, with the *carbunculi* placed between the larger *apostemi* and the smaller and more numerous 'herpeti et altri simili mali'. Unlike the *apostemi*, which formed mostly in the principal lymph nodes (but could form elsewhere according to Puccinelli), the *carbunculi* were less discriminate, appearing in 'diversi parti'.[70] Others, however, such as Francesco Alessandri, divided the signs more or less into two groups. He placed the *carboni* with the *buboni*, *tubercoli*, and other names for the larger swellings—all of which could form in or outside the three lymph principal nodes—and contrasted these to the smaller and more numerous *petecchie*.[71] Regardless of these accidents, Alessandri saw the consequences of the various types as much the same: the illness created a terrible stench, death came in three or four days, and the disease was highly contagious as witnessed by the fact that all or most members of a household died suddenly.[72] Similarly, in his instruction on how to identify plague corpses, the Udinese physician Eustachio Celebrino used *carbone* as a general term for the larger glandular swellings, which he juxtaposed to the smaller spots that spread across bodies.[73] In other places he explored the variations of the larger pestilential swellings, for which he again employed a single term: *carbone*. However, he divided these larger swellings into five types, based on colour, the intensity of burning, and shape: one sort had a blister (*vesiga*) on top and burnt with fire; a second was black on top and red underneath; a third, black and red; a fourth

---

[67] Boerio, *Trattato delli buboni*, 56. Moreover, these tiny black bumps, often called *petecchie* and *carboni*, would persist as ubiquitous and deadly signs of plague through the early nineteenth century: for the plague in Rome of 1656–7, see the letters of Rome's head of plague hospitals Girolamo Gastaldi (Sonnino, 'Cronache della peste a Rome', 51–3, 64–74); for the plague of Marseille, 1720, and of Messina, 1743, see Mead, *A Discourse on the Plague*, 5 and 153; and for the plague at Noja in 1815, see Morea, *Storia della peste di Noja*, 5, 233, 301, 438–9. Also, Tagarelli, *La peste di Noja*, 48–9.

[68] Mercuriale, *De pestilentia*, 3.   [69] Ibid.

[70] Puccinelli, *Dialoghi sopra le cause della peste*, 31v.   [71] Alessandri, *Trattato della peste*, 7v.

[72] Ibid., 44r.

[73] [Celebrino Eustachio], *Regimento mirabile et verissimo*. There was an earlier edition of 1527, which I have not seen.

was full of blisters on top and black underneath; and a fifth, purple surrounded by red. All these were equally deadly, leaving the patient no redemption, except by God's grace and 'the pick and the shovel' (burial).[74] According to Antonio Cermisone, a Paduan physician of the first half of the fifteenth century, whose tract was published for the first time together with Eustachio's in 1555, the *carboncelli* could be green or black, the black ones being deadlier. Unlike the Genoese surgeon Boerio, Cermisone saw these larger swellings regardless of their name or colour forming not only in the principal lymph nodes but in various places on the body. He contrasted them with the smaller, more numerous spots and like late medieval doctors saw them as the most dangerous form.[75]

For other sixteenth-century doctors the various terms for swellings did not relate to any part of the body. *Carbonicelli* could appear in the groin, armpits, or behind the ears just as did the tumours, *apostemate*, and the *glandulae*. A difference, nonetheless, can be discerned: when these larger swellings appeared in the plural or spread over entire bodies, *carbone* and not *bubone* and the like was the term doctors chose. This difference is seen clearly in Niccolò Massa's tract, written during the plague of 1555–6. To make himself clear to a larger audience he used two vocabularies, one for the laity with common terms, the other for the medical profession. For both, the principal distinction was between the singular large *aposteme* swellings (*detti buboni, antraci, & carboni*) that formed in the three principle lymph nodes, and the 'multitude of spots' ('called *petecchie* in this city') that appeared in various colours and 'formed on backs, breasts, necks, arms, buttocks, hips and other parts of the body', which also 'could be pestilential signs'.[76] Agostino Bucci, who taught medicine at the University of Turin, elaborated on this same two-part distinction, seeing different causes or agents for the different skin manifestations.[77] Yet in other places he adopted the three-part division of the pestilential skin disorders, similar to Mercuriale: the plague signs could be swellings (*inguinaglie*) in the lymph nodes, *petecchie* and spots on the skin; or indeed *carboncoli* and black and malign pustules that formed in various parts of the body.[78]

Others made a similar distinction between the larger swellings (regardless of their names) and the smaller spots, but some such as a doctor from Salò saw the *petecchie* in isolation from 'buboni, o carboni', as not so deadly (*più miti*) as when the buboes appeared alone.[79] He seems, however, to have been referring here not to plague but to *petecchie* (what historians now assume was typhus) where the smaller spots appeared without the larger glandular swellings, was less malignant, and took longer to kill as with an epidemic in Milan in 1477–8, when red,

---

74 [Celebrino Eustachio], *Reggimento mirabile et verissimo*, 7r.

75 Cermisone, *Remedii verissimi*, n.p. (not in Edit 16). Also see Ceruti, *Questo sono recepte facte*.

76 Massa, *Ragionamento*, 11.

77 Bucci, *Modo di conoscere*, ch. 2: 'Divisione della peste in due specie; De' segni distinguenti l'una dall'altra' (8r–9r).

78 Ibid., 58r.   79 Gratiolo di Salò, *Discorso di peste*, 34.

as opposed to the more deadly black, *morbilli* formed without larger glandular swellings, and in which victims took two weeks instead of two or three days to die.[80] Detailed descriptions of the signs and symptoms of plague appeared even in verse, as in the long Latin poem of the Brescian doctor Bartolomeo Theani [Tiani]. He described swellings (*phygethlon*) and *carbones*, both of which could form in 'a multiple of glands' in the groin, behind the ears and in the armpits, as well as on the chest, the shins, the sides, the buttock, and crown of the head. According to Tiani the pustules appeared later on victims' bodies in the brief course of this disease.[81]

So what do we make of this array of opinions, definitions, and schemas of plague swellings and other skin disorders? How do they relate to the descriptions by doctors on Milan's health boards? Clearly, words such as *carboncello, tumore, glandula, pustula, morbilli* and others had specific meanings whose subtleties may now be lost, and using later definitions from the nineteenth- or twentieth-century medical manuals is risky. But despite the diversity with occasional contradictions between plague tracts, clearly most were seeing, describing, and categorizing the signs of these plague realities in ways not so dissimilar to those of the practising Milanese doctors of the health boards. There were not two modes of seeing the plague's pathology as Cipolla and others have suggested:[82] one of empirical practising doctors, surgeons, and barbers, some of whom may have sat on health boards; the other of academic physicians, their heads stuck in erudite texts of ancient authorities and who were far removed from the daily chores of clinical observation and care. On both fronts doctors, surgeons, barbers, and the laity needed by law to identify plague victims in their homes and neighbourhoods and to report such cases immediately to gate guards, parish priests, and other authorities.[83] As a result, the sixteenth-century university physician (at least by the time of the plague of 1575–8) added new sections to their plague tracts on 'the ways of recognizing plague', not seen in earlier plague tracts thus far brought to light by Karl Sudhoff. This was no arid academic discourse dependent on ancient texts by authorities who had never seen plague of the Black Death sort.

Why do these terms and distinctions matter? In short, if we interpret the *carboni* or *carbonicelli* of the Milanese plague death reports to have been the same as doctors of the twentieth century have defined them—rashes—or as many of the doctors of the sixteenth-century defined them as the smaller, flatter bumps that could appear anywhere on plague victims, then without further

---

[80] For the statistics on the course of this disease, see below.

[81] Tiani, *De singulari pestilentiae magnitudine*, 9r.

[82] According to Palmer, 'The Control of Plague', the 'terminological dispute' in Venice of 1576 'revealed the continued vigour of the classical tradition in medicine ... [and] also revealed the gulf between academic approaches to the disease and the pragmatism of the Health Offices' (320). He also saw a theoretical divide between members of the health office and the general character of Counter-Reformation culture based on a 'Hebrew tradition' in which plague was understood as God's wrath (280).

[83] See for instance Ingrassia, *Informatione*, 88.

analysis we should conclude that the signs of the early modern Milanese plagues depart significantly from clinical descriptions of 'typical bubonic plague' of the so-called 'third pandemic' in India or anywhere else in the world. The second most common swelling according to the fifteenth- and sixteenth-century plagues in Milan was not a bubo and might not even have been a swelling at all but an elongated rash that could appear in or outside the three principal lymph nodes, constituting almost a fifth of the plague's skin disorders, not counting the third basic category of skin disorders—the small spots or *morbilli*—to which we will turn shortly. With this meaning of *carbone*, early modern plagues would at best fit 'atypical' forms of bubonic plague, such as the 'generalized eruption' type, which afflicted Mauritius in 1925, or the 'angina pestosa' sort seen in Ecuador's largest city, Guayaquil, in 1908. But, these 'atypical' plagues were rare and not nearly as deadly as the typical bubonic plagues of India and elsewhere. The 1908 plague of Guayaquil recorded only 227 cases and of these only 24 were fatal, despite the fact that several of the sufferers developed septicaemic plague from which none recovered.[84] Moreover, in all these Ecuadoran cases, the victims survived longer than a week. Other examples of 'atypical' forms of *Yersinia pestis* also have been extremely rare during the twentieth century (I know of none as yet reported for the twenty-first), and have been even less dangerous than that found for Ecuador in 1908: they have been mild forms of plague with many fewer casualties and longer periods of illness than with 'typical' bubonic plague as seen in India or China in the early twentieth century or Madagascar today.[85] In addition, if historic plagues are pinned to 'atypical' plague, the epidemical puzzle becomes greatly more vexing than before: how do we explain the vastly higher rates of morbidity and especially mortality of the Justinianic, medieval, and early modern plagues on the one hand and these mild and rare forms of plague of the 'third pandemic' on the other?

POSITIONS OF THE BUBOES AND *CARBONICELLI*: THE MILANESE RECORDS

Against what many plague doctors wrote and what the Milanese *Libri dei morti* suggest, let us assume that carbuncles, *carboni*, and *carbonicelli* were essentially the same as buboes, anthraces, apostemes, and *glandulae*; they were neither small bumps nor rashes but resembled the 'gavoccioli' described by Boccaccio in 1348: 'as big as a medium-sized apple or an egg'.[86] Does the evidence from the early modern Milanese plagues then fit 'unmistakably' the signs and symptoms of 'typical' bubonic plague of the twentieth and twenty-first centuries?

---

[84] Chun, 'Clinical Features', 322; and Martinez Vinueza, 'Peste eruptiva'.
[85] Chun, 'Clinical Features', 321–7.   [86] Boccaccio, *Decameron*, 10–11.

Table 2.3 Eight Hospitals from the Presidency of Bombay, 1896–7 (published in 1897)

Position	Number	Percentage
Cervical	42	6.3%
Parotid	23	3.5%
Submaxillary	2	0.3%
Axillary	167	25.2%
Inguinal	213	32.2%
Femoral	202	30.5%
Popliteal	1	0.2%
Supertrochlear	0	0.0%
Sublingual	0	0.0%
other:	0	0.0%
arm	3	0.5%
abdominal	1	0.2%
right calf	1	0.2%
scalp	2	0.3%
mammary	3	0.5%
feet	2	0.3%
Total places identified	662	
Multiple	32	4.6%
Total	694	100.0%
No buboes	180	25.9%

Table 2.4 Eight Other Hospitals from the Presidency of Bombay, 1896–7 (published in 1898)

Position		Number	Percentage
Cervical	neck and behind ears	260	10.3%
Parotid	Knee	42	1.7%
Submaxillary	Jaw	4	0.2%
Axillary	Armpit	616	24.4%
Inguinal	Groin	1068	42.4%
Femoral		524	20.8%
Popliteal	Knee	1	0.04%
Supertrochlear	Shoulder	3	0.1%
Sublingual		2	0.08%
Other		1	0.04%
Total places identified		2521	
Multiple		197	7.3%
Total		2718	100.0%
No buboes		608	22.4%

As we have already seen, outbreaks of *Yersinia pestis* across the globe since 1894 show no simple, standard, or 'unmistakable signs'. Boils, rashes, blisters, exasma, spots, and other signs of necrosis can form anywhere on the body or not at all; fatality rates could be low as with *pestis minor* or high as 90 per cent as witnessed in Hong Kong in 1894 or with pneumonic plague in the Manchurian plagues of 1910–11 and 1922, where it approached 100 per cent.

Records from the twentieth century show variations even for the classic bubonic eruptions of plague in India at the beginning of the century and China (the Tungliao area, Inner Mongolia) in 1928, and could vary from one hospital to the next during the same plague. For instance, at the Parel Hospital in the Presidency of Bombay during the years 1896–7, 6.3 per cent of the buboes were in the cervical region, while at the hospital of Pathare Prabhu the proportion was three and half times higher (22.6 per cent of the swellings). The presence of multiple swellings in these hospitals varied even more radically with 16.9 per cent at the Grant Road Hospital and 0.9 at the Jain Hospital. Nonetheless, even if *Yersinia pestis* has been more variable than historians and scientists of the Black Death and plague often assume, the bubonic form with swellings principally in the three lymph nodes has been overwhelmingly the most common form of the disease since Yersin cultured the pathogen in 1894. Overall, the data from Brigadier-General Gatacre's reports in 1897 and 1898 conform largely with medical textbook generalizations ever since: in India those in cervical region combined with the submaxillary (below the jaw) amounted to 6.6 per cent of the cases (slightly less than the general model); those in the axillary glands, 25.2 per cent (slightly more than the model), and those on the thigh or within the inguinal region, 62.7 per cent (well within the range of the model). Outside these three principal lymph nodes, moreover, only 5.4 per cent of plague swellings formed in minor glands such as under the breasts, behind the knees (parotid and popliteal), or, rarer still, in places which may not have corresponded to any lymph nodes at all. Finally, 27.8 per cent of these Indian cases formed no swellings or skin disorders. Some may have been cases of pneumonic or septicaemic plague, when sudden death allows no time for swellings.

For another eight hospitals of the presidency of Bombay collected for the same plague years but published a year later, the results were comparable: 10.5 per cent in cervical region, 24.4 per cent in the axillary, and 63.2 per cent in or near the groin, leaving less than 2 per cent outside the principal glands, and 22.4 per cent of patients showing no swellings. Cases of more than a single bubo constituted 4.6 per cent for the first eight hospitals and 7.3 per cent for the second.

The series assembled by J. W. H. Chun show patterns roughly similar to those I have calculated from the raw data provided by W. F. Gatacre, although with two slight variations: the multiple cases for the Chinese and later Bombay data were greater, ranging from 7.5 to 13.7 per cent; but the positions in minor glands or outside them altogether were fewer, ranging form 2.4 to 1.7 per cent of cases.

***

Table 2.5   Plague Cases Summarized by J. W. H. Chun[1]

	Chien Chia-tien	Whole Tungkiao Area	Bombay, 1900
Positions			
Cervical	10.0%	9.4%	8.4%
Axillary	25.0%	18.9%	21.9%
Femoral	8.7%	62.3%	30.9%
Inguinal	40.0%		23.3%
Multiple	13.7%	7.5%	12.9%
Other places	2.4%	1.8%	1.7%
No. of cases	80	159	9500

[1] Chun, 'Clinical Features', 314.

On first impression the positions of the swellings from the early modern Milanese necrologies may not seem out of line with twentieth-century bubonic plague. Over the six plague years—1452, 1468, 1483, 1485, 1502, and 1523—19.3 per cent of the larger swellings identified by a bodily position were in the armpits, almost exactly the same as that generalized in the textbooks for modern bubonic plague. Swellings in the cervical region were slightly below the textbook norm with 7.8 per cent but are higher than those found for this area in eight hospitals in the Bombay Presidency in 1896–7. If tumours, buboes, and the like that formed on the throat, beneath the chin, or under the jaw (which the plague doctors of the twentieth century placed within the submaxillary gland) are added to those behind the ears and on the neck, the Milanese total becomes 10 per cent, exactly the textbook norm.

Those in the groin, however, raise questions. If the *coxa* or area of the hip is considered as a part of the glandular region, then this region still does not reach the twentieth-century norm with only 50.2 per cent of the swellings. If those in the *coxa* are considered to be outside the inguinal node (which in many cases they must have been, as with buboes that extended across to the back or side), then those of the groin and femoral duct fall far short of the norm, constituting only 27.4 per cent of the large swellings. These results from Milan, moreover, are strikingly different from the impressions given by the less systematic sources for the Black Death and plague waves of the second half of the fourteenth century and early fifteenth, when according to one doctor's clinical report and plague swellings observed in saints' lives the cervical region was the principal site of pestilential swellings.[87] Had the signs of the plague changed, or does the difference reflect problems with the less numerous and less systematically collected sources for the earlier period?

Despite several similarities in the signs between early modern and twentieth-century plagues, the total percentage represented by pestilential swellings within the three principal nodes for the Milanese plagues, however, fails to conform

[87] Cohn, *The Black Death Transformed*, 77–82 and appendix I: 'Miraculous plague cures'.

to 'typical' bubonic plague. Between 22.3 per cent and 19.8 per cent of the larger swellings during these late Renaissance plagues (depending on where the submaxillary swellings are placed) lay outside the three principal areas[88] and if those of the 'coxa' are considered outside the inguinal ducts, the figure climbs to an astonishing 45.5 per cent of the swellings. By contrast, bubonic plague in India and China recorded less than 2 per cent of swellings straying beyond the three glandular drains, and only in one case—the first eight hospitals of the Presidency of Bombay—did they climb as high as 5 per cent.

Further, the stray swellings recorded in the Milanese necrologies contrast with those from the twentieth century. Unfortunately, Choksy fails to elaborate on the largest of these databases collected from two hospitals in the Presidency of Bombay with 13,600 cases from 1896 to 1908 and 9600 buboes present on patients. From the hospital reports listed of the Bombay Commission, however, the swellings outside the three principal ducts concentrated in other minor lymph nodes. For the first eight hospitals (published in 1897), which present the largest proportion of swellings outside the three lymph nodes (5.4 per cent) and which provide the most detail, 3.6 per cent or two-thirds of them formed in one minor lymph node alone, behind the knees, leaving only 1.3 per cent of the buboes outside the glands altogether: three on the arm, one on the abdomen, one on the right calf, two on the scalp, and two on feet. By contrast, the Milanese plagues produced relatively few swellings or rashes behind the knees (only 0.5 per cent). Instead, the majority of the strays appear in places without significant lymph nodes altogether and where extremely few, if any, have been found for classic bubonic plague in India and China among thousands of published clinical cases. The most significant of the Milanese ones were on the back, sides, shoulders, arms, and shins. Others formed on still more unusual places for modern plague: in eye sockets, on eyelids, lips, elbows, feet, fingers, the vulva, penis, buttocks, and the anus.

In some cases it is difficult to know if these stray swellings were outside glands. For instance, some were specified as on nipples (*puppa*) as opposed to being under breasts in the more minor mammary glands. Others were more vaguely sighted on chests, which could have been in the mammary glands or outside them. Conservatively, I have placed these vague ones in the mammary glands. Still, a rough summary of these swellings shows a significant gap between the 'bubonic' plagues of early modern Milan and those of the twentieth century. For the former, only slightly over 10 per cent of those swellings outside the three principal glands appear to have been in minor lymph nodes.

---

[88] Recently, Carmichael, 'Universal and Particular', 45–6, has tallied the positions of swellings from 2,781 cases of plague from the Milanese records. (It is not clear which plague years she has examined.) Regarding the three principal lymph nodes, her results are similar to mine; however, she ignores completely swellings that Milanese doctors specified in places outside these three nodes, leaving the impression that none formed outside of them.

Table 2.6 Positions of Swellings: The Milanese Plagues, 1452–1523

Positions			
PRINCIPAL LYMPH NODES			
sub aselle	in the armpits	1180	19.3%
post aureum	behind the ears	329	5.4%
Colli	on the neck	143	2.4%
Inguine	in the groin	1663	27.3%
Coxa	on the hip	1405	23.1%
Ancha	on the hip	11	0.2%
Femur	on the thigh	6	0.1%
Subtotal		4733	77.7%
HEAD AND FACE			
gula/gutare		58	1.0%
Maxille		27	0.4%
Alitate	windpipe?	24	0.4%
sub mento		28	0.5%
Fauces	cavity at the back of the mouth	8	0.1%
emontorio cerebri	Nose	73	1.2%
Fronte		18	0.3%
Varghi		3	0.05%
Oculis		11	0.2%
Barbam		14	0.2%
Oris		1	0.02%
Boccio		2	0.03%
Facie		7	0.1%
scia		4	0.07%
Sio		18	0.3%
Uscio		2	0.03%
Supercilio		4	0.07%
Capite		1	0.02%
cornu capitis		5	0.1%
Palpebra	Eyelid	1	0.02%
aur/cartilig		1	0.02%
visonem/post		1	0.02%
f[r]ontenella		1	0.02%
Labro		1	0.02%
Varghi		3	0.05%
Subtotal		316	5.2%
TRUNK:			
Humero		81	1.3%
Pectore		79	1.3%
spatula		64	1.1%
Pomo		4	0.07%
Mamilla		38	0.6%
Cordis		10	0.2%

(continued)

Table 2.6   (*continued*)

Positions			
Renum		15	0.3%
Stomaco		8	0.1%
Ventre		42	0.7%
Latera		17	0.3%
Spleni		2	0.03%
Umbilicum		9	0.2%
Dorsu		105	1.7%
Ypocudero	Liver	5	0.08%
Costis		1	0.02%
Subtotal		480	7.9%
LIMBS:			
Brachio		155	2.6%
Adiutorii	humeris or ulna	18	0.3%
Manu		13	0.2%
Cubiti		4	0.07%
Mandibrilam		1	0.02%
Pulsum		9	0.2%
Genu		28	0.5%
Tibia		184	3.0%
Crucie	Shank	21	0.3%
Circumferentiis	circumflex: knee or elbow	1	0.02%
Pedis		18	0.3%
in police manu		2	0.03%
dito/digito		2	0.03%
Subtotal		456	7.5%
GENITALIA AND BUTTOCK:			0.0%
Vulva		1	0.02%
Nate		27	0.4%
Herneram		1	0.02%
Caudam		1	0.02%
bursu testicular		3	0.05%
anum/cullo		3	0.05%
Scrutum		1	0.02%
Natica		2	0.03%
Membro		1	0.02%
Subtotal		40	0.7%
UNKNOWN PARTS:			
Ratuine		1	0.02%
Nonia		1	0.02%
Verentibus		1	0.02%
Spiritualia		1	0.02%
Sattis		1	0.02%
ote silvestru		1	0.02%
Spadicula		1	0.02%
Spindela		1	0.02%

Table 2.6 (*continued*)

Positions		
super spondilem cuiguli	3	0.05%
Fancilla	4	0.07%
Calonico	1	0.02%
Precie	1	0.02%
Stemato	1	0.02%
ex fistula cavarnoxo	1	0.02%
Pinzio	1	0.02%
diversis partibus corporis	16	0.4%
?	24	0.4%
Subtotal	64	1.1%
TOTAL	6089	100%

Table 2.7 Swellings Outside the Three Principal Glands: Milanese Plagues, 1452–1523

Minor glands	Number	percentage of all swelling	Percentage of stray swellings
Submaxillary	85	1.4%	6.3%
submammary	42	0.7%	3.1%
parotid/poplitcal	28	0.5%	2.1%
total minor gland	155	2.6%	11.4%
Outside	1201	19.9%	88.6%
Unknown	64	1.06%	
total known	6025	98.9%	
Total	6089	100%	
total stray swellings	1356	22.5%	

The comparisons between the early modern data and commission reports from India and China of 'typical' bubonic plague present further anomalies. From the hospital reports of the Bombay Presidency, multiple swellings amounted to 4.6 per cent in 1897 and 7.5 per cent in 1898. From N. H. Choksy's 1909 India data and the Chinese cases from the Chien Chia-tien and 'whole Tungkiao areas', cases of multiple buboes were higher, 13 per cent, 13.7 per cent, and 7.5 per cent, respectively. Yet cases of multiple swellings in early modern Milan were consistently higher: 12.6 (1452), 18.0 (1468), 12.9 (1483), 11.5 (1485), 18.5 (1503), and 22.7 per cent in 1523, collectively almost doubling the proportions found for published data on modern plagues in India or China.

Still more anomalous was the presence of the smaller swellings or bumps (called *morbilli* at Milan).[89] Unlike the buboes and other swellings, these bumps

[89] These constitute at the very least 95% of plague mortalities since Yersin's discovery, and probably closer to 99% of them. I base these estimates on calculations that 95% of plague mortalities since 1894

Table 2.8   *Morbilli* and the Larger Swellings: The Milanese Plagues, 1452–1523

Skin disorders	1452		1468		1483	
morbilli without larger swellings	37	37.8%	47	53.4%	58	47.9%
morbilli	98	53.6%	88	32.4%	121	27.9%
cases with skin disorders	183	97.9%	272	94.4%	433	81.1%
total cases	187	100%	288	100%	534	100%
no swellings or *morbilli*	4	2.1%	16	5.6%	101	18.9%
multiple swellings/no *morbilli*	10	5.5%	7	2.6%	11	2.5%
multiple buboes	23	12.6%	49	18.0%	56	12.9%
total multiple cases	111	60.7%	130	47.8%	166	38.3%
Skin disorders	1485		1503		1523	
morbilli without larger swellings	661	57.0%	37	53.6%	204	42.8%
morbilli	1159	27.0%	69	75%	478	39.5%
cases with skin disorders	4298	98.7%	92	47.7%	1209	84.3%
total cases	4357	100%	193	100%	1434	100%
No swellings or *morbilli*	359	8.2%	101	52.3%	225	15.7%
multiple swellings/no *morbilli*	242	5.6%	10	10.9%	54	4.5%
multiple buboes	493	11.5%	17	18.5%	274	22.7%
total multiple cases	1410	32.8%	76	82.6%	698	57.7%

(as the doctors' treatises also attest) were not localized in lymph nodes (major or minor) but instead covered entire bodies (*per totum corpus*). By contrast, such bumps in modern plagues have been so rare as not to be mentioned in most major texts on infectious diseases. Moreover, the lists of signs for 'typical bubonic plague' assembled by Chun and Choksy do not mention any such bumps or rashes, and from the hospital reports included in Gatacre's Plague Commission, only two cases appear from over 3,000 clinical reports. These, moreover, were not bumps or spots but black blisters, and these did not cover entire bodies but only surrounded the larger plague swellings.

In Milan, such bumps—black, purple, or occasionally red—were a normal feature of plague, as physicians noted in their treatises on how to recognize plague and as the Milanese health board doctors consistently registered them across the plagues of the late fifteenth and sixteenth century. For the plague of 1452, *morbilli* appeared in over half the cases showing any skin disorders (53.6 per cent); in 1468, 32.4 per cent, in 1483, 27.9 per cent, in 1485, 27.0 per cent, in 1503, 75.0 per cent, and in 1523, 39.5 per cent. These skin disorders, moreover, do not appear as separate diseases such as measles (the present-day translation of *morbilli*), smallpox, or typhus without bubonic signs as Ann Carmichael has suggested for the mixed skin disorders that characterized plagues in Florence and

have come from India, where few cases of the atypical plague have been cited. Moreover, no cases of atypical plague observed by Chun, Machiavello, Laforce et al., for India, China, Ecuador, Chile, Nepal, and Iran, resulted in over a hundred dying from this form of plague and, in most of the cases, the mortality rates were far fewer.

elsewhere during the fourteenth and fifteenth centuries.[90] Instead, almost exactly half the plague corpses with the smaller spots (or much less frequently, the stripes and black rashes that covered the entire bodies) recorded in the six plagues of Milan (49.5 per cent) also possessed buboes or similar large swellings primarily in the three principal lymph glands. These victims, moreover, often died at the same time, even on the same day as other plague victims in the same household, and in the same quick fashion within two or three days with the same symptoms as those with only the black spots or only the larger swellings.[91]

Secondly, plague doctors at Milan as well as authors of plague tracts recognized that those with spots alone, especially red ones, could be confused with other diseases that were not 'true plague'. Here the Milanese doctors made their diagnoses based not on a single sign or symptom but on a complex of signs and symptoms, such as the presence of the characteristic plague trio of continuous fever, severe headache, and vomiting, and more importantly on epidemiological criteria: whether the victim died in a house afflicted with plague and whether the death was a quick one, that is, within a week. In 1477–8, Milan was afflicted by an epidemic of *morbilli* that spread over bodies, killing over a thousand in little over a year. But the health board's doctors did not confuse this disease with plague: the bumps were normally red, not the more deadly purple or black; none of the victims was afflicted with the larger swellings in the lymph nodes; and most decisively, the victims invariably took longer to die. In contrast to plague victims of whom less than 2 per cent survived longer than a week once the first signs of illness appeared and on average (medium) died in less than three days,[92] less than 8 per cent of the victims of the red *morbilli* in 1477 and 1478 died within a week: on average they took two weeks to die (14.7 days).[93]

Further, the plague bumps of 'atypical' twentieth-century outbreaks of *Yersinia pestis* signalled vastly different consequences for the afflicted. Chroniclers and doctors of the Black Death and plagues of the fourteenth and fifteenth centuries along with comments seen above from the sixteenth-century doctors point to these skin disorders as among their plague's most deadly signs from which few, if any, recovered. By contrast, the rare appearance of these smaller and more ubiquitous bumps in twentieth-century plagues, sometimes called 'small-pox

---

[90] Carmichael, *Plague and the Poor*, 59 and 82–3. Curiously, she does not suggest the same in 'Universal and Particular'.

[91] See below for timing. Also, if the *morbilli* had been measles, smallpox, or another existing disease in the penumbra of diseases, why would these diseases that had long been domesticated in the medieval West suddenly and only during plague years have infected such great numbers of children and adults (presumably already exposed to these diseases), and why would these diseases have suddenly become so much more lethal and only so in plague years?

[92] For these calculations, see Cohn and Alfani, 'Households and Plague'.

[93] Popolazione, no. 75 (Register I, 1 July 1477 to 18 January 1478). Records from the first half of 1477 are missing. Historians have diagnosed this disease as typhus based on the spots alone. The seasonality of the disease, however, does not conform with typhus, at least when lice were the vectors. Like plague, this disease occurred mostly in summer, when victims were wearing less, not more, clothing.

plague', as in Chile 1903 and Ecuador in 1908, signified the opposite—benign forms of plague scoring few, if any, fatalities, and when fatalities occurred, the period of illness was long (except in still rarer cases when the bumps quickly spread into continuous rashes, and not distinct bumps, indicative of the haemorrhaging of septicaemic plague with death ensuing in a matter of hours).

Unfortunately, neither the Milanese death books nor records for any other place in late medieval or early modern Europe that I know provide statistics on the lethality of various forms of plague. The Milanese books of death, however, lend some credence to the claims of doctors and other commentators on late medieval and early modern plague. Those afflicted with the *morbilli* during plague did not linger long in their illness. In fact, death was slightly more rapid when the smaller bumps spread over plagued bodies than when they suffered with larger glandular swellings alone. In the most severe plague recorded in the Milanese *libri*, that of 1485, those with the smaller spots died on average in two and a half days (2.58).[94] For all other plague cases, the average duration was slightly over a week (7.34 days).[95] By contrast, during the plague of 1523, when doctors more consistently specified the duration of plague illness, those without the *morbilli* survived a fraction of a day longer than the others (3.7 days compared with 3.5 days). However, over the six plagues in Milan recorded in the *Libri* victims with *morbilli* died slightly more quickly than those without them (3.3 days on average compared with 3.4 days).[96] There were no signs that these were two distinctive and simultaneous diseases.

More telling was the testimony of the Capuchin friar Paolo Bellintani, who headed Milan's lazaretto in 1576–7, and soon afterwards similar establishments in Brescia and Marseille. In the 1580s he distinguished between red and black spots. For the black ones he repeated several times: if these appeared, 'no one escaped; all of them died'. From his vast experience of overseeing thousands of plague deaths in three lazaretti, three cities, and three plagues, probably more than that seen by any sixteenth-century doctor, he had never witnessed a single patient recover with these signs. Of the ten signs he catalogued for recognizing plague, this was the only one he claimed led to certain death.[97] Even if by the sixteenth century, there was not a great difference in the rapidity of death between those with or without the black or purple pustules, certainly this smallpox form of plague was hardly the benign plague or *pestis minor* that such bumps have signified since Yersinia's discovery.

In addition to the *morbilli*, the Milanese records describe other ubiquitous pestilential signs found on plague corpses—striped rashes either on the back

---

[94] Of 1,159 plague victims afflicted with the pestilential *morbilli*, the records indicated the period of illness in 423 cases (36.5%).

[95] The *Libri* indicate duration of illness in only 539 of 4,357 cases (12.37%), and doctors appear even less concerned about the duration for those without *morbilli*. Only 116 of these cases were so monitored.

[96] For those with *morbilli*, the doctors recorded the duration in 1,693 cases and for those without them, 581.

[97] Bellintani, *Dialogo della peste*, 127–30.

or covering the entire body (*corpus* or *dorsum vergulentum*) and signs of more generalized haemorrhaging which left the entire body blackened (*tota denigrata* or *totus denigrato*). These were, however, extremely rare. Striped bodies are found in only sixteen of 6993 plague cases, and blackened bodies less frequently: eleven cases, all of which were confined to the plague of 1485. These cases could also include *morbilli* or plague tumours and buboes. Death came quickly with these unusual signs and can be found in households with other plague victims, leading doctors to conclude that the victims had died of plague, even if no buboes or other spots had formed. However, the quickness of death was not strikingly different from that observed with other plague cases. For the 1485 cases of blackened bodies, the average period of illness before death was similar to that for plague in general: 3.4 days. Those with striped bodies died slightly but not significantly faster (in 3.3 days). In neither case was it a matter of hours, as happens with *Yersinia pestis* in septicaemic form. Several even survived for six or seven days, and only one died within a day: a one-year-old girl in 1523 stricken with epilepsy, continuous fever, and a striped back.[98]

PNEUMONIC PLAGUE AND SYMPTOMS

Can pneumonic plague hold the key to explain the swift spread of late medieval and early modern plague? As I have argued elsewhere, modern cases of pneumonic plague (*Yersinia pestis*) either as primary or secondary to the prior formation of bubonic plague was not as contagious as historians have often assumed.[99] Its transmission rates, particularly secondary cases of transmission, were low.[100] But there are other reasons to suspect that a pneumonic form of the plague (much less pneumonic *Yersinia pestis*) was not at work in any of the six Milanese plagues. First, although plague could peak later than is generally seen in Mediterranean places such as Florence in the later Middle Ages or early modern period, all six Milanese plagues were in decline by November and did not rage again until the late spring or summer—not the usual seasonality of pneumonic diseases in general or pneumonic *Yersinia pestis* in particular.

Secondly, the plague seems to have evolved in one critical respect since 1348. One reason historians have identified the medieval plagues as *Yersinia pestis* was because of the two forms the Black Death assumed in 1348, most famously described by the pope's doctor, Guy de Chauliac. In Avignon the new disease struck first in winter (January), when it was characterized by continuous fever

---

[98] Popolazione, no. 87, 7.x.1523.

[99] Cohn, 'Epidemiology of the Black Death', 81–2 and 93–4.

[100] See Gani and Leach, 'Epidemiologic Determinants for Modeling Pneumonic Plague'. For the 1994 outbreak of plague in and around Surat, cases of secondary transmission of the plague were unknown; see Mavalankar, 'Indian "Plague" Epidemic', 548.

and the spitting of blood. It was highly contagious and the victims died within three days. Then in March (according to Guy), the disease took another form, with buboes forming in the three principal lymph nodes. The disease continued to be contagious but the victims took slightly longer to die—five instead of three days.[101] According to other contemporary chroniclers and doctors, however, the two forms of the disease coexisted in the same seasons, as is seen in the plague patients' ledger kept by the Lucchese doctor Ser Iacopo during the third plague in Tuscany in 1373.[102] After the third or fourth wave of plague, however, the dramatic descriptions of plague patients vomiting and spitting blood are difficult to find, and by the 1450s, at least in the Milanese records, this form of plague had vanished entirely.

In addition to recording various pestilential swellings, rashes, spots, and their positions, the Milanese plague doctors often described other 'pestilential accidents' or symptoms (in some plagues, especially 1523, with great consistency, in others such as the first three of 1452, 1468, and 1503, less often and in less detail). Certainly, by the plague of 1483, a set of three symptoms had become synonymous in these reports with 'the pestilential accidents': they were continuous fever, headaches, and vomiting (but not of blood). Perhaps such a plague trio of symptoms may not appear so distinctive; one might imagine numerous diseases when the three are common. However, a glance at the descriptions of non-plague deaths and a reading of the reports from Milan's second most deadly epidemic of the late fifteenth and early sixteenth century—that of the red-spotted 'morbilli' in 1477-8—highlight this trio of symptoms as emblematic of early modern plague. The trio does not characterize any other disease in these records. It is not found among the thousand cases of the red *morbilli* epidemic of 1477–8; however, on 22 September 1478 when cases of this disease were subsiding, plague struck Milan, killing a twelve-year-old girl within one or two days.[103] She was covered with purple *morbilli* 'and worst', 'a notable antrace' formed on the underside (*domestica parte*) of her left arm and another minor one in the curvature of her elbow.[104] Another twelve cases of plague followed, the last one occurring on 16 November. Whether it was a weak strain of the plague, the time of year it struck, or the vigilance and experience of the health board, its doctors, and the public, this plague was contained, never flaring into a full-blown epidemic: all but one of the cases occurred within the zone outside the walls of the parish of San Protasio, which had consistently been one of the most prominent neighbourhoods of plague during all six plagues of the second half of the fifteenth and early sixteenth centuries. No new cases of plague appeared until 12 March 1483.

[101] Guy de Chauliac, *Inventarium sive chirurgia magna*, I, 117–18.
[102] *Il Memoriale di Iacopo di Coluccino Bonavia*, 397.
[103] She died on Tuesday: her illness arose either Monday or Tuesday.
[104] Popolazione, no. 75, 22.ix.1478.

Relying on signs alone, the doctors might have consigned the new cases of plague to have been only the tail-end of the disease of red *morbilli* (which in fact were not always red). However, the new cases differed from the red *morbilli* epidemic in ways other than colour. In addition to the new plague victims dying within a few days instead of two weeks, the new plague cases of 1478 were all distinguished by the plague trio of continuous fevers, headaches, and vomiting as had typified numerous other plague cases diagnosed in the Milanese registers since 1452. In the fifteenth and sixteenth-century death books of Milan, this trio was unique to plague.

The descriptions of 'pestilential accidents' beyond the buboes and *morbilli* did not, moreover, end with this trilogy of symptoms. Plague doctors paid attention to urine, complexion, eyes, places of pain, colour and character of the tongue, and other conditions, such as sleepiness or deep sleep (*sumno profundo*), loss of appetite, irascibility (*colirico*), high heart rates (*passione cordis*), and the possible failure of organs such as the kidneys (*passione renali*). Plague victims' urine was often described as *confussa* or confused or disorderly, which may have meant cloudy, *citrona* (or pale yellow), *turbina, cum flussu, subiugalis* (under the yoke), *urina cara* (fleshy piss ?), *urina malla* (bad piss), *vissis* (stinky), retention of urine (*reptentione urinae*), burning urine (*ardore urina*), thick and turbulent urine (*urinarum grossitie et turbulentie*), and in at least one case, bloody urine. Exactly how these terms now translate into modern clinical terms is sometimes difficult to imagine. The tongue was described as *alba* (white) *spissa* (thick), and *spinoxa* (prickly),[105] the eyes as grave and *collegacione* (drawn together). Pain was described first and foremost in the head but also in parts of the body such as the groin, the *coxa*, underarms, and other areas where swellings had not yet formed but perhaps were subcutaneous. Pain in the stomach, abdominal bloating, and nausea were also common and led to vomiting.

Other conditions and perhaps other diseases may have accompanied plague. As with twentieth-century plague, pregnant women frequently aborted.[106] Epilepsy accompanied thirty-eight cases, almost all of whom were children under six; the oldest was eighteen. Pleurisy characterized only three plague victims, all between one and six years old, all during the plague of 1485. Worms were slightly more common, 42 cases or (0.6 per cent); again mostly with young children, although four were over 18. Perhaps, these conditions depicted the general conditions of plague victims as living in squalid conditions in the most overcrowded and impoverished parishes of Milan.[107] Other conditions depicted

---

[105] Also with twentieth-century bubonic plague, 'the tongue is thickly coated with white fur'; Chun, 'Clinical Features', 311.

[106] Ibid., 311.

[107] A number of the plague tracts also pointed to worms as an accompanying affliction of plague; see for instance Fumanelli, *De compositione medicamentorum*, 315; Gratiolo, *Discorso di peste*, 33; Mercuriale, *De pestilentia*, 3; Baravalle, *Praticam medicinam protitentis de peste*, 13; Napolitano, *Trattato di mirabili secreti* [1576], 13; Bellicocchi, *Avvertimenti*, 414r (BAV).

in the early accounts of the Black Death and to a lesser extent in successive plagues of the Middle Ages—delirium and crazed frenzies—are still less apparent in the Milanese doctors' reports. A frenzied state (*frenixi*) was used to describe four victims and 'delirium', once. *Alenacione* or *alienatione mentis*, possibly meaning crazed or having lost one's mind, was used slightly more often but still extremely rarely (in five cases). In 1485 one plague patient was characterized as *freneticus* and *spasanatus*,[108] and in two cases—one in the plague of 1483, the other in 1485—the victims were described as irascible (*colirica passione*). More often than these crazed and perhaps violent states and fits, the victims were described in nearly the opposite terms: somnolent or caught in deep sleep (at least thirty plague victims). *Abbominatione et subetia* may have been another psychological trait found in one 1485 case. *Cum subetia* are found in another sixteen cases (all but one from the plague of 1485) and may have also expressed a certain state of mind but more probably referred to the physical state of oozing pus. Perhaps these bits and pieces of fifteenth- and sixteenth-century clinical evidence point to states of mind that resemble those of twentieth-century plague victims more than the violent frenzied conditions chroniclers attributed to victims in 1348. By the mid-fifteenth century such violent fits, as with pneumonic symptoms, appear no longer to have been a common feature of plague (although the former may have arisen again with plagues of the seventeenth and eighteenth centuries).[109]

These varied descriptions of conditions, signs, and symptoms could often fill six or more lines per victim in the Milanese death books. In addition to recording clinical traits, the doctors frequently stated the course of the disease, charting the timing in days, even hours, from the onset of fevers to certain pains, to the formation of buboes or other skin disorders to death. This attention to the succession of various symptoms and signs even for the extremely short periods of the plague's duration can be spotted in the Milanese registers before 1523, but in that plague year, as with other clinical reporting, the doctors' accounts became more precise and consistent. For instance, on 21 August, 1523 a forty-year-old man died within a day (*a die heri*). First, a *carbonchulo* formed on the right part of his mouth (*in sio*), then during the night a fever and headache ensued; the next morning a bubo formed in his right groin, and he died.[110]

However, usually fevers heralded the disease before more specific 'pestilential accidents' became evident, when families and the health board would have taken notice. On Saturday, 22 August 1523, a husband and wife died of plague on the same day. The first signs of the husband's illness had arisen only on that day (*infirmatur a die hodie*)—a *carbunchulo* on his right arm and pain in his right

---

108 Popolazione, no. 77, 8.iv.1485.

109 See for instance the descriptions of the surgeon Giuseppe Balestra at Rome's lazaretto on the isle of Tiberino during the 1656–7 plague, who described cases of delirium and frenzy (Conforti, 'Peste e stampa', p. 145); and the comments of Morea, *Storia della peste di Noja*, 8–9, who described plague symptoms in 1815 as fevers with delirium, diarrhoea, nausea, etc.

110 Popolazione, no. 87, 21.viii.1523.

armpit. His wife's illness had begun two days before on Thursday: she had a fever accompanied with back pains, and on the following day, she aborted her baby. Finally, on the day of her death, two *carbonchuli* appeared on her right arm along with a *bubo* in her right armpit.[111] On Wednesday, 4 September, a twenty-seven-year-old woman immigrant died. On the previous Monday she had become ill with a fever, on Tuesday she aborted her baby, and 'today' (the day of her death) black *morbilli* began spreading over her body along with a 'tumore' that formed in her right groin.[112] A thirty-year-old *magister*, probably a master artisan, from Pavia, was one of the few to have been ill for more than a week before succumbing to plague. Thirteen days before his death he had a fever, but it was intermittent until Wednesday (two days before his death), when it became continuous with the emergence of a *bubo* on his left hip (*coxa*).[113]

Another long struggle with plague is found for 18 August. This is one of the few cases in these plague-time records of a doctor dying of plague (as opposed to barbers, who by the 1485 records were one of the most afflicted professions during plague). By the sixteenth century, doctors had evidently learnt how to protect themselves, probably by sending barbers and others to do much of the dirty and dangerous work.[114] This doctor, Lord Gaspar Conte, moreover, was an important one, *Prestantisimus illustrissimus*, doctor of Milan. He became ill on 1 August with vomiting and *cum fusione urinarum*. With certain remedies, however, he improved. On Wednesday—six days before his death—he was attacked (*invasit*) by fever again, this time of a more serious sort (*cum rigore*), which was also continuous. On the Sunday, three days before dying, the 'same' milky urine returned along with red *morbili*. Finally, on the day of his death, black *morbilli* appeared, and on the basis of this last affliction, despite his unusually long illness and temporary recovery, he was judged (*advertendum est*) to have died of plague. Curiously, the doctor added to the end of this entry as the one giving the judgement was Magister Gaspare de Comite himself. (Was this a scribal error or his last diagnosis for the Milanese state?)[115] Although rare, other equally lengthy reports can be found in these registers.[116]

Yet, despite this attention to clinical detail, incomparable with any from late medieval records, the infrequency of any signs of respiratory illness associated with plague are striking. While coughs (*catarrhi* or *tussi*) were often described in these records for other deaths especially during winter, they vanished as a condition of early modern plague in Milan or elsewhere in early modern Italy as far as I can discern. Of 6,993 cases, the doctors noted only one plague victim

---

[111] Ibid., 22.viii.1523.   [112] Ibid., 4.ix.1523.   [113] Ibid., 9.ix.1523.

[114] According to Pomata, *Contracting a Cure*, 66, matters of the 'inner-body' went to the highest in the hierarchy of healers—physicians—whereas care of the 'outer body' was the responsibility of barbers and others lower down the medical hierarchy. Contagion was considered a matter of the outer body.

[115] Ibid., 18.viii.1523.

[116] See for instance Popolazione, no. 76, 6.ix.1483, 11.ix.1483, 8.x.1483; no. 77, 30.xi.1485; and no. 87, 23.viii.1523.

with coughs—a forty-year-old man *cum tussi gattariosa* who died in four days on
3 March during the plague of 1503. But this was not a case of pneumonic plague
or at least of primary pneumonic plague (of the *Yersinia* or the early modern
variety): the victim was also afflicted with a tumour in his right groin and took
four days to die after the appearance of the pestilential swellings; yet the cough
had preceded it![117]

Further, although vomiting was a usual symptom of the Milanese plagues,
it was accompanied by nausea, abdominal bloating, emissions of fluids (*fluxu*)
and stomach pains—not the spitting or vomiting of blood. Of the 6,993 cases,
only two involved bloody vomit: a twenty-year-old woman during the plague of
1485, who died with black *morbilli*, continuous fever, and 'vomito sanguineo
sine emotoyca passione',[118] and, a five-year-old boy, who in the plague of 1523
died in four days with continuous fever and bloody vomit, but 'without any other
sign'.[119] Other than the three cases of pleurisy cited above, the closest indication
of any possible respiratory illness accompanying plague were cases of snotty and
bloody noses (*cum fluxu et sanguinis narium* or *fluxu sanguinis narium*). These
too, however, were rare: 16 of 6,993 cases. Instead, vomiting, stomach ailments,
and their effusions suggest that by the mid-fifteenth century the intestinal tract
had become a principal conduit of the plague's diffusion.

The sixteenth-century plague tracts convey the same impression, even though
these academic physicians on occasion strove to reach universal evaluations, not
only about plague but about common traits and causes of epidemic diseases. In
observing their own plagues they relied on theoretical and historical evidence,
citing both antique and Arabic texts—Hippocrates, Galen, Avicenna, Averröes,
Rhazes, and others—and chroniclers, commentators, and plague doctors of the
later Middle Ages and Renaissance: Matteo Villani,[120] Giovanni Boccaccio,[121]
Gentile da Foligno,[122] Guy de Chauliac,[123] Tommaso del Garbo,[124] Saldino
Ferro Ascolano,[125] and especially the Florentine humanist Marsilio Ficino,[126] as
well as contemporaries such as Giovanni Battista Da Monte, Andreas Gallo, Oddo
degli Oddi, Giovanni Battista Susio, Girolamo Mercuriale, Alessandro Massaria,
Niccolò Massa, Girolamo Fracastoro, and many others.[127] For instance, after
describing in great detail the various types of pestilential swellings and where they

---

[117] Popolazione, no. 80, 3.iii.1503.   [118] Ibid., no. 78, 29.iii.1485.

[119] Ibid., no. 87, 10.ix.1523.   [120] Mercuriale, *De pestilentia*, 68 and 70.

[121] Alessandri, *Trattato della peste*, 27r and 44r; Mercuriale, *De pestilentia*, 70; Ingrassia, *Informatione*,
10; Bucci, *Reggimento*, n.p.; Susio, *Libro del conoscere la pestilenza*, 51.

[122] Borromeo, *La peste di Milano*, 25; Sassonia, *Praticam medicinam*, 6v (not in Edit 16); Pasini, *De
pestilentia Patavina anno 1555*, 15r.

[123] Gallo, *Fascis de peste*, 217.   [124] Razzi, *Modo di conservarsi sano*, 5.

[125] Gratiolo, *Discorso di peste*, 2, 22, and 91.

[126] Daciano, *Trattato della peste*, 14; Razzi, *Modo di conservarsi sano*, 5; Ingrassia, *Informatione*, 10;
Puccinelli, *Dialoghi sopra le cause della peste*, 13r, 26v; *Cause et rimedii della peste*, 6; Gratiolo, *Discorso di
peste*, 2, 74, and 91; Bucci, *Modo di conoscere*, 5v.

[127] See, among others, Sassonia, *Praticam medicinam*, 3v, 6v, and 19v.

appeared on the body, Mercuriale turned to other symptoms such as changes in excrement brought on by plague *mutatione* and bloody drops (*stillae*) and noses. But he did not point to respiratory complications and specified that the vomiting of plague victims was of food (*vomitus ciborum*).[128] The Genoese surgeon Boerio identified seven signs of plague along with a catalogue of pains. He further devoted an entire section to vomiting (the seventh sign) but said nothing about the spitting or vomiting of blood or other clear signs of pulmonary illness.[129] Similarly, Andrea Gratiolo di Salò's general description of plague symptoms with various places of pain, mental disorientation, colour of the tongue, vomiting, the nature and various colours of urine and excrement, pulse, breathing, and much more, made no mention of respiratory complaints or vomiting of blood.[130] Further on, he turned with greater attention to bloodily effusions, seeing no cases of the spitting of blood in his plague practice, even though (he commented) it was common with numbers of other patients not afflicted with this disease. Moreover, bloody noses were not common: he had heard of only three plague cases with it during his entire career. On the other hand, he recorded plague patients with coughs, but these were children whose spittle was almost entirely black, and unlike plague victims of 1348, not even they vomited blood.[131]

Few other doctors in their plague tracts mentioned the spitting or vomiting of blood, and those who did, did so when citing other, earlier authorities, such as in a long list of plague symptoms, catalogued by the Veronese doctor Fumanelli, who cited the seventh-century compiler Paul of Aegina;[132] or with Vittore Bonagente, who cited Boccaccio 'atque alij scriptores pestis anni 1348'.[133] One exception might have been the Tridentine doctor who practised in Frankfurt, Andreas Gallo. In the mid-sixteenth century, he dedicated an entire treatise to pneumonic plague, 'from whence coughs with bloody sputum ensued, along with difficulty in breathing (*inde tussis cum sanguinis sputamine subsequebatur . . . anhelandi difficultate*)', but his testimony came exclusively from historical sources, especially from the popes' famous doctor during the Avignon plagues of 1348 and 1362, Guy de Chauliac, and not from his own practice or from citations to other sixteenth-century physicians.[134] With the plague of

---

[128] Mercuriale, *De pestilentia*, 3.   [129] Boerio, *Trattato delli buboni*, 52.

[130] Gratiolo, *Discorso di peste*.

[131] Ibid., 36. For others who described symptoms including vomiting but related it to the stomach and nausea, see Susio, *Libro del conoscere la pestilenza*, 51; Bucci, *Modo di conoscere*, 58r, 74r; Alessandri, *Trattato della peste*, 54r; Iordan, *Pestis phaenomena*, 62; by contrast he described excessive spitting (*Sputa cruenta*) with the sweats (308). Agricola, *De peste libri tres*, 26; Borromeo, *Pratica per i curati*, 36r; Somenzi, *De morbis*, 2r.

[132] Fumanelli, *De compositione medicamentorum*, 315.

[133] Bonagente, *Decem problemata de peste*, 5v.

[134] Gallo, *Fascis Aureus*, 216–7. Tomai, *De medendis febribus humoralibus*, 18v, mentioned coughs as a possible symptom, but only with pestilential fevers in general. Agricola, *De peste libri tres*, 102–3, described pulmonary plague 'with coughing, a great deal of spittle (*sputa cocta*), and the spewing of liquids'. But his was a long historical account of diseases reaching back to ancient Egypt; there was no sense that he was here describing his own clinical experience. Also, Bennassar, *Recherches sur les grandes*

1575–8, Alessandro Massaria even questioned whether the plague of his own day was 'true plague' because the symptoms of spitting blood and respiratory difficulties were no longer present as had been described by Boccaccio and Matteo Villani in 1348.[135]

The plagues of late-fifteenth and early sixteenth-century Milan were bubonic or pustular (whether or not its agent was *Yersinia pestis*). Except for the plague of 1503, in which slightly more than half the cases had no evidence of skin disorders, the other plagues showed higher proportions of victims afflicted by either the larger swellings or the smaller *morbilli* than has been seen with any modern plague, in which as much as a quarter of plague deaths show no notable skin disorders.[136] By contrast, in 1452, only 2.1 per cent of victims' bodies bore no cutaneous signs; in 1468, 5.6 per cent; in 1483, 18.9 per cent; 1485, 8.2 per cent, and 1523, 15.7 per cent. The proportions of cutaneous signs for these early modern plagues, moreover, were without doubt higher than these statistics reveal. When cases came from closed or locked houses, where other household members had been previously stricken, the health-board doctors did not generally feel obliged to describe the cases in detail; instead, they appear as one-line listings that included the victim's name and parish followed by 'decessit peste'. Similarly, when members of the same household died of plague on the same day, the doctors occasionally saw little reason to prove their point with longer clinical reports. Moreover, the care in registering plague cases was sometimes abandoned, as with the last months of the plague of 1523, when the health board had ended its separate booklet of plague deaths: from 17 September to the end of that year, 101 of the remaining 421 plague deaths, nearly a quarter of them, were listed simply as 'decessit peste'. When we consider only those cases in which physicians specified that the victims died swiftly, perhaps within plagued households or with 'the accidents' of continuous fever, headaches, and vomiting, but stated specifically 'sine alio signo', the proportion of bubonic or pustular plague climbs higher. For 1523, instead of 15.7 per cent without cutaneous signs, the proportion falls to 1.5 per cent (21 of 1434 cases).[137]

épidémies, 44–5, finds no evidence for the spitting of blood in plagues of northern Spain at the end of the sixteenth century, even for villages as high as 1,200 metres when plague peaked in February.

[135] Massaria, *De peste*, 31v. Morea, *Storia della peste di Noja*, 441, continued to see vomiting as a plague symptom associated, however, with diarrhoea and not the spitting of blood.
[136] In Gatacre's two reports for the Bombay Presidency, 22.4 and 27.8% of cases showed no cutaneous signs.
[137] Such cases when neither buboes nor *morbilli* had time to form did arise as in 1468 when two sisters died in rapid succession on the same day, one within eighteen hours of her first signs of fever; the second, in sixteen hours without any skin disorders; Miscellanea Storica, no. 1, carte no. 167; and no. 149.

CONCLUSION

The judgement that the European plagues of the late Middle Ages and early modern period were the same as the rodent-disease *Yersinia pestis* has hinged largely on the supposed 'unmistakable' signs and symptoms of the two plague pandemics. Detailed clinical reports from Milan's health-board physicians during six plagues from 1452 to 1523 provide unparalleled clinical evidence for plagues before the nineteenth century. Their reports on deaths within the city walls of Milan sought to diagnose and distinguish plague deaths from all others, detailing the symptoms leading to death, the duration of illness, the signs left on corpses—the position and number of swellings and other skin disorders—along with occasional reports on the daily, even hourly, progress of the disease. To what extent does this evidence match clinical descriptions of the bubonic plagues from the end of the nineteenth century to the present? First, similarities can be seen. In the Milanese records a tripartite set of symptoms associated uniquely with plague were continuous fever, headaches, and vomiting. All three are also seen from clinical reports of modern plague (but modern clinicians have never reported them as the distinctive symptoms of plague as sixteenth-century doctors did).[138] Other symptoms such as pains in places where buboes were forming subcutaneously, white or spiky tongue, nausea, and delirium are also seen in cases from both plague eras. More importantly, the principal criterion for evaluating the two diseases as the same—the plague signs—shows further parallels. For both, the groin was the most common place for pestilential swellings, and if the 'coxa' is interpreted as within the same lymph nodal drain as the groin, the frequency of early modern swellings in this most important place falls short, but not excessively far from that expected with recent 'typical' bubonic plague.[139] Further, the second and third most common lymph nodal zones—the axillary and the cervical—were closer to *Yersinia pestis*'s mark.

But here the similarities end. The published data on plagues in China and India during the late nineteenth and twentieth centuries show little more than 2 per cent of swellings, and often less, located outside the three lymph zones. By contrast, a quarter of the late fifteenth- and sixteenth-century Milanese plague swellings formed outside the three—on shoulders, backs, eyelids, shins, arms, hands, the crown of the head, ankles, testicles, toes and other places (and this not

---

[138] As Carniel, 'Plague Today', comments: 'Vomiting is considered a usual symptom by some physicians, but not so by others' (118).

[139] Unlike late medieval chroniclers and doctors, who never mentioned that most of the glandular swellings formed in the groin, several doctors of the sixteenth century maintained they did; see for instance Massaria, *De peste*, 76r: after listing a number of places where the swellings formed, he concluded: 'sed maxime omnium in inguine'.

counting the smaller bumps). Secondly, multiple swellings with plague cases in early modern Milan were consistently higher than that found with *Yerisinia pestis* in the twentieth century, ranging from 12 per cent of cases in the plague of 1485 to almost a quarter of them in 1523, while in the twentieth century they usually hovered around 5 per cent. Finally, smaller pustules outside the three principal lymph nodes have been negligible with modern plague; for sixteenth-century plagues, as indeed earlier, such bumps covering entirely plague victims' bodies was a common plague characteristic. For the Milanese plague of 1452 these smaller bumps marked over half the corpses and in 1503, three-quarters of them. For the plague of 1485 they were less in evidence but still afflicted over a quarter of plague corpses. When coupled with the multiple boils, between a third and four-fifths of the plague cases had multiple swellings in early modern Milan. Furthermore, in the extremely rare incidences of twentieth-century plague when such pustules were present, the consequences were the very opposite of that seen in late medieval and early modern plagues. For the latter, these pustules were among the deadliest signs, bringing certain death, while for modern plague they have signalled benign plague with long periods of illness and few deaths.

Thirdly, few records of these atypical plagues in the twentieth century have been published. Where they exist, their case numbers and mortalities have been small. An example of twenty-three plague cases from a village in Nepal in 1967 was surmised to have been spread by the human flea, *Pulex irritans*. Unlike classic bubonic plague, the disease spread person to person and had a high household clustering. In addition, a high percentage of these plague victims formed no buboes (more than two-thirds), and their distribution did not concentrate in the groin. But, while these 'atypical' Nepalese cases might correspond with the person-to-person contagion of medieval and early modern plague (at least within tiny villages, but not between villages), their signs differ even more radically from those of early modern plague in Milan than do the skin disorders seen with classic bubonic plague in India, China, and Madagascar. Pinning medieval and early modern plagues to twentieth-century 'atypical' plague, moreover, creates further difficulties: the epidemiological differences between these plagues—mortality rates and the rapidity of spread over vast territories—make historic and modern *Yersinia pestis* even more difficult to square.

Finally, the differences between the two plague periods may have been greater than our statistics indicate: much depends on assumption about terms for parts of the body such as *coxa*, and about the precise meanings early modern doctors had for skin disorders such as *carboni* and *carbuncelli*. Certainly, not all the boils were Boccaccio's well-formed ones as big as pigeon eggs. If *carboni, carbuncelli*—the second most common term for the swellings at Milan, constituting a fifth of all cases—were more of surface rashes and of smaller size than the apostemes, tumours, and buboes as most of the sixteenth-century plague tracts suggest, then the cutaneous differences between the twentieth century's plagues and the early modern ones were greater still.

Beyond the comparison of signs and symptoms, this chapter has made a second point regarding observation and possible differences between academic physicians who wrote plague treatises and those engaged in the daily clinical evaluations of plague corpses on health boards. To be sure, these treatises with their new sections 'on how to recognize the plague' often placed their diagnoses within scholarly frameworks, giving various names of buboes and other skin disorders in Greek, Latin, Italian, and regional dialects. Their discussions embraced ancient doctrines with copious references to Hippocrates, Galen, Avicenna, and other medieval and Arabic compilers, as well as to diseases from the plague of Athens to their own first-hand experiences in the sixteenth century. This bookish framework, however, did not blind them from observing their own contemporary diseases as historians often allege.[140] There was a shared medical universe combining book-learning and experience, not a radically divided one. As our comparisons have shown, physicians' definitions and evaluations of pestilential glandular and non-glandular swellings in various parts of the body, their descriptions of symptoms, listing as many as fifty-two characteristics,[141] correspond closely with the clinical information seen from thousands of individual plague cases diagnosed in Milan's books of the dead. Physicians on health boards and those writing academic treatises (sometimes one and the same) strove to distinguish diseases,[142] particularly 'true plague' from other ailments, and they did so not principally with theoretical constructs taken from antiquity but from observation in their own practices of the signs, symptoms, course of the disease along with epidemiological traits.

Both sources—doctors' theoretical treatises and the health office records— suggest that certain aspects of the plague had remained more or less the same from 1348 to the sixteenth century: it continued to be highly contagious; deaths clustered in households; buboes and other sorts of swellings formed mostly within the three principal lymph nodes but also often strayed to other bodily parts and even into strange places as far as modern *Yersinia pestis* goes. The more ubiquitous and numerous black and purple pustules continued to accompany the larger swellings and were among the plague's most deadly signs. Yet at least one difference separated the plagues of 1348 and those of the late fourteenth century from plague by the middle of the fifteenth century and afterwards: no longer did the theoretical literature or the clinical death records report a bimodal division of the plague into a pneumonic form with spitting blood and a bubonic one. Despite sixteenth-century doctors' knowledge of and reverence for sources such as Boccaccio and Guy de Chauliac, they described the pneumonic form as part of their plague's Black Death past and not a feature of their own times. Not

---

[140] See Introduction, n. 8 and n. 82 above.   [141] See Ingrassia, *Informatione*, 86–8.

[142] Fracastoro's *De contagione* was the most famous of these tracts that defined and distinguished a wide array of different contagious diseases—measles, smallpox, the English sweats, plague, *Lenticulae* (now assumed to be typhus), *phthisis* (possibly tuberculosis), rabies, syphilis, elephantiasis, leprosy, scabies, and more—all calling for specific and different treatments.

only does modern plague (*Yersinia pestis*) show protean characteristics across time and space: historic plague also was not as stable with fixed characteristics over its near five-century history as historians and scientists assume.[143] It was a disease that continued to evolve in its pathology (if less dramatically than diseases such as syphilis or tuberculosis) and more so in its social and demographic consequences, as we shall see.

Even if scientists may one day agree (and at present they do not) that the so-called second pandemic that struck Europe in 1347 and the bubonic plague of the end of the nineteenth century first cultured by Yersin had the same pathogenic agent, such a finding would not solve the problem of understanding the character of the Black Death and its successive waves of plague during the so-called 'second pandemic'.[144] Not only was the epidemiology of the two plagues drastically different, but descriptions from sixteenth-century theoretical texts and detailed clinical reports show the clinical traits of the two far from being 'unmistakeable'. If the agent of the two were the same, then the wide discrepancies in the clinical and epidemiological characteristics would cry out for new biological explanations. We now turn to physicians and other intellectuals of the sixteenth century to see how they dealt with the threat from and changes in their most mortal enemy, and how their approach and evaluation of plague evolved from the Middle Ages to the early modern period.

---

[143] Most recently see Maclean, *Logic, Signs and Nature*, 268, who describes historic plague as 'unvarying' in its clinical pattern.

[144] On this difference in the disease even if the agent may have been the same, see Cohn, *The Black Death Transformed*, 250–2; Nutton, 'Introduction', 12–14: 'Indeed, one might argue that the identification of the agent of the Black Death with *Yersinia pestis* adds very little to what the historian could gain from the sources themselves. Where they agree with modern descriptions, the identification is unnecessary: where they do not, the identification is unhelpful and potentially misleading' (12). On the theoretical level of understanding what a disease is, see Temkin, 'The Scientific Approach to Disease'.

3

The Impetus from Sicily

With Italy suddenly seized by fear of a pandemic spreading simultaneously from north and south in 1575, the number of plague tracts soared vertiginously: almost half of them for the entire sixteenth century were penned in two years alone and their language switched from a predominance in Latin to nearly 90 per cent in the vernacular. Changes in the tracts' form and content were as striking. These years witnessed a new genre of plague writing, what in Milan, Verona, Padua, and Venice would be called *Successo* or *Progresso della peste*. They were written mainly by those outside the medical profession but who were involved in administrating services either for the Church or State during the plague. Although this break from the traditional plague tract became manifested more in cities of northern Italy and by those outside the medical profession, a physician from the south led the way, transforming the plague tract from abstract definitions, causes, cures, and preventatives to a detailed chronicling of the disease's progress from its entry into a city or region to its liberation. This tract, like others that sprang up simultaneously and independently in the north, was based on data collected by states and their health boards (in this case, newly founded with the plague in 1575) and was lodged within the concrete political and social realities of a region's struggle to survive. To understand this transformation, we turn first to Sicily after a glance at the traditional plague tract as it had evolved in the sixteenth century.

THE SIXTEENTH-CENTURY PLAGUE TRACT

Plague tracts had a multiplicity of forms: some written by university physicians mobilized immense erudition to discuss differences between pestilential fevers and true plague, and the universal causes of plagues from astrological movements and signs to changes in climate, winds, and earthly disasters, mostly earthquakes, which produced poisonous vapours. In good Galenic fashion, they discussed the reasons for the putrefaction and corruption of air and linked these atmospheric and celestial causes to terrestrial ones such as rotting corpses of animals and humans caused by war or the fumes emitted from earthquakes or stagnant and polluted water. They then connected these poisonous vapours to the bodily humours of individuals, explaining how the 'atoms' of such vapours penetrated the body and how persons of different conditions, complexions, ages, sex, social conditions, diet, behaviour, and states of mind were more or less susceptible to these atmospheric poisons. They discussed the differences between epidemics that were 'simplex', of one disease, as opposed to 'compositus', of several diseases, and what defined a disease as 'popular', 'morbus comunis', or 'pandemus'. While Galen was their most prominent source, it had become an alloy of other tendencies from antiquity, Arabic physicians and compilers, and Christian philosophers and theologians. As with plague tracts since the Black Death, the sixteenth-century ones continued to search for the portents of plagues in signs from the celestial and natural spheres, citing Aristotle and astrologers from antiquity to their own times and repeating clichés from the early eleventh-century Persian physician Avicenna on birds leaving nests flying to the ground and animals that resided underground such as snakes, scorpions, and mice rising to the surface. Most fundamentally and in contrast to Galen and Hippocrates, the sixteenth-century physician almost invariably began with God and man's sins as plague's first cause. Finally, these doctors turned to their own theorists, most importantly, the Veronese physician Girolamo Fracastoro (1478–1553), whose *De contagione* (1546) became an essential text of Italian plague medicine, especially with the plague of 1575–8.

Other tracts were more pragmatic, and many by the sixteenth century possessed a more or less standard organization. They might begin with universal causes but spend little space on them, simply repeating the truism that God's vengeance provoked by man's sins was the first cause. Quickly they turned to definitions of plague and then moved to the signs and symptoms by which doctors and the laity could recognize the disease. Sometimes short separate chapters were devoted to the bubo, to the *carbunculo*, and to various forms of pustules. They then revealed preventative remedies during plague to protect the healthy, concentrating on diet and behaviour, known as the six non-naturals.[1] Classical references, usually starting with Hippocrates, cautioned moderation in exercise and sex, and following Galen, chapters were devoted to anger, gaiety, sadness, and melancholy that made individuals more or less susceptible to plague.

Finally, the tracts addressed cures and were filled with 'experience' and 'experimentation' on various concocted drugs, syrups, purgatives, and plasters to be applied to various forms of swellings. Often, recommendations for such drugs and recipes were divided socially: those for princes and *gran signori*, ones for

---

[1] These followed closely Galen's lines on hygiene; see Temkin, *Galenism*, 102–3; Niebyl, 'The Non-Naturals'; Nutton, 'Medicine in Medieval Western Europe', 141; Porter, 'The Eighteenth Century', 417; Maclean, *Logic, Signs and Nature*, 252–3; and most recently Fabbri, 'Treating Medieval Plague', 248–9. They were often listed as 'air, food and drink, motion and rest, sleep and waking, inanition and repletion, and accidents of the soul' (Niebyl, 'The Non-Naturals', 488). Baths and coitus also featured. Also, see Rawcliffe, 'The Concept of Health' on the six non-naturals as central to the *Regimen sanitatis* and Nicoud, *Les régimes de santé au Moyen Age*, I, 5–6 and 153–84.

merchants and the rich, others for the poor. Doctors of the late sixteenth century claimed that one reason for the poor dying in greater numbers than the rich was because of their lack of access to doctors and medication. They may have been correct, but in hindsight the strong and peculiar drugs sometimes prescribed to princes and the rich might cast doubts on this claim. Based on the theory of fighting poison with poison—Galen's notion of the *antidotum*—doctors turned to ancient and medieval pharmacological recipes as well as devising their own, calling for pastes and solutions known as theriac (whose origins reached back to the third century BC) concocted from the poisons of venomous snakes, oils from scorpions and even crocodiles.[2] Other procedures for the rich could be equally bizarre, such as a method recommended by a Bolognese doctor who practised at Rome's most prestigious hospital, Santo Spirito: 'To cure an aposteme and remove its poison, get a young hen that has never given birth to chickens; pluck it well to the tail, then press its sexual organ over the aposteme and leave it there until it dies. In this way the hen will draw out all the poison; the aposteme will dry up, and the patient will be liberated from the danger (of plague).'[3] The Sicilian doctor trained at Padua who became the head of Palermo's health board and medical service of the kingdom of Sicily (*Protomedico del Regno*),[4] Giovanni Filippo Ingrassia, recommended the same but with a capon, cock, or hen, adding that the hen was least desirable.[5] A Milanese doctor, Archileo Carcano, modified the procedure calling for the bird's anus, instead of its sexual organ, to be plucked and pressed against the bubo.[6] Not until the beginning of the seventeenth century did doctors invent (or at least recommend with academic authority) the cheapest and most readily available tonic for the poor in plague time—the drinking of human urine.[7] After these lists of purgatives and other pharmacological recommendations, surgical procedures might follow. However, as discussed above, such interventions as phlebotomy that had dominated plague tracts of the late fourteenth and fifteenth centuries had by the sixteenth century become rare.

---

[2] See for instance, Arellani, *Trattato di peste*, 91: 'Prendino due vipere il mese di Maggio, alle quali toltone via le teste, le code, la grassa, e le interiora; si riempirono di buona theriaca, d'aglio pesto, di cepolla rossa forte, e contusa, di zafrano, pepe, garifoli, canella, zenzare . . . .' He then details how to cook the ingredients.

[3] Pisanelli, *Discorso*, 118. Later, another Bolognese doctor, Rivetti, recommended the same treatment (*Trattato sopra il mal delle pettechie, peste è gianduissa*, 48).

[4] King Martin introduced this position for Sicily in 1397; however, it was usually not entrusted to a doctor. See Nutton, 'Continuity or Rediscovery?', 32 and 45; and Pitrè, *Medici, barbieri e speziali*, 40 and 162. By contrast, Palmer, 'Physicians and the State', 57–8, maintains that the post was originally held by the royal physician. In the sixteenth century the office of state physician spread to other parts of Italy. Also, see Gentilcore, ' "All that Pertains to Medicine" '.

[5] Ingrassia, *Informatione*, 154.   [6] Carcano, *Trattato di peste*, 12r.

[7] Settala, *De peste*; Panseri, 'La nascita della polizia medica', 168. At the time of the plague of 1630, Settala was considered among the best medical doctors in Italy; see La Cava, *La peste di S. Carlo*, 43, 52, and 164. This 'drug', however, was not novel with Settala. See Chapter 4 for the therapies being sold by the Flemish merchant at the height of Venice's plague in the summer of 1576.

These sixteenth-century medical writings, even ones in the vernacular and intended for a wide lay readership, were often supported by copious references to Scripture, Thucydides, Hippocrates, Avicenna, Averröes, Cornelius Celsus (called the Latin Hippocrates) and even Homer as well as to more modern authorities such as the fifteenth-century Florentine humanist Marsilio Ficino, and their own contemporaries of the sixteenth-century. Before 1575 these tracts rarely hinted at prevention or remedies beyond the frame of the individual patient's bedside. Despite governmental efforts to control plague since the Black Death with ordinances such as those of Pistoia published in 1348 and increasingly with the formation of permanent health boards in various cities of Italy from the mid-fifteenth century on, physicians, at least in their tracts, largely ignored the social and political ramifications of plague.[8] The closest they came to community-wide advice was to cite Hippocratic legend via Galen when a fifth-century BC epidemic from Ethiopia threatened Greece.[9] Heroically, Hippocrates supposedly successfully intervened ordering the burning of massive community-wide fires of scented woods to 'mutate the air'.[10] Even though doctors had served on health boards at Venice and Milan since the mid-fifteenth century, had gathered evidence on plague mortalities, and had diagnosed plague victims in new city-wide death books, their tracts across Europe offered little if any advice on community action or public health before 1575.[11]

GIOVANNI FILIPPO INGRASSIA AND THE SICILIAN PLAGUE OF 1575

To judge from their published treatises, the crisis of 1575 fundamentally altered doctors' approach to and thinking about plagues from the individual patient to the community. The first of these works was Giovanni Filippo Ingrassia's *Informatione del pestifero, et contagioso morbo*. Published in 1576 it clearly began (as his dated reports within this treatise indicate) the moment plague threatened Sicily from North Africa and spread to Messina and towns south of Palermo early

---

[8] On the literature on health boards, see Chapter 6. To date, no one has plotted the pace or geography of the formation of permanent health boards. The period from 1575 to 1578 may have proved an important stimulus, with the formation of health boards in Palermo and Florence for instance (where this plague never hit).

[9] Instead, the disease may in fact have come from the north of Athens; the Ethiopian origins of this plague became a part of the Hippocratic legend later on; see Pinault, *Hippocratic Lives and Legends*, 37.

[10] See for instance Boccalini, *De causis pestilentiae urbem Venetam*, 8 and Arellani, *Trattato di peste*, 46 and 52. No such actions or recommendations appear in the works of Hippocrates; instead the legend evolved sometime between 366 BC and the first century BC and came to late medieval doctors through the works of Galen, Aëtius, and Oribasius; see Pinault, *Hippocratic Lives and Legends*, ch. 2.

[11] See Chapter 8.

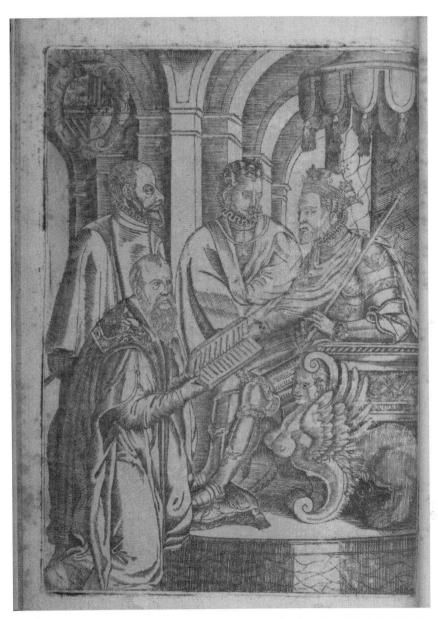

Illustration 1. Giovanni Filippo Ingrassia presenting his book to King Philip II of Spain.

in 1575, finally, striking Palermo at the beginning of June 1575. Two departures from previous plague writing distinguish this work: (1) it was chronological in structure and relied on weekly health board reports of mortality and the spread of plague (which in fact Ingrassia had initiated); (2) it addressed the state for community-wide action.

Unlike the new forms of plague writing that sprung up almost simultaneously in northern cities, often called *Successo della peste* (to be explored in Chapter 4), Ingrassia's *Informatione* was that of a physician who dealt with theoretical problems such as definitions of plague and encased his work in abundant citations to ancient and contemporary authorities. From his introduction, the reader might anticipate the usual physician's plague tract of the sixteenth century. After defining the essential cause of plague as God's wrath against human sin and beginning 'with the honour and glory of God', its early chapters distinguished 'true plague' from other pestilential fevers, then turned to causes, followed by symptoms of plague ('i segni pathognomonici').[12] Later chapters, while original, also did not break the mould significantly, although it recommended the first 'medical regimens' intended for the health officials ('reggitori & Ufficiali') who ran the risks of becoming infected. This discussion, however, followed lines of previous plague tracts with considerations of diet, behaviour, and numerous recipes and preventative measures to protect the individual. Other chapters prescribed curative measures, again from the individual patient's perspective—various purgatives, plasters, diets, medications, and surgery.

However, the bulk of Ingrassia's 566 pages broke new ground: it described the administration of the sick ('governo e reggimento') 'for preserving the city' recommending rules and decrees the duke and the city's health board should follow to extinguish plague ('ammorzare il pestifero'). He discussed the organization of the seven hospitals of Palermo and the construction of a new lazaretto, along with two new hospitals for convalescents. These books made recommendations to King Philip II (to whom his first plague tract of 1576 was dedicated) and to his lieutenant in Sicily, the duke of Terranova, to mobilize resources and enact laws to combat the plague's spread in Palermo and through Sicily. His recommendations include decrees and designs for building hospitals, enactments of general quarantines, sequestering the infected and suspected, cleaning streets and disinfecting houses, regulations for butchers, killing of domestic pets and animals such as hens and roosters suspected as carriers, severe punishments with theatrical executions to deter the theft of infected goods, and more.[13]

---

[12] Ingrassia, *Informatione*, 3–4.

[13] Such punishments can be seen in the early plague statutes of Palermo promulgated in 1575, inspired, if not enacted, by Ingrassia; see *Bando et ordinationi per . . . città di Palermo*. They begin with those who have entered the city without an authorized *bollettino*. Such violators were to be tortured with four pulls with the cord, payment of fines, and imprisonment in the royal prison for seven years. If the violator was a commoner, poor, or a woman, the penalty was four pulls and mandatory service in Palermo's plague

The attention to the detail of hospitals is at a level unmatched in previous medical tracts and later ones at least until the seventeenth century or even later. Ingrassia discussed his ideas and medical debates over the choice of possible sites of the hospitals, reported popular protest coming from the neighbourhoods where the new pesthouses were planned, the duke's intervention and change of mind, the reasons for different plague hospitals, the adaptation and conversion of older monasteries and the lepers' hospital into new hospitals, reasons for placing the newly constructed plague hospitals at least a half-mile beyond city walls, details of the main plague hospital, Cubba, with drawings of its thirty-four sections divided into rooms for infected women and men and others for convalescents, divided by sex; the dimensions of each; the positioning of windows; number of beds per room; maximum numbers per bed for men, women, and children; the capacity of each room; the building of chapels; the place and procedures for baptizing offspring of the infected and for performing the sacraments; the charitable roles of various religious orders in the hospitals; election of hospital rectors; the place, dimensions, and importance of gardens; why the lazaretto should point north; and ten conditions for deciding who should be taken from locked houses (*barreggiati*) to the new plague hospital.[14] Later, Ingrassia tallied the public expenditures for these new institutions with financial details for new clothing of inmates and other necessities, building costs, and charity.[15]

In addition, Book Two discusses the reasons for a separate convalescent hospital within the city walls to be built in the Borgo di Santa Lucia. Given the prejudices of the populace, Ingrassia argued, if those who had recently recovered were immediately sent back to their working-class districts, they would be isolated and die of starvation. He detailed the expenditures for this convalescent hospital, for good beds with well-stitched covers and regular meals 'with good chicken, or at least *buona carne di genco*, veal in abundance, and good bread'.[16] He then turned to the administration of the locked houses of the plague infected and suspected, the declaration of martial law in Palermo ('di poter procedere assolutamente a modo di guerra') with four podestà to be appointed by the duke to enforce new decrees, use of soldiers to guard the locked houses, the number of plague deputies and their various tasks, the recruitment of midwives (*donne levatrici*) and barbers to serve the *barreggiate*, punishments for those violating the decrees of the locked houses—torture, whippings, and the death penalty. Separate chapters dealt with quarantine, the purification and burning of goods found in the locked houses, purification and quarantine of horses and other animals found there, various means for washing and airing goods thought to

---

hospital for four months (2r). Those who escaped from a sequestered house (*casa barregiata*) faced the death penalty (3r). Women of any age or condition were not permitted to spend the night outside their homes. The rich were fined; the poor publicly flogged (7v).

[14] Ingrassia, *Informatione*, 138–54.   [15] Ibid., 235.   [16] Ibid., 230.

spread the contagion—dirty wool, furs, and leather—recipes for various soaps, expenditures to be solicited from the duke, keeping of registers of the interned in the locked houses to include names, ages, sex, and descriptions of all their pestilential signs.

Ingrassia used these records, which he initiated, to argue for or against various policy proposals for combating the disease. For instance, many thought that its spread in Palermo depended on the city's design—its numerous neighbourhoods comprised of small courtyards and aggregations of small houses (*casuzze*), in which all residents entered through the same gate and shared a communal well and common sink or sewer (*pila*), what in Naples were called *fondachi*. These co-residents, they argued, interacted closely with one another, thereby 'amplifying' the contagion. To lessen the spread of plague, certain deputies proposed banishing these inhabitants from the city. Ingrassia's first argument against them was the expense and complex logistics such a move would require; such compounds were in great abundance within this city of 'no less than 100,000'. Then, turning to the new plague records, he argued that in only one of a hundred such compounds did the disease spread from one house to infect the rest and concluded: 'Neither via the well, nor the cats, nor the mice [*topi*[17]] nor the chickens did the disease spread to the neighbours.'[18] With these records, he also initially refuted claims seen in other urban places that the disease was spread by women and children, and argued against their forced removal from the city.[19]

Despite the heavy reliance on classical sources and citations, Ingrassia's plague book created from the start a new structure and approach. Intermeshed within detailed descriptions of historical plagues from Thucydides, Hippocrates, Livy, Galen, and others to the sixteenth century, Ingrassia's structure is narrative, charting the plague's progress in Palermo, its possible origins and first infections within the city, its mounting mortality figures, changes in thinking on what the disease may have been, debates and administrative action on public health, and reactions to the imposed governmental measures. Beneath a traditional structure of topics outlined in his introduction, the reader finds a chronological arrangement dated precisely to the day at three points when Ingrassia sent his reports to the king's lieutenant in Sicily, the duke of Terranova.

The first section ends on 18 June, two weeks after cases had been discovered in Palermo. At that point, Ingrassia's text centred on heated debates among the city's physicians on whether their disease, 'morbo contagioso', was 'true plague' and what to do about the grand hospital of Palermo—the 'confusion' arising from mixing newly afflicted cases with other hospitalized patients. As with

---

[17] *Topi* could mean mice or rats.   [18] Ibid., 228.

[19] Ibid., 240. Unfortunately, Ingrassia does not show the numbers and, as far as I can ascertain, these records do not survive; see Aymard, 'Epidémies et médecins en Sicile'. For places where women predominated as victims, see Bennassar, *Recherches sur les grandes épidémies*, 49; Alfani and Cohn, 'Nonantola 1630', 108–10; Calvi, 'L'oro, il fuoco, le forche', 433; and Morea, *Storia della peste di Noja*, 219.

the reactions of some academically-trained physicians that arose a year later in northern Italian towns, Ingrassia vigorously argued that the disease was not 'true plague' and was hardly contagious. It was not transmitted, he claimed, through merchandise, clothing, or to doctors who took the pulse of the afflicted. Only those who cared closely ('strettamente servivano') for the ill, 'embracing them, taking in their breath', were at risk. His criteria derived from Fracastoro, not antiquity, and the disease did not meet his three modes of contagion characteristic of pestilential fevers. Nor did it supposedly meet an older elementary rule of contagion, infection clustering within households.[20] For these reasons, he refused to support the inconvenience and inhumanity of locking families in their homes (*barreggiare*).[21] Yet he saw the disease spreading at the same time in Messina differently because there it was amassing greater casualties and appeared to be contagious: 'many had died in the same household in a short period', eleven dying in the same household within a week.

Ingrassia then turned to the controversies over the origins of the plague in Palermo. He brushed aside rumours that a cursed galley ('maladetta Galeotta') arriving at Messina from the Barbary Coast disembarking at Palermo and other ports was the contagion's secret carrier.[22] Another popular rumour (according to Ingrassia, one of madness) saw the plague's first victim as a Maltese prostitute working in Palermo. He argued that her signs 'clearly' matched those of malign pestilential fever but not 'true plague'. Small bumps (*petecchie*) had spread over her body, and she had died on the fifth day of illness.[23]

In Galenic fashion, Ingrassia instead turned to atmospheric conditions and to astrological signs of the previous year, heavy rains of the winter months that had caused flooding and had led to an epidemic of small pox (*varole*) that killed many children that winter, the over-fishing of tuna in the Bay of Palermo and the bloody sea that ensued from the fish slaughter, the city's filth and in particular the rotting animal corpses from butchers' shops. These had led to the putrefaction of the air, causing the present disease. According to Ingrassia, neither a foreign agent nor a carrier had been responsible.

By the beginning of the month, Ingrassia and his colleagues, however, began to change their tone. Cases began to mount in the artisan neighbourhood of Seralcadio, called Celuaccari. During June, Ingrassia had known the symptoms of those dying from the disease only by rumour, since the stricken were either 'lower class' artisans or peasants who had come from Palazzo Adriano or Sciacca. In July, he began examining the afflicted himself and described their malign fevers as accompanied by the 'cruellest symptoms': 'beyond the buboes and the spots (*petecchie*), the victims died suddenly, in two, three, or four days'. The disease in his city was certainly more serious than he had initially thought in June and as a result changed his mind, upgrading the disease's nomenclature to the 'son of plague', as 'God's declaration of war against our sins'.

[20] Ingrassia, *Informatione*, 32.   [21] Ibid., 33.   [22] Ibid., 25.   [23] Ibid., 30.

Nonetheless, he continued to raise doubts that the disease was 'true plague', arguing that it shared symptoms with many other ailments and was not terribly contagious. Seemingly, it was not capable of spreading from the working-class quarter of its origins across the city. In contrast to Palazzo Adriano, Sciacca, and Messina, where the disease had been spreading by *fomites* (using Fracastoro's categories), that is, by clothing and other merchandise, it was not spreading by these means in Palermo. However, as the month progressed and death rates rose, Ingrassia changed his mind again: now the sale of infected rugs, leather, and other animal skins from the infected three towns above 'fed' the disease in Palermo. Although he still refrained from calling it 'true plague', because it lacked in his opinion the one cardinal characteristic—'contagion at a distance' (again relying on Fracastoro)—he nevertheless speculated that it was spreading because of the air, first the climatic disturbance of the past winter and secondly the putrid smells arising from the city, enhanced by the butchers' failure to clean their streets of animal carcasses. 'As a remedy', Ingrassia proposed to the city's governors regular street cleaning, at least two or three times a week, removing all things causing stench and not just throwing thin layers of straw over them (as must have been the previous method).[24] He charged that the city was littered with dead animals, especially cats and dogs, and that their carcasses should not just be swept from one street to the next but should be thrown into the sea or, better, buried appropriately. He also raised suspicions about warehouses where tuna was salted, from which 'a gigantic stench' gushed. On his recommendations, a commission of two gentlemen 'with good eyes and noses' was appointed to search the streets for sources of stench, not only in Palermo but in its suburbs three to four miles beyond the city gates. Others from the College of Physicians were also asked to follow their noses. They found that the two most troubled, smelly parts of the city were the new and old squares of butchers' shops.

In addition, Ingrassia criticized the state of Palermo's public latrines, which emptied into the bay and which he alleged had not been cleaned for the last two months. Stagnant ponds had turned green, and a ship filled with human excrement sat in the bay.[25] He recommended that the city's lords establish guards to patrol the city against increasing pollution, that the spread of the disease could increase by transmission—*fomite* and even *ad distans*—thereby becoming 'true plague' if the status quo continued. Finally, Ingrassia's recommendations went beyond sanitary patrol to the amelioration of social conditions: he advised rulers to help the poor—the chief victims of the disease. Their hardship, he claimed, fuelled the spread of the disease. He advised extended charity and cheap loans, and the suspension of sales taxes (*gabelles*) imposed on the poor. In their place, the rich and 'doctors ourselves' should pay extra taxes (*collete*).

With rising death tolls 'first from two or three in the city to the tens and now hundreds', he now contradicted his earlier judgement and proposed strict

---

[24] Ingrassia, 43.   [25] Ibid., 43–4.

separation of infected persons and goods from the healthy, especially within the city's grand hospital, where infected peasants arrived causing 'great confusion'. He proposed clearing the infected from this hospital and building a new one for them, 'what in Italy is called Lazaretto'.[26] In the meantime, those showing 'the pustules' or buboes would be attended in a room of the Monastery of San Giacomo. He submitted his appeal backed by the College of Physicians to the Spanish administrators, soliciting funds from the duke and crown to build new hospitals for the infected. As we have seen, his entire second book was dedicated to their planning and financing.

Ingrassia's actions and thinking about plague continued to develop within his tract as the disease progressed. No previous plague writing by a physician or anyone else had shown such attention to the chronology of a plague or an author's intense intellectual wrestling with it, recording changes of mind as the disease unfolded. To discover the origins and nature of the disease, he proposed that two trusted men—a nobleman and a physician from the College of Physicians—be sent to Palazzo Adriano to investigate why the disease there was killing as many as in Palermo (ten to twelve a day) in a town less than a twentieth Palermo's size. As the month progressed and victims mounted, Ingrassia changed his mind also about other aspects of the disease. Against his initial chiding of the populace's vulgar beliefs, he now began to take their lead: the disease, after all, may have entered from 'foreign contagion', and not just from the skies. 'As a major caution' he advised city officials to patrol their gates and separate the sick from the healthy. Yet he still questioned whether the disease was 'true plague' or indeed had been imported from outside, since it remained confined to the poor in the neighbourhood of Celuaccari and may have arisen from that locale's smells and corrupt air. Moreover, he continued to believe astrologers' reports of planetary conjunctions and signs that had appeared in March. Because of increasing mortality in Sciacca, however, he also speculated that it might have been carried to Palermo by winds and hence could be 'true plague'.

In July, he became more suspicious of the stench from the Bay of Palermo: the over-killing of tuna had turned the sea bloody red, adding putrid humidity to the air. Further, polluted streams and fountains washed all the waste (*bruttezze*) from butchers' and leather shops, along with 'all the trash (*sporchezze*)' from the city's cloth production into the bay. Reflecting on previous illnesses in Palermo, such as after flooding in 1557, he believed that diseases did not originate solely from the air but could arise from water spill-offs after flooding or heavy snows in the mountains. These contaminated wells and washed pollution from the ground and from gardens filled with excrement and could cause diseases to spread including the present *mal contagioso*.[27]

His next section from 18 July to 3 August reported the duke's authorization of Borgo called Santa Lucia outside the gate of San Giorgio as the place to

---

[26] Ibid., 49.   [27] Ibid., 63.

sequester the afflicted along with other plans to build new lazaretti. (The funds were received and, as far as I can establish, these new hospitals were built.) Based on Ingrassia's recommendations, further decrees were passed in Palermo and other cities and villages of the kingdom to kill all cats, dogs, and other household animals to control the spread of the disease. From the registers that he had earlier initiated, Ingrassia reported the numbers of those who had died from the disease—150 in the past twelve days, the same number felled during the first seven weeks from 1 June to 18 July.

From 3 August to 28 September the death tolls continued to rise at an increasing pace: 750 died over these 56 days, a rate of 13 a day. As troubling to Ingrassia, the deaths now were city-wide. A law was passed requiring anyone falling ill of the *mal contagioso*, with spots, black pustules, or buboes, to report immediately to the deputy of the neighbourhood. Against Ingrassia's thoughts in June, houses of the inflicted would now be boarded up ('barreggiata & sequestrata') and placed under guard with the infected sent to the lazaretto. Those violating the ban were sentenced to death. In addition, the disease had spread to neighbouring villages on Palermo's outskirts, Monreale and the Terra di Carini. He asked the rulers to authorize money for their assistance.

The next report to the duke, from 4 to 28 September, was more positive. Ingrassia described a religious procession of 6,000 men; women had been excluded to avoid scandal since it had been held at night. He succeeded in convincing the duke that another hospital for the purification of convalescents was needed, and funds were allocated for its construction in Borgo Sant' Anna, a place just within the city walls but containing few inhabitants. The reasons for it were more social than medical. Because of the 'cruelty and iniquity of the plebs', those who had recovered from the disease in the lazaretto were not welcomed back in their homes from fear of contagion. A second place was needed to feed and care for them without social exclusion and to prove their good health to their neighbours.

Ingrassia praised Palermo's officials in separating the afflicted from the healthy and especially their administration of the new plague hospital and the sequestrating of the contaminated belongings to a place that had been the duke of Bibona's garden. Already 140 had been cured in the lazaretto and had returned to the city with 250 still interned and another 200 cured, ready to leave. In the first days of November the disease declined, 'such that neither doctors nor servants in the hospital died as before', and the majority of patients were recovering. In 54 days from 28 September to 21 November, 900 had died from the disease, averaging 17 a day within the city, borgo, and the new lazaretto, Cubba, and the majority of these had died in October. Now hardly ten arrived at this hospital. On the feast of San Martino (10 November) not a single person died, and only two were admitted to the lazaretto.

From 21 November to New Year, Ingrassia's interwoven narrative of the disease's progress and the corresponding administrative developments to combat it became less clear and less optimistic than on Saint Martin's day. Although he does not count victims as he did for the first five months, the disease must have picked up momentum in late November and December with another thousand deaths (as can be calculated from Ingrassia's final tally in his dedication of the four books to Philip, king of Spain and Sicily). The now renamed *pestifero contagio* 'fed on and spread through the city and outside it' beyond the working-class quarters where previously it had been largely confined.[28] In addition, the city's social controls appear to have declined: gravediggers were stealing the clothing of plague victims and thereby spreading the disease.[29]

The final chapters of this book also allude to problems among the doctors of Palermo and their failure often to recognize the disease. Ingrassia sympathized: it resulted from their inexperience because an epidemic of this sort had not afflicted Palermo for a hundred years. To assist these doctors as well as the heads of neighbourhoods and the general public (who needed to recognize the disease for deciding whether a house should be locked),[30] Ingrassia's tract ends with the most extensive description of plague signs seen in any tract of the sixteenth century or before, a list of fifty-two characteristics, the last two of which were crucial in distinguishing pestilential fever or the more serious *morbo contagioso* from 'true plague'. Both concerned contagion: 'no. 51: when one catches the disease, all or most in the same house die quickly with some of these signs (seen in the previous fifty points) and especially these four—'cioé, bubboni anthraci, papole, & petecchie'. And 'no. 52' clearly indebted to Fracastoro: 'when it is passed from one house to another and from one person to another by contact, or through the infection of things [*fomite di robe*], and, worst of all, over distance'.[31]

The worst moment of this plague, at least for Ingrassia, came at the end of November, when 'the ignorant and ungracious plebs (*la sciocca & ingratissima plebe*)', whom he called 'the wicked and misfortunate masses (*lo sciagurato & mal avventurato volgo*)', accused him and his doctors on the health board of prolonging the disease to collect their salaries, filling their pockets and pilfering from the public purse. Ingrassia never specified who these 'ungracious plebs' were, but his plague tract launches into a long defence of his services 'to Omnipotent God, his master, the duke, and his country': from the beginning of the plague in June when he accepted the position of *Protomedico* and chief adviser to Palermo's health board, he allegedly had endangered his life in the service of the plague-stricken. What is more, by assuming the new post, he was forced to abandon his private practice, caring for the city's aristocracy, who were not infected with the disease. By forgoing his private practice, his earnings dipped well below what he now received from his public duties. Moreover, this public sacrifice had alienated his

---

[28] Ingrassia, 268.   [29] Ibid., 242.   [30] Ibid., 88.

[31] Ibid., 87–8. Earlier, doctors such as Fracastoro pointed to the exceptional contagion of 'true pestilence' and that its germs 'invade so very quickly' (*De contagione*, 112–13).

better-heeled patients, and Ingrassia feared a further loss of income once plague had passed. He found the commoners' slurs more injurious still because they questioned 'his honour as a philosopher, for whom avarice was a grievous sin'.

To quell the plebs' mumbling, he wrote a letter (copied into his tract) to the duke and the deputies on the health board stating his refusal to accept his salary any longer. The letter summarized his previous duties as the region's chief consultant on the disease, which included his advice to the health board, the periodic accounts he sent to the duke, and weekly visits to the city's principal lazaretto and the two convalescent hospitals. In addition, he 'made frequent rounds throughout the city' ('per la Città facendo la ronda & in ogni luogo tante volte'). After refusing his salary, Ingrassia insisted on continuing his fight against the *morbo contigioso*, even if some of his previous tasks no longer continued. He no longer made (or at least did not include them in his plague tract), for instance, his periodic accounts (*ragguagli*) on the state of the city's health.

Not only did the plague continue through the winter but it was still lingering on when Ingrassia finished his first tract in April 1576. The dedication to the king signed that month, however, returned to a note of optimism and praise of his city, its administration and medical corps. Unlike the smaller agro-towns of Sciacca and Palazzo Adriano and the city of Messina, Palermo had averted the worst. Of a population of over 100,000, Ingrassia boasted, only 3,100 had perished. He saw this as vindicating his policies of sequestration and *barreggiatura*, building new plague hospitals, and enacting social policies that extended charity and tax relief to the poor. It was a victory of medicine, administration, governance, social control, and religion from charitable assistance to prayer, processions, and fasts.

Heavily indebted to Galen and other antique authorities as his copious citations reveal, Ingrassia's plague tract went beyond them in placing the particular modes of contagion as the central premise for diagnosing plague. Here he was indebted to Fracastoro's seminal work of 1546. But like other physicians in 1575–8, Ingrassia also went beyond Fracastoro in his approach and remedies for fighting plague and other epidemic diseases. Ingrassia and his generation now addressed public health issues and social policies, making specific recommendations to the prince as opposed to prescribing drugs and other remedies for the individual patient alone. Furthermore, his tract is remarkable not only in exposing a range of issues, especially in public health never before addressed at length in any plague or medical treatise, but it revolutionized the genre of medical writing, structuring the plague tract as a narrative of unfolding events, ideas, and attitudes about the plague, including those of the author. The tract's narrative in fact is more a story of Ingrassia' changes of mood and opinion, of experimentation and learning as the disease progressed than it is a didactic treatise on medical procedures.

***

Certainly, it is not difficult to find plague tracts of the fourteenth to the sixteenth century that had been sparked by a particular plague in a physician's town or locality or one that threatened from outside. Usually, however, in the tract's dedication or prologue, before the medical aspects of the tract itself commenced, the physician signalled only briefly that a plague had recently struck. For example, a late fourteenth-century tract by Doctor Stephen from Padua informed the reader that plague had hit Padua, leaving the doctor and his wife deadly ill, but nothing more, not even the date of that plague or the other regions it struck.[32] Instead, the tract delved immediately into recipes and cures, revealing nothing about the plague's arrival and transmission or the development of the author's ideas as the plague progressed. The prologues and dedications to plague tracts of the sixteenth century, perhaps because of printing, became longer than manuscript ones of the later Middle Ages, but before 1575 little more was revealed in these tracts about the plague that had prompted the physician to draft his treatise. Physicians and others revealed plague secrets on diet, preservation, and remedies, but rarely even indicated the origins of a plague other than configurations of planets, distant earthquakes, or perhaps the weather. Observations, government reports, and rumours noting human transmission from one town to another, the mobilization of troops, or the transport of specific items of merchandise were apparently not seen as pertinent to the physician's practice. These doctors made no attempt to discuss or trace the disease from outsiders to particular neighbourhoods or from one section of a city to another; nor did any see the plague tract as a space to detail the plague's progress with city-wide death counts, admissions to plague hospitals, rates of recovery, or administrative actions as plague tolls mounted.

By the sixteenth century and especially with the plague of 1555 and 1556 in Padua and Venice, these introductions to present calamities became more extensive, but despite titles such as *De Pestilentia Patavina anno 1555* by the Paduan professor Lodovico Pasini,[33] these tracts continued to portray their present plague predicaments only within short prologues and not within the bodies of their texts, which instead centred on general questions of causation, types of fevers, various forms of contagion, and preventative measures and cures for the individual. Pasini's tract may have had an unusual section comparing the venom of plague with the snakebite,[34] but on the specific details of the plague in Padua in 1555—which towns it struck, its possible avenues of entry to Padua, the mounting of casualties by month, week, or even the day—his tract narrated little: we learn only that it started in June and lasted to September and its first case was one with a tumour in the throat.[35] A tract entitled *Il Consiglio sopra la peste di Vinetia l'anno 1556* by the Paduan professor Bernardino Tomitano

---

[32] 'Ein Paduaner Pestkonsilium', 355–7.

[33] He was born in 1500 and died in 1557. According to Edit 16, he published only this work, located presently in only four libraries in Italy.

[34] Pasini, *De pestilentia Patavina anno 1555*, 8r.   [35] Ibid., 3r and 4v.

supplied even less; instead of dates and places of the plague's spread, it jumped immediately to speculation about plagues' remote causes.[36]

Unusually, the beginning of the plague tract of the Venetian physician Niccolò Massa published in 1556 gives the context for writing. The Venetian government had called him and others of the city's College of Physicians to diagnose whether the current contagion was plague. He tells us that at the time he was home, ill from being overworked by attending so many of his aristocratic patients (though none had been afflicted with plague).[37] With copious references to Galen, Hippocrates, Plato, Philo, Homer, and others, the learned Niccolò then expounded on pestilential airs, symptoms, plague signs and their bodily positions, humours, and contagion. He speculated about bad fish and food poisoning as causes of plagues in general, entered debates on whether all animals were susceptible to plague, and whether a disease confined to the poor could be plague. He ended with personal recipes and remedies, but gives little hint about the then current plague of 1555–6 and nothing on its progression or his own intellectual or emotional development during the disease's turbulent months (although comparison with his earlier tract written before 1540 shows that somewhere along the way his thoughts about plague, its causes and cures had changed).

The preface to a tract by an Augustine friar and doctor in Naples published in 1556 informs us that plague was present in this 'illustrious' city', that he had been afflicted with the disease but had recovered, that others among the city's nobility had been infected as well as noble friends in Rome and other places in Italy, and that he had been elected by the governors of the city ('dalli magiori') as head of the hospital to care for those afflicted by the present disease. Yet here the friar was clearly not talking about 1556 but instead repeating his thoughts of 1527 when he was first elected as hospital head, although no dates are supplied in either edition.[38] After this preamble, moreover, as with others before 1575, he launched into definitions of plague, the preservation of the individual against it and secret recipes on cures. Other tracts, such as that of the Messer Giovanni da Vigo, Pope Julius II's personal physician also published at the end of this plague in 1556, do not even mention whether plague was present in their cities or threatening from nearby places.[39] The tract that investigated furthest the precise

---

36   Tomitano, *Il consiglio sopra la peste*. On Tomitano, see Palmer, 'The Control of Plague', 110–12, 115–16; Zitelli, 'Catalogo: le teorie mediche sulla peste', 59–60 and 118; Panseri, 'La nascita della polizia medica', 162–3; Laughran, 'The Body, Public Health and Social Control', 107–23; and Davi, *Bernardino Tomitano*, 40–6 (on his plague writing). Similarly, De Forte's *Il trattato de la peste* related only a few facts about the current plague: that it had first 'devoured the inhabitants of Capo d'Istria' and struck Venice in early July, and that Angelo, 'an investigator of nature and medicine', had practised and 'philosophized' for many years in Venice.

37   Massa, *Ragionamento*, 2v-3r.

38   Napolitano, *Opera et trattato che insegna* [1556], 4v. In 1527 he published a tract of the same title that differed slightly from the 1556 edition; yet here the details were mostly the same (1r).

39   Da Vigo, *Secreti mirabilissimi* (not in Edit 16).

local conditions, circumstances, and progression of a plague before 1575 was one in verse by the Piedmontese 'scholar in medicine' Christoforo Baravalle (Baravalo), *L'Historia della Peste di Padoa del'Anno MDLV*. From it we learn that the plague came to Padua from Venice, began in March, lasted six months, reached its peak in August, and that almost all Paduans fled the city. With the declaration of liberation from plague on 19 October, the city rejoiced with processions, games and feasts; but we are told little more; nothing comparable to the specific details of Ingrassia's 566-page narrative, on the course of the disease based on health board death counts, shifts in medical debate, government action, changing beliefs of doctors, the populace and the author himself.[40]

PHYSICIANS AND POLITICS

Before the appearance of Ingrassia's tract of 1576, doctors stuck mainly to their trade as philosophers and physicians. To be sure, it was a wide remit, including pondering philosophically on the universal causes of all diseases with attention to astrology and theology and reflecting on problems such as God's purpose as a mass killer of humanity, the innocents included. On occasion these doctors also could become briefly historians, listing previous plagues in history. Guy de Chauliac was the first I know of to use history to give a comparative context for his own plague experience. His historical survey and comparisons, however, were limited to part of one long sentence, naming four epidemics in world history, those of Thrace, the Philistines, one cited by Hippocrates, another by Galen, and a fifth in Rome at the time of Gregory IX (1229).[41] By the sixteenth century the historical canvas had enlarged, and, as Nancy Siraisi has shown, history became an important tool for medical science.[42] In addition to mining the Bible, Hippocrates, and Galen far more thoroughly than doctors had done in the later Middle Ages, they also tapped Homer, Aristotle, Plato, Thucydides, Livy, as well as modern writers, such as Boccaccio and Matteo Villani.[43] In 1576, one tract was completely dedicated to the historical chronology of plagues, tracing them in Italy for a purported 2,309 years, back to 735 BC, the time of Rome's first king Romulus, in an attempt to investigate the relationship between plague and astrological and climatic forewarnings.[44]

Furthermore, I know of no doctors' tracts before 1575 to engage at any length with the governmental side of prevention, advising on the mechanisms and management of quarantine, sequestrating, locking houses, constructing new

[40] Baravalle, *L'historia della peste di Padoa*, 509r–19v (BAV).
[41] Guy de Chauliac, *Inventarium sive chirurgia magna*, I, 118.
[42] Siraisi, *History, Medicine, and the Traditions*.
[43] For the Black Death, Boccaccio leads the list of cited authorities, followed by Guy de Chauliac, then the chronicler Matteo Villani. For the sixteenth-century authorities, Fracastoro was the most often cited.
[44] Tranquilli, *Pestilenze che sono state in Italia*.

plague hospitals and homes for convalescents. Before Ingrassia's tracts, none addressed public finances, the needs of the poor, or the means for provisioning for them as a part of a disease's remedies. Although doctors had served on health boards and as *Protomedici* of city-states, regional territories and kingdoms as early as the fifteenth century, their preventive and curative measures presented in thousands of plague tracts dating back to the Black Death had not extended much beyond patients' bedsides. They refrained from addressing questions of law, community control, charity, and, most importantly, public health. With Ingrassia's treatise the doctor's intellectual remit suddenly widened, his focus changing as the genre itself was transformed; now politics were central. With the plague's simultaneous assault on the north, the same intellectual change in social, political, and medical thought was happening but on a larger scale and over a wider social and professional horizon. We now turn to these genre shifts in plague writing.

4

The Successo della Peste

To claim that plague narrative or that the analysis of plague according to a chronological development was new with the crisis of 1575–8 may appear exaggerated. Despite its brevity, the first half of the introduction to Day One in Giovanni Boccaccio's *Decameron* set the historical context for the following hundred stories and ranks alongside Thucydides' description of the plague of Athens as among the most influential of any historical or imaginary account of a disease.[1] Sixteenth-century Italian doctors, in fact, cited Boccaccio more than any physician for evidence on the Black Death of 1348. Moreover, on the Black Death they relied on another non-physician, the Florentine chronicler Matteo Villani. Neither source, however, plotted statistically or dramatically the sequence of events during plague, the mounting of plague deaths or concomitant changes in legislation, ideas, and attitudes, health care policies, figures on what was spent, and other interventions and innovations, including those of the Church, its public prayers, processions, and its secular health measures. In Boccaccio's memorable account, the plague in Florence lasted from April to July. Within that time, he describes the swellings, called *gavòccioli* in Tuscan, that formed in armpits and the groin and dark blotches that spread over the multitude of corpses; the abrupt end to customary mourning and burial practices; the crassness of gravediggers; the lamentable abandonment or absence of care for the ill; the emotional divide between those who suddenly became more pious, and the majority who took to drink and debauchery as a better way to ward off plague; the fear of venturing outdoors; the story of two pigs tossing the infected rags of a pauper and dying suddenly; the failure of medicine; and a total number of deaths of 100,000 (which may have been taken from statistics collected by the archbishop that pertained to the diocese and not the city proper as historians have thought).[2] Yet Boccaccio treats this four-month carnage as roughly a single incident in time, without chronological development. Much the same can be said of Matteo

---

[1] Lorenzo Valla's translation of Thucydides' histories into Latin, commissioned by Pope Nicholas V between 1448 and 1452, brought the plague of Athens to scholarly attention, but its wider dissemination resulted first with the Aldine edition in Greek in 1502, then with an Italian translation in 1545. On the long historical importance of Thucydides' description of the Plague of Athens, see Nutton, 'Introduction', 1.

[2] Boccaccio, *Decameron*, 10–19. For Thucydides' plague account as non-narrative 'protohistory', see Gordon, 'The City and the Plague', 68.

Villani's contemporaneous account, even though he traces the plague's origins to heathen sin in India and China. But once the plague arrived in Florence, he says little about its development, either epidemiologically or in human reactions, except that Florentines initially helped one another and many were cured, but as mortalities mounted they adopted the 'the cruel inhumanity' of the heathen: mothers abandoned their babies, husbands their wives, and so forth.[3]

Nor do we find much temporal detail or development with other chroniclers. English ones such as Geoffrey le Baker speculated on the plague's entry into British shores, but once arrived, a narrative progression of events all but ended.[4] The only chronological detail of a plague year from the Middle Ages that I know is Gilles le Muisit's second chronicle, devoted almost exclusively to the year 1349.[5] This account portrays competition among various penitent groups for ritual space within Tournai over the year but hardly mentions the plague or relates this religious and emotional history to the disease.[6] We are told nothing about its epidemiological progression, the trajectory of deaths, the reactions and decrees city officials passed, the attitudes and debates among doctors and others as plague deaths climbed or declined; nothing approaching detailed reports of plague spread, governmental policies, debates, or ideological or psychological developments of the author himself. We do not even know from Gilles's account when the disease ceased in Tournai.

In the sixteenth century to the plague of 1575–8 other individually published descriptions of plagues were extremely rare.[7] Most notable of these was Niccolò Machiavelli's *Descrizione della Peste di Firenze dell'anno 1527*, one of his lesser-known essays.[8] Written in the last year of his life, Machiavelli's narrative opens with him roaming the abandoned streets of Florence, once 'clean and beautiful, full of rich and noble citizens', now 'emptied, smelly and ugly'.[9] He crosses the Ponte di Santa Trinita, where he nearly stumbles over a plague corpse and then, in the church of Santa Trinita, chances upon a beautiful widow who has just lost her husband to plague. He dwells on her beauty and contrasts it with the stench and wretchedness of Florence's present condition. He fears, however, that she could be harbouring the plague. Overcoming these fears he converses with her and (in his

---

[3] Villani, *Cronica*, I, 9–17. See Carmichael, 'Universal and Particular', on chronicle descriptions of the Black Death: 'Plague narratives conflated the events of three years' duration into one great mortality report, just as Agnolo [di Tura of Siena] here could no longer even distinguish between the days of a long brutal summer' (40).

[4] On le Baker's and other English accounts of the plague's arrival in England, see Cohn, *The Black Death Transformed*, 102.

[5] *Chronique et annales de Gilles le Muisit*.

[6] Technically Gilles cannot be considered an eyewitness to these events since he was blind during the plague years; see Guenée, *Between Church and State*, 76.

[7] The most notable exception is Baravalle's history in verse, *L'historia della peste di Padoa*, discussed in the previous chapter.

[8] Machiavelli, *Opere*, V, 34–50, which since 1831 has not been included among his collected works. As a legitimate part of Machiavelli's oeuvre, see Radicchi, 'Descrizione della peste di Firenze'.

[9] Machiavelli, *Opere*, 35.

fantasies) marries her. This description, however, pertains to one day alone, May Day, and gives no sense of the plague's progression, even whether this moment was near the plague's origins, its crest, or end.[10] With the plague of 1575–8 a new genre of plague reporting came into being, penned principally in the north.

THE GEOGRAPHIC DISTRIBUTION
OF PLAGUE TRACTS, 1575–8

As far as the published records go, Ingrassia's was the only report to detail the progression of a plague in Sicily or even for the south of Italy during the sixteenth century. The 1575–8 plague in the north, however, sparked almost simultaneously a new trend in plague writing that followed lines similar to Ingrassia's (although clearly not influenced by him). Even more decisively than Ingrassia's, the northern writings broke with previous academic plague discourse going back to the Black Death. Moreover, the explosion of plague writing in general in 1575–8 took place overwhelmingly in northern Italian cities: 148 of them, or fully three-quarters, were penned by authors experiencing plague and drafting their tracts north of Tuscany; less than 8 per cent were written south of Rome.

My calculation of these places of plague writing does not rely on place of publication but where the authors practised or wrote at the time of the plague. Doctors and other authors often were published outside their own localities of practice, and not only when they resided in small towns such as Camaiore and Massa Lombarda, which were without presses.[11] Even those from metropolitan centres of printing might publish their works elsewhere, as was the case with the Augustinian Giovanni Battista Napolitano, whose various editions of *A treatise teaching the most worthy secrets against the plague* were all published outside his home town: two in Venice, the others in Pesaro, Brescia, and Turin. Neither Giovanni Battista nor others discussed the reasons for choosing a particular press (or vice versa). Even those experiencing plague in the most prominent centre of printing in sixteenth-century Europe—Venice—might publish elsewhere, as did

---

[10] Carretto's unpublished *De pestilentia cohorta Agrigenti* is another exception. However, it relates little about the plague's avenues of entry or chronology of transmission. We learn only that the plague reached Agrigento in May and that its death toll mounted in June from ten to sixty a day, reaching its peak sometime in July with a hundred deaths. But this is a short paragraph with no corresponding narrative of changes in plague ordinances, the psychology of the city, or that of the author. Instead, claims of wickedness, adultery, incest, and fear encapsulate the whole of this plague experience without chronological development.

[11] Giudici, *Il trattato della peste*; Sorboli, *Discorso del vero modo di preseruare*. According to Edit 16, neither Camaiore nor Massa Lombarda had presses in the sixteenth century. On the other hand, Genoa had 15, Palermo, 36, Naples, 128, Florence, 137, Milan, 192, Rome, 234, and Venice, 1,018. Other plague publications, such as Daciano, *Trattato della peste*, cannot be pinned to places from their titles alone, but the text makes them clear. Daciano was *Medico fiscio stipendiato* of Udine and his tract was dedicated to the town's city council. Its letter of dedication reviews the history of the city's most recent epidemics—plague in 1556, and *delle Petecchie* in 1560 and 1572.

Table 4.1   Origins of Plague Tracts, 1575–8[1]

Northern	Central	Southern
Alessandria 1	Bagnoregio 1	Naples 8
Bologna 8	Camaiore 1	Palermo 5
Brescia 4	Chieti 1	Salerno 1
Correggio 1	Fermo 1	
Cremona 1	Florence 8	
Ferrara 1	Lanciano 1	
Forlì 1	Lucca 2	
Genoa 3	Macerata 3	
Mantua 3	Perugia 2	
Massa Lombarda 1	Rimini 1	
Milan 33	Rome 16 (Papal 9)	
Padua 7	Siena 1	
Pavia 1	Pieve Santo Stefano 1	
Piacenza 1		
Turin 1		
Treviso 1		
Udine 1		
Venice 45		
Verona 32		
Vicenza 2		
Total 148	39	14

[1] I have not included the broadsheets. I have, however, added a few, such as Tranzi's tract that was stimulated by and pertained to the plague of 1575–8 but not published until a decade later. I have used the present-day divisions of northern, central, and southern Italy as defined by the Touring Club Italiano.

the Venetian notary Rocco Benedetti, whose *Raguaglio minutissimo del successo della peste di Venetia* was published at Tivoli in 1577.

The northern predominance might be seen as more pronounced than the table above suggests: litanies, prayers, supplications, and ordinances of the papacy pertained to the whole of Italy and not just Rome, as I have labelled them. In addition, several collections of verse in 1575–8 contain the works of a number of authors, several with over a hundred stanzas. I have counted these (all found in the north) by the collection and not by the individual poem or author.[12] Nonetheless, despite this northern dominance, no previous plague in Italy, or any afterwards, produced such a pan-peninsula presence in plague writing or publication as did the pandemic of 1575–8.

***

The plague of 1575–8 sparked the creation of a new form of plague writing: works often with 'progesso' or 'successo' in their titles. These tracked plague within

---

[12] See for instance, *Raccolta delli componimenti*. Also see Ceruti, *Prosopopeia amphitheatri*; *Rime di diverso a gli habitani di Venetia*; and Maganza, *Canzone . . . nel calamitoso stato di Venetia*.

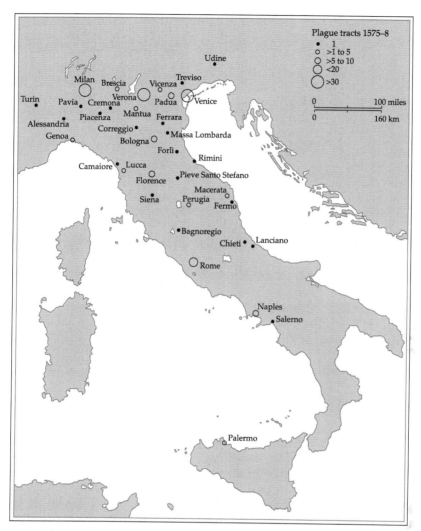

Map 4.1. Plague Tracts, 1575–8

regions, cities, and neighbourhoods with unprecedented chronological rigour by employing statistics gathered from health boards and government magistracies on mortality, morbidity, and financial expenditures. Unlike earlier plague tracts of the sixteenth century, discussion of remote causes hardly figured.[13] Instead, these writings centred on the transmission and contagion of plague by investigating the

[13] In 1575–8 some physicians shunned the standard sections on definitions, causes, and future signs of plague as unnecessary 'pompe'; Contardi, *Il modo di preservarsi*: 'lasciando da parte che cosa sia Peste,

flow of goods and persons from distant lands where the plague first erupted to first victims within an author's city. They then traced meticulously the plague's 'progress' until their cities' declared 'liberation' from the disease.

This new model of plague writing came from northern cities—Milan, Padua, Verona, and Venice—and none as such were penned by a physician. These writings cut across a broad spectrum of the literate population, written by a priest, a bishop, a gate guard, a gentlemen administrator, a merchant, humanists, and, most prominently, notaries. Other titles without the words 'progesso' or 'successo' might, however, be added to the list of these new plague narratives and these included new works by physicians, such as the *Discorsi e Ricordi* of the Venetian Jewish doctor and biblical scholar David de Pomi (1525–*c*.1593). Interspersed with theory and recommended remedies, his three letters to his city counsellors and the health board, published as a single work, were in effect a chronological account of the plague in Venice from 15 February 1576 to 28 February 1577. Another doctor, Leone Crotto (although he described himself as a gentleman and foreigner), published what he called a brief history of the plague in Venice based on his dated communications with the health board and the doge.[14] And as we shall see, other doctors in 1575–8 began their medical tracts with in essence short *successi*, detailing in narrative form the complex paths by which they tracked the contagion of 1575 as it snaked through northern Italy to their home towns. Let us start with Milan and those outside the medical profession.

THE *SUCCESSI* OF MILAN

Written by the Jesuit priest Paolo Bisciola, *Relatione verissima del progresso della peste di Milano* is divided into three parts: the progress of the plague (*questo funesto male*), the provisions of Cardinal Borromeo for 'spiritual welfare', and the ordinances and 'remedies' promulgated by the governors of Milan for 'temporal well-being and health'. Despite these topical divisions, the structure of the pamphlet throughout is chronological. It begins with the uncertainty of where and from whom the contagion entered the city, reporting various rumours: first, a woman from the village of Marignano (today on the south-eastern outskirts of the city) carried it within the gates. She had been caring for her sister, married to an innkeeper in the village, when a carriage of noblemen from Mantua arrived afflicted with the plague. City officials immediately carted off the innkeeper and

---

da quali, e quante cause ella provenga; di quante sorte ne sia alle volte stato, gli segni della futura peste, & altre pompe, fuori di ogni vostro bisogno e fuor di tempo' (3–4).

14 Crotto, *Memoriale delle provisioni generali*, 3r–v. According to Edit 16 he was a doctor, but nowhere in this, his only publication, does he specify his profession, although his text shows a wide reading of medical classics, especially Hippocrates and Ficino, and knowledge of Fracastoro's modes of contagion. Instead, he calls himself 'libero'.

his family to Milan's lazaretto, where they died, but the woman, 'not knowing any better', roamed freely through the city. Others believed that the plague had been consciously spread by 'certain ones' who wiped city walls and gates with a plague poison they concocted. The next morning, others 'confirmed' that almost all the doors and door handles of the street leading to the Porta Nuova and walls in various places had been smeared with the substance. A city ban, however, prohibited the spreading of these rumours and replaced them with the counter-claim that Spaniards trying to raise havoc had unwittingly spread the disease. Yet young wild ones (*scapestrati*), delighting in frightening others, continued to spread these rumours.

Still others claimed the disease had entered the city when a nobleman fled the plague in Mantua. His brother, then staying with the monks at the Certosa, invited him to Milan, but the prior refused him entry. Constrained to sleep on hay in a peasant's house, the nobleman died that night. Having spotted his purse, the peasants stripped him, stole his goods and secretly and carelessly buried him in a nearby field. Among the peasants present were several of their relatives from Borgo degli Ortolani—Milan's first neighbourhood to be afflicted on 2 August. Without believing firmly in this or any of the other stories, Bisciola suggested another possibility: the plague may have had another noble component. When the plague entered Milan, tournaments, jousts, and festivals were being held there to honour Don Giovanni of Austria. Many foreigners were in attendance and especially noblemen from Mantua, who 'could have spread the disease [*mal seme*]'. On the night of San Giacomo (25 July), several watching the tournament died unexpectedly. Bisciola reported yet another theory: the plague's contagion had been more slow-moving, festering over the early spring and summer, when ones expelled by Milan's health board unwittingly spread the disease in the village of Paruzer or Parular near Rho[15] in March, and from there on 2 August the disease entered the city's Borgo degli Ortolani.[16] Bisciola's uncertainty and reports of multiple stories of the plague's spread should sound a cautionary note to modern historians, who readily accept any single tale of plague infection as unquestionably the route and moment when a disease first entered a city or village.[17] As the more discerning Bisciola concluded:

Given this variety of origins, it is difficult to know which opinion was closer to the truth. One story does not necessarily rule out another; all the cases might even be correct. Ultimately, God will make the final judgement.[18]

Like chroniclers such as the early fifteenth-century Giovanni Morelli, the Jesuit priest, recognized the difficulty of plotting the spread of plague in its early phases,

---

[15] Rho is 15 kilometres to the north-west of Milan. It must be Paruzzaro.

[16] The Venetian ambassador stationed in Milan, Ottaviano di Mazi, reported cases at this and surrounding villages on 9 April and at the Borgo degli Ortolani on 12 August (Mutinelli, *Storia arcana*, 306 and 312).

[17] See Chapter 6, n. 177.   [18] Bisciola, *Relatione verissima del progresso della peste*, 1v–2r.

when the disease secretly smouldered in a neighbourhood and then leaked out to others:

> It was not as if the taking of the first brick in a building suddenly brought the building's collapse; instead, once it had appeared in the foundation, it began to feed on the material with little to stop it from spreading through the city from one place to another such that no place could be certain that it was not infected.[19]

Yet, despite these difficulties, Bisciola saw this tracking of crucial importance for understanding the plague. No previous chronicler, including Morelli, or any medical treatise before the 1575 plague, paid such care in tracing the plague's transmission or that of any other disease.

Without turning to God, man's sins or other moral judgements, the Jesuit continued the story of the plague once inside Milan's city walls. By the end of August, most of the nobility of Milan had left the city; commerce began to decline and provisioning the city became difficult. In September the number of deaths reached three hundred a day but were erratic; yet once the disease had taken root it tended to increase and did so until the middle of December, when some hope of 'liberation from the misery' appeared. He then reported the death counts in various monasteries and religious orders within and outside Milan: some, such as the Monastery of the Inconronata, counted only two, while a convent in Brescia lost all but one of its occupants. In his own house of San Fidele, Bisciola observed that the dying were mainly those who had assisted the plague-stricken.

Much in the vein of Daniel Defoe two centuries later, Bisciola then felt an impulse to narrate stories against this backdrop of mounting plague fatalities taken from the city's registers.[20] One was of a barber who became infected after treating many plague patients. Seven times he appeared to have passed away. Finally, taken for dead, he was tossed into a plague pit, where he remained in a heap for over twenty-four hours. When the bodies were gathered for burial, he awoke, rose to his feet, and sent the plague cleaners (*monatti*) flying, frightened out of their minds. Without pause, he continued caring for the afflicted. Another man left for dead in a plague heap awoke on hearing a priest passing with the Holy Sacrament. He rose to his knees, pleaded with great passion for communion, and 'gave up the ghost' ('fra poco rese l'anima a Dio').

Part two of Bisciola's *progresso* again proceeded chronologically, though the topic was different; now he turned to 'the spiritual provisions of Cardinal Borromeo for the souls of the city'. As soon as cases were reported in the region, the cardinal began to pray and by a miracle held the plague at bay for some time. He encouraged the heads of households to make their last wills and testaments. At his own expense, he cleaned up the lazaretto and, once plague struck, dispensed charity, 'warmly and lovingly' to the afflicted. Under the papal bull *In coena*

---

[19] Ibid., 2r.   [20] Defoe, *A Journal of the Plague Year*.

Domini he endowed the priests of Milan with powers to absolve the afflicted of their sins at the altar of the lazaretto and granted indulgences to enjoin spiritual and medical assistance to the afflicted. Among those granted various indulgences were priests who offered the afflicted last rites, doctors who took their pulse, nurses ('le comadre') who assisted them, wet-nurses, who cared for the infants left as orphans by the plague dead, barbers and their assistants who treated the infected, and lowly plague cleaners who transported the stricken to plague huts, hospitals, or their graves.[21]

Bisciola reported further sacrifices the cardinal made for the secular welfare of his Milanese flock. On 1 October he assembled all the priests and religious orders of the city to beseech their help. The Capuchins were given the task of maintaining the lazaretto; other orders were given responsibility over the plague huts. Parish priests were instructed to hear confession and grant communion to the afflicted in their homes. Borromeo published a pamphlet with detailed rules for assisting the souls and bodies of the ill under these conditions.[22] He ordered priests to accompany the plague cleaners into the houses of the dead and with crosses and candles to escort them to the grave to assure proper Christian burials. He forbade indecent transport of victims heaped in carts or carried on shoulders. For this task, he recruited priests from the Swiss valleys within his diocese 'who were by nature robust'.[23]

For the first week of October, Cardinal Borromeo granted a full indulgence (*un 'Indulgenza plenaria*) in the form of a Jubilee to those who fasted for three days and marched in three processions. Carrying the relics of the city, he processed barefooted, hooded, and dressed in mourning with a great rope tied round his neck, his gown dragging on the ground. A thousand flagellants followed, similarly dressed, who beat themselves continuously. 'But what moved the lower classes most' was a large black cross bearing 'the Holy Nail' and the blood that gushed from the cardinal's feet.[24] He established prayers for forty hours; altars were built in streets and religious festivals celebrated with singing and music to console the people ordered not to participate but to stay by their windows. He accompanied the city's priests, administering communion door to door. He placed fires and incense (*profumi*) outside these houses so that the priests following communion could protect themselves by cleansing and perfuming their hands.

Bisciola's narrative then skipped to February when 'the embers of plague began to rekindle'. The cardinal went from parish to parish visiting and blessing his

---

[21] These indulgences are detailed in other documents issued by Cardinal Borromeo; see *Constitutiones, et decreta sex prouincialium Synodorum Mediolanensium*; idem, *Ordini d'orationi*, n.p.; idem, *Pratica per i curati*, 7;. and *Gregorii PP. XIII [S.D.N.D.] Iubileum ad avertenda pestis pericula*, n.p.

[22] Borromeo, *Cause, et rimedi della peste*.

[23] According to the Venetian ambassador, the cardinal deputized two Swiss priests on 3 September 1576 to hear confession in the Milanese lazaretto; Mutinelli, *Storia arcana*, I, 321.

[24] Bisciola, *Relatione verissima del progresso della peste*, 4r.

flock, giving communion in the streets; one day to men, the next to women. He administered the sacraments to the plague-stricken and continued to visit daily the lazaretto and plague huts. While in the homes of the afflicted, he stood in a wooden cage ('un seraglio di legno') to avoid being touched by the sick. He also visited infected villages outside the city, offering them 'spiritual and temporal help'. At this time, the city began the restoration and enlargement of the church of Saint Sebastian, one of Milan's early Christian martyrs, and making a silver casket to hold the saint's relics. Bisciola now expressed mixed sentiments: on the one hand he praised Milan as 'a heaven [*un cielo*] adorned with so many beautiful stars, angels, and heavenly citizens; our city glittered with great numbers of illuminated candles and was perfumed with wonderful scents, and the mouths of all men and women of every age was full of praise for the Lord'. On the other hand, he told less luminous stories of his citizens, such as of a nobleman who hid the death of his plague-stricken child from city officials, which then led to the 'ultimate ruin' of the family.

By May the plague had almost ended. With relief and joy, Bisciola reported new processions of thanksgiving. Those of the Holy Nail performed with 'magnificent happiness and triumph' contrasted with the morose dirges of previous months. The women of the city, however, were still deprived of this glee. Along with children under fourteen, they were kept locked in their homes, their participation confined to viewing the triumphal processions from windows. Bisciola praised other temporal provisions 'grandissimi & utilissimi' decreed by the 'Holy Pastor', such as cleaning the walls of the rooms and homes of the poor, requiring priests to shave their beards and cut their moustaches, and implementing regular cleaning of all the streets and houses of the city and especially rubbish dumps 'which obviously were a major cause of the plague's spread'. Further, Borromeo ordered the killing of dogs and cats, which through children's play were believed to carry plague from one house to another. He gathered all the homeless poor of Milan—those who stayed in taverns or inns, servants and boys who had been laid off by their lords from fear of contagion, those who lived hand to mouth on charity, and those who practised unskilled trades ('qualche arte leggier') which at present provided no employment—and brought them to a place called Vittoria, eight miles from Milan, which earlier had been built by Francis I of France ('Re Christianissimo Francesco'). The cardinal dressed them in red and purple cloth and the youngest were taught to sing and play musical instruments so that when they returned to the city they would be able to collect charity and 'bestow the greatest consolation to all'. In addition, the 'good pastor' worked tirelessly to comfort the afflicted, those who would die in only a few days.[25] In October (1576), he began constructing new plague huts just outside the city gates for those who had recovered in the lazaretto, to be cleansed and placed

---

[25] Biraben, *Les hommes et la peste en France*, II, 170, seems to think that such practices began only in the seventeenth century. His only examples come from Montpellier in 1629.

under quarantine. But the growing numbers of the plague-afflicted changed his plans: quickly new plague cases filled the huts.[26]

Bisciola provides less on the secular side of control and intervention during the plague in his third section. From his account the true innovator was the cardinal. His narrative of secular controls and assistance concentrates on the general quarantine of 29 October 1576, which confined almost all to their homes. Licences were required to open shops and for heads of families to go out of doors. Those who were infected were not permitted to stay in the city except in locked houses designated with big white crosses painted in lye. Others were sent immediately to the plague huts. The city provided ample food to the poor and to those who could not survive without work or trade: they were given more than their daily requirements in bread, rice, salt, and once a week small change ('qualche parpaiola').[27] 'It was a great sadness to see such squalid poverty . . . people broken, totally defeated [*macilente & tutta disfatta*], and deprived of freedom.'[28]

By mid-September the city had begun to 'purge' infected houses and goods but to little effect: when the afflicted returned to their homes, they re-infected them. Nevertheless, the government learnt from its mistakes, reformed its practices, and began whitewashing the walls of these houses, which proved more effective. Once the quarantine had been imposed, provisioning the city became much more restricted, with designated distribution points within neighbourhoods and officials appointed for the tasks. The government passed decrees against those hiding plague-infected goods and offered rewards to those who revealed the culprits. Bisciola illustrated these crimes by telling the story of two young gentlemen who made a business of robbing the goods of abandoned plague-stricken houses. Many plague cleaners (*monatti*) were prosecuted for 'their evil acts', and the penalties were harsh. On 28 March the quarantine was relaxed to allow men and women to go to church.[29]

Bisciola reported the city's need to hire foreign barbers and doctors to assist in caring for the plague-afflicted. He praised the German barbers, who succeeded 'benissimo' in their treatment, but (like other Milanese observers) was less favourable towards the seven hired French 'doctors': according to Bisciola, five of them died quickly and the other two refused to work until the city granted them the extortionate wage of 500 *scudi*.[30] He ended his tract with statistics covering Milan's plague experience from 3 March 1576 to 20 July 1577, such as the city's expenses and purging of 1,589 houses.

[26] Bisciola, *Relatione verissima del progresso della peste*, 6v.

[27] *Parpagliole* were small coins of common exchange minted in Provence that entered Milan in the sixteenth century, then worth two and a half *soldi*; *Grande dizionario*, XII, 638.

[28] Bisciola, *Relatione verissima del progresso della peste*, 6v.   [29] Ibid., 6v–7r.

[30] Ibid., 7r. The Venetian ambassador reports in detail the hiring of the French staff (actually one physician, a surgeon, four barbers, and three other servants) paid collectively 1,600 *scudi*, their refusal to take victims' pulses, the failures of their secret drugs, and the eventual death of all except the surgeon; Mutinelli, *Storia arcana*, 336–8.

Not only is Bisciola's brief tract strikingly different from previous plague writing in any form before the Italian threat of 1575–8, but it also differs in certain crucial respects from Ingrassia's *Informatione* published a year earlier. First, despite Bisciola's praise for the 'buon pastore' Cardinal Borromeo, God hardly enters the frame, while Ingrassia's and other earlier medical plague treatises of the sixteenth century began almost invariably with God and man's sins as the plague's first cause. Nor did Bisciola entertain long-term or remote causes such as speculating on planetary configurations, seasonal peculiarities, or mutation of air.[31] Instead, his first concern was tracking human infection and contagion to trace the disease from previously infected regions and then chart its mortalities within the city. Secondly, unlike earlier plague writing, the individual patient was not Bisciola's frame. Instead, his focus was on public health: solutions to plague came first from the innovative health policies of the 'buon pastore' and then the state; both addressed the spiritual and the temporal needs of a large metropolitan region with charity, laws, processions, fasts, the building of churches, hospitals, and plague huts, the purging of infected houses, quarantine, and provisioning large populations deprived of work and the freedom to circulate within their neighbourhoods. Bisciola narrated the progress of these two governmental forces over the seventeen months of his plague chronicle. Thirdly, its structure was chronological and narrative, not didactic and topical as with the traditional physician's plague manual. Finally, in anticipation of later classics of plague literature, he slotted individual stories into a chronological and quantitative structure of plague deaths taken from governmental registers—stories of hope, despair, and the near miraculous efforts of unknown masses to combat plague's gruesome realities.

***

Two other narratives of Milan's plague crisis of 1576–7, written in the same years, differed from Bisciola's in several essential ways: they were longer, attributed far more to the secular arm of the state than to Cardinal Borromeo's spiritual and secular initiatives, and examined in greater detail and with more documentation events within the city walls as well as showing greater concern for the plague's spread within Lombardy. They devoted attention to the communication between various city-states and Milan and compared Milan's reactions and solutions with measures taken in Verona and Venice.

Giacomo Filippo Besta, a notary and gate guard during the plague, published *Vera Narratione del successo della peste* a year after Bisciola's *progresso*. It was seven times the length and began, not with Milan, but with Trent, a pivotal place recognized by most plague commentators as northern Italy's plague port of entry in 1574 or 1575. Based more closely on the Milanese state's own records and tracking of the plague, Besta's version of the plague's origins and trajectory

---

[31] For an example of an earlier sixteenth-century text heavily indebted to Galen with copious citations to him and other ancient and Arabic authorities, see the 326-page tract of the Veronese doctor Fumanelli, *De compositione medicamentorum.*

differed from Bisciola's. Besta reported other stories and rumours of plague entry into and through the Milanese state: while the plague infected Trent in the summer of 1575, it did not penetrate the Milanese territory until 14 March 1576 when it struck Paruzzaro, north-west of Milan,[32] killing 205 there by the end of September. By Besta's tracking, this outpost was not, however, the plague's point of entry into Milan. Instead, its route was more circuitous: first, it struck Venice and Mantua in the summer of 1576, and Milan's infection came later from communication with these metropolitan centres. Like Bisciola, Besta saw the Mantovani as the culprits. On 27 July several of them stayed at an inn called the Falcon in Melegnano, 10 kilometres south-east of Milan. They carried the disease infecting servants at the inn and eventually killing ninety-seven in the village.[33] Within a few days a house in Borgo di Rancate, 28 kilometres north-east of Milan, was infected by a woman from Melegnano, who left 'before officials could lock her up'.

Besta then details the city's reactions and preparations. Doctors, surgeons, barbers, and others were immediately called into service to fight the plague's spread. Dogs and other animals found in the houses of the infected were killed. Borromeo issued plenary indulgences, not only to the plague-stricken, but to those who served them spiritually and bodily. He observed that many who administered the Eucharist to the afflicted became infected and died, and as a consequence, he initiated the practice of sticking the finger that gave the host to the infected into the flame of a candle, which he contended protected from infection. With city-wide quarantines, trade and industry came to a standstill. These conditions led to poverty and famine, further fuelling the death tolls. Besta described the actions of the cardinal and the clergy, which he saw benefiting the city psychologically, with the erection of crosses and the enactment of Christ's passion along with larger projects such as the dedication of a chapel to San Rocco in a public street near the church of San Simpliciano in one of the city's worst afflicted areas.[34] Besta described the processions that took place over four days: the cardinal dressed in black, his head covered as 'a sign of sadness', in bare feet, the cord around his neck, the Holy Nail raised in the air. Unlike the Jesuit's account, however, Besta's emphasized the participation and organization of the civic hierarchy in these processions. Following the cardinal the governor of Milan with members of the Senate and all the magistrates processed; the people along with the clergy followed, 'all in tears, beseeching God's mercy for their sins'. They returned to the cathedral, where the Holy Nail was exposed for forty-eight hours; charity was distributed: 600 *scudi* given to the Hospital of Victory and a plenary indulgence to all participants.

[32] By today's roads Paruzzaro is 41 kilometres from Novara and 66 kilometres from Milan.

[33] The Venetian ambassador in Milan tells a similar story; Mutinelli, *Storia arcana*, 311.

[34] From the Milanese necrologies of the late fifteenth and early sixteenth century, the parish of San Simpliciano consistently counted among the highest numbers of plague victims.

The major reforms for provisioning the city, moreover, came from Milan's governor and its city council, which organized the importation of grain, vegetables, rice, and wood from uninfected regions and especially from the countryside of Lumelina. The city spent 70,000 *scudi* on these provisions, which the treasury (*Fisco*) resisted, but the cause of the 'suffering of the poor' accentuated by shortages going back to 1570 prevailed. Nonetheless, the plague's 'male progresso' outpaced the city's efforts. Early on, the lazaretto of San Gregorio reached capacity with its 388 rooms divided into three sections. Besta describes in detail the plague huts, how they were provided with water from nearby fountains, the placing of crosses, how the plague-stricken were led in prayers, daily celebrations of mass, and registers that no longer survive containing the names of the interned, their parishes, house numbers, and dates of entry.[35] He further describes the procedures for the entry of the infected or suspected into the huts: first stripped, then washed and given new clothes. When they died, the huts were either perfumed or burnt. Barbers or the recently employed French health carers, who had first been in Venice 'to liberate that city from plague', first examined the stricken. These doctors also treated the infected at San Gregorio and were paid the extraordinary salary of 1,600 *scudi* a month as well as living expenses. Like Bisciola, Besta found their services less than satisfactory: 'they were inexperienced in their duties, renowned solely for their greed, profiting as much as they could. Ultimately they paid for their arrogance and vanity either by death from plague or imprisonment.'[36]

Elected by the College of Physicians, physicians were consigned to the huts and paid 45 *scudi* a month to visit victims daily. The cardinal delegated two friars from each gate to celebrate a daily mass at the huts. These and other friars, priests, and secular officers who visited the huts were granted plenary indulgences. 'Despite the great fear of catching the contagion', many took on the tasks, 'crossing the fence'. Besta detailed the daily portions of food doled out to the healthy and ill; for men it was 28 ounces (*onze*) of bread, a full measure (*schietto*)[37] of wine, and 29 ounces of rice soup but was less for women and children. The Milanese senate granted authority to redact last wills and testaments to those registering entrants to the huts, even though they were not public notaries.[38] The number of straw huts grew to 3,188, but a further 599 were needed, and the senate ran out of straw.[39]

Besta reported changes in social services, attitudes, and dress. In a large home, where wet nurses and other servants were employed, public funds provided for children and infants left parentless by plague. Senators and the rich abandoned their togas and the 'great diversity of other pompous and ornate clothing' previously worn 'lasciviously throughout the city' in exchange for shorter and simpler dress, which they thought would make them more resistant to contagion.

---

[35] Besta, *Vera narratione*, 18–19.   [36] Ibid., 20r.   [37] *Grande dizionario*, XVII, 1,009.

[38] Besta, *Vera narratione*, 20r–22r.   [39] Ibid., 22v.

However, not all was so rosy. Besta describes scenes and records the voices of the poor: the plague cleaners with their carts full of the dead, stretchers transporting the stricken to the huts with poor women dressed pitifully who followed. Even at the beginning of the plague city coffers could not meet the costs of feeding the mounting numbers of poor for more than four days. Therefore, the government had to call for contributions from citizens and collected over 18,000 *scudi*. According to Besta, their motives did not spring solely from altruism; they gave from fear that 'la plebe' would revolt. The citizens exhorted their magistrates and nobles to take on new measures for public welfare; otherwise their own health would soon suffer.[40] Later, he confessed that he would never have believed that the poor of Milan could have become so wretched with such numbers incapable of maintaining themselves. Besta's authority on these matters came from direct experience (as he informs the reader): he had been delegated to visit the poor in his parish of San Lorenzo, registering plague cases and issuing licences (*bollette*) to leave their homes for essential business within the city.[41]

By the end of October conditions worsened. Besta, like Bisciola, described (but in greater detail) the draconian public health measures taken by the city: the general quarantine, the closing of shops and commerce, except those that sold essential items for survival, the new organizations and procedures for cleaning streets and dumping waste in specified places beyond city walls, the specifics proposed by the College of Physicians for 'purging' suspected houses, clothing, money, and other items; the cleaning of books and other written materials including merchants' account books, doctors' tracts, and notarial instruments.[42] During the quarantine, he described the cardinal's measures to strengthen the city spiritually and psychologically: seven times a day he summoned parishioners to come to their windows to hear prayers, the mass, and sing the litany and other songs. In the face of their misery 'the city at his bosom took heart and in their every need showed their loving gratitude'.[43]

By January 1577, the heads of families were allowed to process during feast days with their guild flags, and in February commerce resumed, but Besta warned, if caution was not taken, 'the city would return to the same misery and infection'. Unlike Venice, Milan was cautious, and the plague failed to re-emerge as it had done the previous spring. With the city's 'liberation' from plague, Besta put its death toll at 17,329 (taken from the health board's records). He described triumphantly the festivals and jubilees of thanksgiving to God that accompanied the official declaration of the plague's end and concluded his tract in praise of the administrative structures and decisions that had carried Milan through 'these darkest days of its history'. He especially praised the diligence of those *visitatori* of the parishes (like himself), delegated to guard the city's gates. Public health and administrative rigour had prevailed. As with others writing during the 1575–8 crisis, Besta's analysis, advice, and lessons were framed in a narrative,

[40] Ibid., 22v–25r. [41] Ibid., 36v. [42] Ibid., 25v–29r. [43] Ibid., 38r.

and he exposed his changing sentiments as the plague progressed, a feature that does not appear in previous physicians' manuals. Other *successi* of the 1575–8 plague embody similar shifts in form and sentiment.

***

The cavalier Asciano Centorio Degli Ortensi, another administrator during the plague, penned a third journal of Milan's plague experience in 1576–8. Dedicated to the president of Milan's health board in 1576, his was an even grander and lengthier compilation of governmental decisions and administrative reactions to the plague; comprised of 454 small-print pages, it almost quintupled Besta's and was twenty-eight times the length of Bisciola's.[44] Not only was the cavalier's account more detailed, especially on plague decrees passed by the Milanese state, but it took a more Italian, even international, view of the events in Milan. Asciano plotted the twisted path of the plague's infection in 1575 through the Swiss cantons from Zurich to Bellinzona to Trent and to Venice. To Bisciola's and Besta's stories of the plague's spread, he added others, asserting that Jews carried it from Trent to the Ghetto of Venice, and that in Mantua a Jew transmitted it through the sale of infected second-hand clothing from Trent.[45] With these reports, Milan stationed guards at its gates. Asciano also reported in greater detail the arrival of plague in the territory of Milan. The first to be infected was not Paruzzaro but the village of Castelletto Momo, 'four miles distant from Paruzzaro'. A cleric fleeing the plague stayed in the house of the village's parish priest and within four days of his arrival, the priest, his servants, and a woman died.[46] Moreover, Asciano charted other entries and trajectories of plague within the territory before it reached Milan, such as the infection of a village called San Pietro, where a mother, child, and others died within four days of the plague's arrival, and another case at Villa Torre di Menapace. He described the signs and symptoms of many of these early cases[47] and the means by which the plague was thought to have arrived. At Monza, for instance, reports sent to Milan pinned the spread to a woman from Mantua selling coral and other goods; she died in the same house 'with many other people'. Immediately, Milan sent a doctor to confirm the report and investigate the causes. Plague huts were constructed in the Borgo of San Biagio, an isolated zone outside town. By 19 July eighty from the town had been sent there, and 150 died within fifty-six houses in Monza.[48] Even before plague reached Milan, its lazaretto had become full of victims from surrounding towns and villages. Then Asciano traced the plague into the city. As in the reports of Besta and Bisciola, its entry point was

---

[44] Centorio Degli Ortensi, *I cinque libri degl'avvertimenti*.

[45] On Centorio Degli Ortensi and accusations against Jews in 1576, see Besozzi, *Le magistrature cittadine milanesi*, 23–4.

[46] These observations contradict the claims of Scott and Duncan (*Biology of Plagues* and *Return of the Black Death*) that early modern plagues had incubation periods as long as a month in order to spread so rapidly.

[47] Centorio Degli Ortensi, *I cinque libri degl'avvertimenti*, 4–6.   [48] Ibid., 8.

given as the Borgo degli Ortolani, and from there it infected the parish of San Simpliciano. Again, Asciano's tracking, as in country towns, gives no evidence of any lengthy incubation period. Immediately after the first victim's entry into the city, other residents began catching the disease and dying. Unlike Bisciola or Besta, Asciano also traced the plague meticulously through the city: 'from Borgo Sant'Anna, towards San Marco and into the parishes of San Carpoforo, Marcellino, Tommaso, and Protasio'. By 17 September 800 had died, not counting those sent to the lazaretto. Unlike the other two plague chroniclers, Asciano did not lose sight of the countryside or Milan's subject towns once the plague entered the city; instead, his eye followed the plague's continuing and twisted progress, tracking its advances.[49]

The bulk of Asciano's *Cinque libri*, however, reported the efforts of local authorities, the health board and the cardinal, the numerous *gride*, or laws, and announcements decreed during the plague years 1576–7 to combat the plague. For instance, the first decree on street cleaning in Milan also aimed at removing scroungers, rogues, and similar people ('scrocchi e furfanti & simili genti'). The government saw these as the primary sources of contagion because of the dirt they left behind and their stench. Anyone caught throwing dirty water, urine, or other rubbish from their windows into a public street was fined a *scudo*.[50] Similar fines were issued against throwing dead dogs or cats in public places; they were to be dumped beyond the city walls outside the second ditch. Porters, mountain people, and other low life, who lodged in single rooms and whose filthy clothes were never washed, were suspected, and new laws prohibited more than four staying in a room or two to a bed.[51] Jews were not allowed to take lodgings in the city without a licence from the health board, and afterwards their houses along with 'the poor of San Pietro' were to be inspected frequently to see that they were kept clean. The sale of all dead fish, frogs, and eels was prohibited within the city and markets for large animals shut down. On 30 August 1576, an ordinance prohibited the city's nobility from leaving.[52] The health board kept a careful listing of 'suspected' and 'unsuspected' regions of Italy. Along with tricksters, rogues, beggars, prostitutes, and other low life ('furbi, cingari, ghitti, furfanti, herbolari, cantainbanco, commedianti, meretrici e simil sorti'), those from regions 'suspected' of harbouring plague were barred from the city, and those coming even from 'unsuspected' places registered meticulously by name and place of origin.[53] According to the health board, these migrants along with beggars and the poor in general were 'very capable of generating the disease'.[54] Asciano listed the detailed instructions on recognizing plague given to soldiers who patrolled Milan's gates. Finally, he described the official liberation of Milan on 20 January 1578—its songs, prayers, processions, and ensuing gaiety.[55]

---

[49] Ibid., 9–12.   [50] Ibid., 13–14.   [51] Ibid., 15.   [52] Ibid., 101.
[53] Ibid., 21.   [54] Ibid., 331.   [55] Ibid., 421.

His examination of plague laws and decrees then reached beyond Milan: he compared plague laws passed by health boards in Mantua, Venice, Rome, Sicily, Modena, and Bologna.[56] His tract detailed instructions to doctors and parishioners on how to cleanse and perfume houses distinguishing which items were to be burnt or purged. He ended with his own advice on how to avoid the plague, from perfumes to tips on how to stay happy and young.[57] Despite its length, parts of this tract were translated later in the sixteenth century into Latin for German physicians and was republished in its entirety during the plague of 1630–1.[58]

***

Olivero Panizzone Sacco's *progresso della peste* presents a different view of the plague in Milan from August 1576 to the end of 1577. Unlike Bisciola, Besta, and Centorio Degli Ortensi, he was not an insider, part of the city's administrative machinery; rather, he was a merchant from Alessandria, an outsider caught in Milan at the plague's start and prohibited from leaving. He was on the receiving end of those laws and bans implemented by the Milanese state, facilitated by Bisciola, Besta, and Centorio Degli Ortensi. As a result, his perception of the stringencies imposed in 1576–7 differed from that of those writing and enforcing them. He complained personally about not receiving the assistance he expected from city officials, regional rulers, or those of his own city, who refused him permission to leave plague-ridden Milan. Although from a privileged background with access to those at the highest echelons of Milan's ruling elites, Panizzone Sacco, because of his present straits, assumed the voice of the ruled:

It seems impossible that the cities and regions of my country (*del mio Dominio*)[59] could have treated me so cruelly: how could they have imposed this ban on me and not desired to help if the Lieutenant, my Governor, the Marchese d'Aimonte, had not constrained them. O, I beseech you, the cries and laments of my people have been ignored by most of the nobility. We have been mistreated by officials, commissioners, soldiers, doctors, barbers, those who cleanse our belongings, gravediggers, and others . . . It is unsupportable how many of my duchy have been refused travel, kept at bay by the road guards, such that no one can visit me, bring me provisions . . .[60]

No doubt, the change in his predicament coloured his view of the charitable and administrative landscape of Milan and probably gives us a better insight into the plague experience of the majority in Milan than the three previously described plague chroniclers, even though two of them were not at the top end of Milan's chain of command. Although these ones might complain about the greedy and incompetent French doctors or the stench of the poor, Panizzone Sacco's 'lament' targeted Milan's cruel and inadequate administration, the officials, who enforced

---

[56] Centorio Degli Ortensi, *I cinque degl' avvertimenti*, 57, 65, 67, 72, and 77.   [57] Ibid., 425–7.
[58] See Chapter 8.   [59] Alessandria was part of the Spanish-controlled Duchy of Milan.
[60] Panizzone Sacco, *Pianto della città di Milano*, 6r.

the city's health laws badly or failed to carry out them humanely. In Panizzone Sacco's words:

O woe, how little there was to praise; everywhere I saw many, many of the poor infected and mistreated. They died in part from fear, in part from necessity. Alive or dead they were taken away brutally, mixed together in the same cart, one thrown on top of the other. The dead were badly buried, their belongings stolen and hidden. As if to maintain and conserve the very disease, their houses were poorly cleansed. . . . The officers came to these houses not from charity but only to enforce their ordinances and take away their goods. Many came from infected places bringing the disease to add evil to evil. But how many of the poor were given any relief? In reality, very few, I believe, at least of the truly poor. Instead, charity was distributed mostly to the well off [*ben fornite*]. Everywhere I looked I saw ruin and destruction.[61]

From the city's material conditions Panizzone Sacco then lamented its moral decay: illicit sex, games, drunkenness, and dancing went on in the locked houses, the lazaretto of San Gregorio, the plague huts, and other places. Crimes of adultery, rape, incest, murder, theft, blasphemy, and other shameful acts compounded the city's sinfulness. He implored Cardinal Borromeo to expose the sins at San Gregorio and the regional governor, Serbelloni, to visit the huts and punish transgressors.[62] At the same time, he complained that officials were lax in distributing licences to enter the city, permitting those from infected places to fan the flames of the plague; gate guards failed in their duties; the poor in the huts and at San Gregorio were treated badly; commissioners, soldiers, gravediggers, plague cleaners and washers stole or burnt the little the poor possessed. Goods were not properly inventoried; rivalries exploded among officials squabbling over the spoils of the plague dead.[63]

While Bisciola, Besta, and Centorio Degli Ortensi praised the tireless and courageous devotion of doctors, barbers, and others who risked their lives to serve the plague-stricken, Panizzone Sacco reported the darker side: 'Oh, you physicians and barbers, who have abandoned us, where is the charity you owe these poor afflicted ones? Where is your love of country when you have abandoned us in our greatest need?' Even those who stayed, he charged, refused to visit the plague-stricken or enter their deadly locked houses.[64] These observations, moreover, do not appear necessarily as the exaggerated cranky reactions of an outsider: they find resonance in the earliest Milanese plague legislation in 1576, which also accused members of Milan's College of Physicians of escaping town or refusing to treat patients suspected of plague: the laws also charged them as being without charity for their countrymen and called on the Senate to compile a register of doctors who had left and ordered their immediate return.[65]

Panizzano Sacco's complaint continued down the administrative hierarchy. He described the plague-cleaners (*monati*), who carted the plague-ill or suspected

---

[61] Ibid., 4v–5r.   [62] Ibid., 8v–9r, 12v.   [63] Ibid., 12v, 14v–15r, 24r.
[64] Ibid., 16r, 27v.   [65] *Gride diverse*, no. 75, 1576.x.24.

to plague huts, dumping them there, throwing them on the ground, leaving them without proper provisions and, worse, stealing their few and miserable belongings. Further, the huts were badly constructed and cleaned. The merchant sided with the masses: 'my people and the poor . . . you are led to the huts as if to the butchers, where you find little love or charity, but great cruelty, avarice, iniquity, tyranny, vengeance, derision, and theft.'[66] But in the end, he went beyond the rulers, officers, and administrators of the city and health board to attack the Milanese population as a whole: 'O my citizens, noblemen, merchants, men and women of every station, with your sins you have caused my sad predicament and then you have abandoned me. God has treated you well enough while you have played amongst yourselves, one swindling the other.'[67] Stories from other Milanese commentators lend further credence to these legal, political, and cultural horrors of plague.[68] With the next plague in 1585—this one afflicting north-western Italy—Milan's plague experience of 1576–7 had become well known and not only for Carlo Borromeo's sanctity. In giving guidelines to officials in Turin, the physician Francesco Alessandri recalled Milan's negative side—a lesson now to be avoided in his region. By his account, Milan had been 'full of tribulations, conflicts, shouting, complaints, and moaning'.[69]

A year after his first tract, now in the wake of Milan's joyous celebrations of its liberation from plague announced on San Sebastian day, Panizzone Sacco published a second tract on the plague in Milan. This one turned about-face. Although his opening showed signs of his earlier complaint—'no more plague deaths, no more arrogant plague cleaners, no more commissioners, no more soldiers, no more plague huts, no more inspections, no more disgraceful burials, no more purges, an end to the many officials and their assistants, no more wagons carting off the infected, no more houses with the sign, the end of sadness, and terror, and grief'—he now was full of praise.[70] First he thanked God for the city's 'liberation' after seventeen months of suffering, in which commerce had been prohibited. Then he celebrated individually a long list of Milan's rulers and servants of its health board, many of whom less than a year before had been the butt of his harsh accusations: Cardinal Carlo Borromeo; Don Antonio de Guzman, Marchese d'Aimonte, Governor of Milan, 'for quelling the protests of the city'; Gabrio Serbelloni 'knight of Jerusalem', 'for making frequent visits to the plague huts, the lazaretto, and anywhere else where the plague-stricken were found', Count Pietro Antonio Lonato, 'who helped me and my people and served so many of the poor'; Girolamo Montio and Galeazzo Brugora, who presided

---

[66] Panizzone Sacco, *Pianto della città di Milano*, 27v.   [67] Ibid., 17r.

[68] *Gride diverse*, no. 36, 1577.ii.12; 40, 1577.i.6; 68, 1576.x.19; 82, 5.xii.1576; 85, 7.xii.1576; and 97, 1576.ix.12; on other tales and complaints of the evil deeds of the *monatti*, see Bisciola, *Relatione verissima del progresso della peste*, 7r and 8v, reporting the executions of *monatti* in Milan for spreading plague and theft. Also Carlo Borromeo warned his clergy about commissioners, parish elders, *monatti*, and other officials robbing or extorting money from the plague-stricken (*Pratica per i curati*, 29r).

[69] Alessandri, *Trattato della peste*, 21r.   [70] Panizzone Sacco, *Giubilo della città di Milano*.

over the health board in 1576 and 1577; Sigismondo Picinardo, 'my senator and podestà of Pavia, who 'with such hardship and sweat diligently punished all transgressors and watched over his people'.

As against his previous spite and condemnation of the foot soldiers of Milan's health board and servants working to control the spread of plague, Panizzone Sacco now changed his mind, praising those who ran and served the lazaretto, 'miraculously untouched by the pestilential contagion', those who provided food, clothing, and medication to so many people, who had given so much of every sort of provision for 'your people', to the physicians and barbers who had not fled but cared well for the afflicted, bravely taking their pulse. Finally, he 'congratulated' the citizens of Milan, 'all of you' who suffered from such grief (*frezza*) and fear. He praised the merchants for casting aside their vanities and ostentatious dress and the teams of men and women servants of the state and the health board, 'who never became arrogant but diligently performed their duties'.[71]

***

Beyond published *successi della peste* of the 1575–8 plague others can be found in the archives, such as the account by the notary (*scrivano*) of Venice's health board, Cornelio Morello, *Raccolte di deliberazioni prese durante la peste del 1575–1577* composed almost ten years after the plague.[72] More remarkable was an account by a young Milanese artisan,[73] resident of the neighbourhood Borgo degli Ortolani, where on 12 July 1576 (by his account) plague was first to enter.[74] It was one of the poorest areas of the city, and the orthography and style of this tract set it apart from other plague writings.[75] The extent to which other such accounts can be found in Italian archives is uncharted territory.[76]

As with other lay writers of 1575–8, the artisan Giovanni Ambrogio de Cozzi (de Chozis), despite intense piety, saw the source of this plague (at least

[71] Ibid., 11r–18r.

[72] On details of this account, see Rodenwaldt, *Pest in Venedig*; and Preto, *Peste e società a Venezia nel 1576*, 14ff.

[73] At the end of his diary dated 4 August 1577, Giovanni Ambrogio says that, at the age of twenty-five, he married a seventeen-year-old girl; 'Le "Memorie" di Giovan Ambrogio', 14. This 'diary' was not published until the end of the nineteenth century. Other unpublished plague tracts can be found in state and municipal archives, such as one by a Pistoiese physician practising in Venice during the plague in 1576, Galeatius Carius, who urged that a school and an academy be founded to study the plague; see Thorndike, 'The Blight of Pestilence', 470. However, such findings may not be numerous. For instance, a survey of Sicilian libraries by Dollo, *Filosofia e scienza in Sicilia*, finds only one unpublished sixteenth-century work on plague, Carretto, *De pestilentia cohorta Agrigenti*.

[74] By September, in fact, conditions within the borgo appear to have deteriorated and continued to be worse here than elsewhere, as evinced in an ordinance issued by the health board that rescinded licences to those of the borgo to circulate through the city or visit others in houses within the neighbourhood; *Gride diverse*, no. 96, 1576.ix.6.

[75] For instance, see one of Giovanno Ambrogio's opening sentences: 'Io facia memoria che dapoi la calastria fu una mortalità de person e ne moriva più de queli che aveva da mangiar che queli che non aveva e che pativa fame; e questo fu lan de 1571'; 'Le "Memorie" di Giovan Ambrogio', 9.

[76] In the Archives of Verona, I found only one and it was an eighteenth-century hand-copied version of Valier's *Commentariolus* that was published in 1576.

initially) within the human and historical sphere and not with the divine or the atmospheric. He dated the plague's origins as early as 1570 with a great food shortage ('una gran calastria de viver') in Lombardy, followed by a disease the next year when 'those who had the means to eat died in greater numbers than those who suffered from famine'.[77] His account then jumped to 12 July 1576 when plague struck the Casina outside Milan's southern gates, where those from his neighbourhood went to work the fields and mixed with the local population.[78] By his reckoning, a woman from Borgo degli Ortolani visited her cousin there and on returning home, which she shared with another family, infected the wife of the second family; the two died with pestilential signs within a day of one another.[79] The health commissioners locked the house, and all their children were taken to the lazaretto of San Gregorio.[80] Between the date of these two deaths (12 July) and 16 September, Giovanni Ambrogio counted two hundred plague deaths in the city and recorded that the city had to solicit barbers and doctors not only from Milan but from many countries ('de molte paes') to treat the plague victims in the huts, and many of these carers died quickly. By 27 October he estimated a thousand plague deaths in Milan, and a general quarantine was called. His detailed account of the city's ordinances on cleaning and perfuming goods and places and the tallying of plague deaths for his Borgo suggests that Giovanni Ambrogio may have been a petty officer such as a guard or assistant of the gate. He provides rare information from which the lethality of the disease can be calculated. No other narrative accounts for Milan or elsewhere during the 1575–8 plague gives such figures with any apparent precision: from 12 July to 7 December the plague infected 83 houses or apartments ('ciové stanceij') with 773 cases and 700 deaths,[81] a fatality rate of 90.6 per cent. By this date the plague had run its course in his neighbourhood but continued in other parts of the city. In early January the city began to terminate its contracts with the plague cleaners and gravediggers ('li monate'). As Giovanni Ambrogio and others realized, the plague-infected had better chances of recovery in the winter months. From data collected by the health board, he estimated that '1,400 between men and women' had either not been infected or survived and 700 had died, a mortality rate of one-third—almost three times the rate for Milan as a whole (17,000 in a population that may have exceeded 150,000).[82] Although the artisan began with purely secular reasoning he ended with the divine, alleging

---

[77] Also, Besta, *Vera narratione*, 18r, noted this famine as weakening Milanese resistance; the city spent 70,000 *scudi* feeding the city's poor in that year.

[78] The Venetian ambassador does not record the spreading to the Casina until after 5 August (Mutinelli, *Storia arcana*, I, 311).

[79] Clustering of household deaths within twenty-four hours of one another was a common plague pattern; see Cohn and Alfani, 'Households and Plague'.

[80] Also, see Bugati, *L'aggiunta*, 148.   [81] 'Le "Memorie" di Giovan Ambrogio', 13.

[82] See Besta, 'La popolazione di Milano', I, 596–7, who calculates Milan's population in 1592 as being between 142,000 and 150,000, including those recovering in hospitals and ecclesiastics. Before the plague of 1576–7 it was certainly greater.

that a serious plague returned to a particular place every fifty years because of God's need to punish.[83]

PADUA

Milan was not the only northern city to produce this new genre charting almost daily the 'progress' of plague to investigate attempts to cure and prevent it within the societal frame of government and Church. The notary Alessandro Canobbio tracked the progression of the plague from Trent through north-eastern Italy and then focused on his town, Padua, in 1576.[84] Unlike the Milanese writers, he introduced his pamphlet within a scientific and community controversy then brewing in Verona and Padua and soon to rage in Venice. His opening letter to the reader attacked the basic tenets of late medieval and Renaissance academic medicine:

I have sought to prove that the present pestilence has not proceeded from a malign influence [by which he meant the configuration of planets or other astrological events], nor from the malign constitution of air, despite what the scholars have said; rather I will rely on the experience of all that I have observed at this time . . . [85]

To do so, like the Milanese writers, Canobbio adopted a narrative approach. His five 'books' are divided chronologically and not by definitions, causes, preventative cures, diet, remedies, and the like. As with the Milanese, he saw Trent as the Italian source of this plague and its dissemination through northern Italy to the principal cities of Verona, Venice, Milan, and Padua. Canobbio, however, paid greater attention to developments in Trent than did any of the Milanese writers and gave an earlier starting point for its arrival. By his account, the exact moment and cause of the plague's entry was not certain. 'According to some', a foreigner selling various merchandise carried it there at the end of March 1574. Others argued that about the same time, merchants from Trent went to a fair at Bolzano: one died immediately and his goods carried the disease back to Trent.[86] But no more was heard of it until the following May when a merchant's wife died of plague and within three days others with whom she had been in contact died with the same symptoms. At first Trent managed to hide the infection from the outside world:[87] only after Saint John's day (June 24) 1575, when the disease had already spread to many houses, did Verona, Venice, and other places realize that plague had struck.

---

[83] 'Le "Memorie" di Giovan Ambrogio', 13.

[84] Canobbio, *Il successo*. He was a prolific writer with twenty-eight publications. His *Il successo* was published three times by three different presses in 1576 and 1577.

[85] Ibid., n.p.   [86] Ibid., 1r–v.

[87] Ibid., 1r: 'fra Trentini fin all'hora tenuta cosi secreta, che fuori non se ne sapeva cosa.'

The cities of northern Italy set barriers and guards against the importation of goods and the movement of people from Trent, which according to Canobbio had some success, but eventually plague spread to Verona in 1575 when a Tridentine soldier (*bombardiere*) at night swam across the Adige under chains guarding the city and passed into a house of a Veronese soldier in the parish of San Zeno. The Tridentine soldier died of plague in two days and infected the wife and two children of the Veronese, who died suddenly with the same pestilential signs. Immediately the magistrates of Verona locked the houses in the neighbourhood (*contrada*) of San Zeno, barricading it from the rest of the city. Nonetheless, 'within little time' more than twenty died and more than seventy houses in San Zeno were locked up. The citizens, 'full of incredible fear, began to flee in the thousands', peasants refused to supply the city, and with the flight of wool and silk manufacturers, the poor were left without work.[88] Soon death tolls mounted to twenty and twenty-five a day, and three hundred houses were locked.

Despite the rapid spread of the contagion with the usual signs, various doctors and others disputed that these were the results of 'true plague'. Canobbio added sarcastically: 'While they disputed what to call it, Death raged, striking one place then another'; the lazaretti filled up with the afflicted and the poor. Verona was abandoned by her neighbours, blocked from trade and travel.[89] On the other hand, Canobbio described favourably the initial rapid responses of Verona's magistrates, who initiated the necessary measures, regardless of what the doctors called the disease: charity was distributed to the poor, pressure was put on peasants to deliver produce to the city, two lazaretti were built outside the city, and doctors and barbers visited the plague-stricken regularly. By his account the moral reaction to plague was the opposite of that described by Panizzone Sacco for Milan: concubines left one another and returned to their legitimate partners; other sinners changed their ways, and many enemies 'voluntarily made peace'. Canobbio praised Verona's bishop for his diligence in organizing prayers and devotions through the city,[90] and at the end of October Verona was 'liberated' from plague.[91] With only two thousand deaths recorded in the city from all causes, Canobbio calculated that the city had weathered the storm well, noting that this annual mortality was not markedly above the average for a city Verona's size, a population of 90,000. At that moment, Canobbio reckoned that the contagion had passed to Venice, where the story became markedly different. Here it spread 'like fireworks [*un fuoco artificiato*]', its death

---

[88] Ibid., 2v. Canobbio's view is corroborated by legislation passed by Verona's Council of Twelve on 10 October 1575, which described the same consequences for the city's artisans and textile workers and which solicited charity from citizens to ease workers' plight; Archivio di Stato, Verona (hereafter ASVr), Archivio di Comune no. 89, 109v.

[89] Canobbio, *Il successo*, 2v.   [90] Ibid., 3r.

[91] The Venetian senate accepted Verona's liberation only on 2 November 1575; ASVr, Comune no. 89, 111v.

counts mounting from eighteen to thirty a day between December 1575 and May 1576.[92]

Book two, like most of the remainder of his tract, examines the transmission of plague more microscopically to and within Canobbio's home town, Padua, in 1576. By April it had spread through every place and neighbourhood in Venice as Padua looked on in 'fear of and sadness' for its 'mother city' but managed to keep plague from its doorsteps. According to Canobbio, this resulted from the city's vigilance, posting its best citizens ('*da' primarii cittadini*') as guardsmen.[93] Finally, on 3 April the plague slipped in, carried by a Venetian visiting a Florentine living in Padua, who died in three days. The case, however, was contained: by sequestering those with whom he had had recent contact, only a few cases of *petecchie* were recorded for the remainder of April and May.[94]

Canobbio then followed different stories in describing various means by which the plague may have seeped into the city. As his account suggests, all the reports may have been true. In a city Padua's size with its manifold and complex relations with the outside world, he reasoned, one single pathway of the disease's spread was unlikely. One report had it that a mattress infected with plague was brought into the city. By another, two lascivious women ('femine dishoneste') came to live in the parish of Santa Croce, where 'liberamente & inhonestamente' they mixed with the population spreading plague to 'a large portion of the borgo'. By Canobbio's reasoning these were not the plague's only sources: Venetians carrying the disease, especially noblemen and their servants, easily gained permission to enter, contributed to the contagion.[95] The plague then infected many other neighbourhoods.

By June Padua had locked more than twenty-five houses, and with temperatures rising Canobbio feared the worst. Schools were closed, religious feasts and processions banned, the city's saint's day fair cancelled, guild meetings prohibited, and the law courts closed. Beautiful furniture was piled high on streets and burned as infected goods. In these days a pamphlet circulated widely in the city, claiming that wicked ones (*sciagurati*) were spreading the disease intentionally with infected clothing and poisonous ointments (*untioni*) rubbed on door handles and knockers. Conobbio cast aside these rumours as arising from superstition and ignorance. Every day more cases of plague were discovered, especially in the neighbourhoods of the Jews. Conobbio did not, however, jump to anti-Semitic conclusions. Instead, he attributed the rise to their social conditions: they lived in the worst and most overcrowded quarters, 'squeezed into cramped and poorly aired houses (*in un'aria malinconica*) and were supplied corrupt water'.[96]

---

[92] Canobbio, *Il successo*, 3v–4r.   [93] Ibid., 5v.   [94] Ibid., 5v.   [95] Ibid., 5v–6r.

[96] Ibid., 7r–v. Similarly for the plague of 1656–7 in Rome, higher rates of plague mortality arose in the Jewish Ghetto: 13.8% versus 7.4% for the non-Jewish population; Sonnino, 'Cronache della peste a Rome', 39.

Canobbio gave details of the city's administrative structures during the plague and its allocation of charity. On 27 June the city passed ordinances hiring officers to control the plague and to care for the ill. On 1 July the city bought carts to transport the dead and afflicted, employed extra gravediggers, appointed other officials, and held elections to the health board.[97] He praised city officials for their 'grandissima carità' in caring for 'the poor plague-stricken' and those suspected of the disease. He described the mounting economic problems as direct and indirect consequences of plague: the commercial losses that resulted from cities cutting trade with Padua; mounting expenses for charitable contributions to the sequestered poor and to hospitals; the costs of employing new plague officials, which by August totalled one hundred counting cart drivers, gravediggers, plague cleaners, gate guards, but not those employed at the lazaretto.[98] Despite these darkening clouds, Conobbio again noted that doctors and many others in Venice continued to deny that the 'mortality' was 'peste', even though the numbers of *sospetti* grew daily.

Already, walled towns and villages in the *contado* along with 'the rest of the world' had abandoned Padua. Within the city, relatives and friends no longer visited one another, reluctant to enter their homes. When people walked the streets, they carried sponges soaked in vinegar in their mouths or hands.[99] Like Bisciola, Canobbio knitted stories of personal drama into his narrative of the plague's relentless death counts: a tailor whose two children died but had escaped was ordered to be sequestered; conditions were so bad in a tenement (*un Torazzo*) where fourteen families had resided in the Jewish quarter 'that not even the cats survived'. By July most citizens, merchants, and many well-off artisans left the city for nearby villages. 'Only the most miserable, deprived of all means of survival, remained, and most of them died. They lived in wretched houses [*casuccie*), locked up, and readily spread the disease to one another'.

With the summer's extreme heat came an 'insupportable stench'.[100] Canobbio recounted his rounds through the city, finding daily four to six houses per quarter where the doors had to be broken down to enter: 'all the residents were found dead in various positions displaying their last gestures, pleading for mercy'. In one he found a father still alive, transfixed holding his two dead children, one between his arms, the other lying on his breast. In others, he described infants still sucking the cold breasts of dead mothers; in still others, miserable children were kissing their dead parents or crying out for them. In contrast to the massacre within the city walls, where Canobbio claimed that of twenty plague victims only one survived, he praised the treatment of the plague-stricken in the city's lazaretto, where 'almost half the afflicted recovered'.[101]

---

[97] Canobbio, *Il successo*, 8r–v.   [98] Ibid., 9v–10r and 17v.   [99] Ibid, 9v.
[100] Ibid. 11v.
[101] Ibid. 13r. Similarly, the Venetian ambassador at Milan lauded the treatment of patients in Milan's lazaretto at least with the arrival of new servants at the end of September 1576; Mutinelli, *Storia arcana*, 326.

In August, the plague gained momentum: the plague dead rose to seventy a day, and the disease now spread to all neighbourhoods. Prominent citizens as those of the Stefanelli family, doctors, druggists, and city officials began to succumb.[102] Canobbio's initial optimism waned further; he described the miserable spectacle of the plague, the frequent transport of the poor suspected of plague to the lazaretto. At this point his text transformed into a personal diary centred on his own emotions as opposed to the previous clinical chronicling of plague. He pictured himself lost in a bad dream: 'for those like myself, writing in these times, it is as though I am writing a fable; something of make believe, or completely exaggerated, for nothing of these sad happenings could appear to be true'.[103] He described the miserable scenes that passed his door on a street that in one direction led to the lazaretto and in the other to the port where the infected were carried away. A father, his eyes cast down, was constrained to put his seven children in the boat to be transported from the city to the lazaretto. Two died on the way, another that night, and the other four within two days: 'I know no other scourge that could be so terrible'.[104] Conobbio continued:

Every hour I see little children of two or three years old, whose parents had just died, slowly marched away by city guards who paused at every step. Continuously I saw these miserable sights pass my door. Often I did not know whether I was dead or alive, healthy or plague-stricken. If I saw any bite of a flea anywhere on my body, immediately, I thought I had come down with the plague. If my children began crying, immediately I believed they had been afflicted, a little headache for an instant or some other plague symptom and immediately I thought the worst: the disease had struck.[105]

At this time, some doctors and druggists went round the city pushing their newly invented medications on desperate plague victims even though such practices had been prohibited. The dying no longer received the tears even of their relatives.

Book three describes further horrors of September when plague casualties reached ninety a day, the city reduced to habitation by the poor alone, the streets deserted. Again, Canobbio attacked the claims of academic physicians that the plague's cause was corrupt air. He countered that as plague deaths soared the air in Padua circulated freely with beautifully clear days and serene skies, that the climatic conditions 'famous authors' cited for the rise of plagues—humid, cloudy, and dark conditions with winds from the south ('venti d'Austro')—would finally come with the rains in November, the very moment when in 1576 a steep decline of the plague began.[106] Canobbio further concluded that one thing was beyond doubt: for this plague there had been no malign configuration of the planets.[107] The notary then made his own medical analysis based on 'experience and human reasoning', arguing that 'the contagion was so intense and subtle that it passed invisibly from one body to another, and, more amazingly, from animate bodies

---

[102] Canobbio, *Il successo*, 13v.   [103] Ibid., 13v.   [104] Ibid., 16r.
[105] Ibid, 16r.   [106] Ibid., 18r–v and also earlier in book I.   [107] Ibid., 19r.

to inanimate ones. Experience shows 'as if against human reason' that it also passes from inanimate bodies to animate ones'.[108]

Canobbio also challenged current Galenic thinking about comportment, humours, and complexions, observing that many of the poor with bad habits and complexion ('male diretti & male complessionati'), who from necessity had to care continuously for the plague-stricken, did so without falling ill. He raised medical mysteries that he could not explain such as why so many of the poor died, while those who served the afflicted—gravediggers, plague cleaners ('i smorbateri'), cart drivers and other officers in the city and at the lazaretto—for the most part survived.[109] He wondered why those who had isolated themselves in their homes, in monasteries, or in their villas nonetheless had fallen prey to the plague.

In the face of these complexities, Canobbio first turned to God but also observed that it was mostly the wretched, cripples, and similar sorts who were afflicted and of these only one in a hundred survived. He did not draw the conclusion that God had declared plague against the poor, that they somehow deserved such punishment. Instead, he focused on the way they were treated and attributed this to their plight: piled on plague carts head to toe, unclothed like beasts, and thrown onto public streets filled with filth and excrement. Fires that burned their corrupted goods harassed them further. With few to fight the fires, often they blazed out of control. At the same time, robbers made off with the rest of their property. Nor could city officials do much about these 'horrible spectacles'; already 'worn down and afflicted by fatigue and sadness . . . all remedies appeared now in vain'.[110] 'Neither science nor experience' seemed to make a difference; no matter what was tried, despite 'the thousands of ideas of Padua's head of state (*clarissimo Capitano*), various discourses, and many ordinances proposed and passed', matters worsened.[111]

Nevertheless, Canobbio continued to express confidence in doctors, druggists, and city officials. When the poor were sequestered outside the city and given food and medication, many survived. These methods, he estimated, had saved more than six thousand.[112] He reaffirmed that most of the afflicted were cured in the lazaretto, which he praised as being well governed and served by medicine. He lauded its governor and his officials, its location, architecture, and organization, and the Franciscans, who diligently tended to the spiritual needs of the infected.[113] He again contrasted this rule and discipline of the poor within the lazaretto, where food and other basic necessities were supplied, with the ill fate suffered by those who remained in the city. There, 'because of their unfortunate circumstances, wretched virgins, married women, and recent widows broke every rule of decency, exposing their most secret parts in public'. 'Out of necessity', they engaged in every sort of scandal and indecency.[114] He speculated that those

---

[108] Canobbio, 18v. Whether or not he had read Fracastoro's *De contagione* is uncertain; he does not cite him.

[109] Ibid. 19r.   [110] Ibid., 20r.   [111] Ibid., 20v.   [112] Ibid., 20v.

[113] Ibid., 21r–22v.   [114] Ibid., 22v.

cured in the lazaretto would have died had they remained in the city. Canobbio seized on one remedy that seemed to work—separation of the plague-afflicted along with their property from the healthy. Nonetheless, at the height of the plague in late September, his book three ends in near total desperation: 'now all could expect to die'.[115]

Book four continues 'with the calamities of this unhappy city', with great acts of devotion and saintly thoughts mixed with petty scandals. On the last day of September, plague even struck Padua's leader against the plague assault, its Capitano, Signor Alvigi Giorgio. One of Padua's most famous doctors, Capodivacca, was called to his bedside. Canobbio described almost hourly the Capitano's suffering, the course of the disease, his medical and spiritual treatment, and the stages of his convalescence. With the Captain's recovery, the city made immediate plans to build an oratory in the church of the Carmelites for its most holy icon of the Virgin. Work began on 11 October, 'bringing happiness for the first time in months to the miserable people of this unhappy city'.[116] For Canobbio, the occasion was miraculous: after months of not seeing more than two people walking down a street together and thinking most had died or fled to their villas or villages, he now saw four thousand men and women suddenly processing with the icon to its new home. Gun salutes (*artigliarie*), the ringing of all the city's bells, and the frail poor (*poverelli*) strumming all sorts of musical instruments accompanied the procession. That night the Podestà, city magistrates, and the deputies of the health board led a candlelit procession to place the Virgin's image on the high altar, and on that day plague deaths sank to fewer than thirty with no new cases of affliction. Canobbio read this as a second miracle. He also observed that many more were recovering from the illness than had been the case earlier.[117] On St Andrew's day (18 December 1576), the magistrates declared the end of plague, 'filling the *popolo* with incredible happiness'. Before describing the many festivals and processions of thanks that followed, Canobbio could not resist a second dig at the academics and their theories. The change in climate, of unusual hot and heavy air, humidity, and rain, that should have proved *molto maligna* and ripe for the spread of plague, instead marked its diminution and demise.[118] Although not a doctor, Canobbio wrote with confidence of what he had learnt from his medical experience of plague. His diagnosis turned on the plague's 'infallible signs', which matched closely working definitions seen in many sixteenth-century plague tracts as well as in the daily diagnoses of Milan's fifteenth- and sixteenth-century necrologies:

first vomiting, headaches, and fiery fever, then great thirst, backache and sometimes delirium. On the other hand, many cases of glandular swellings may arise without headaches or with little fever. In these cases the disease can be easily treated. Such cases

---

[115] Ibid., 24v.   [116] Ibid., 30r.   [117] Ibid., 30r–v.   [118] Ibid., 32v–33r.

have occurred often at the lazaretto, with two hundred or more returned safe and sound to their communities. The same has been observed in Venice.[119]

His fifth book began precisely on 29 October 1576 with the virtual end of the 'contagious disease', celebrated with three processions that required the participation of the 'entire *popolo*'. However, those from the countryside did not begin supplying the city with food or coming to market until 18 December. Around the same time, citizens who had left town began to return.[120] His final account of the composition of plague mortalities is more detailed than any Milanese account or even Ingrassia's painstaking survey. Plague deaths in the city, territory, and the lazaretto numbered 12,388; 179 were clerics; 96 nobles, 3,018 men of every age; 3,800 women, 220 Jews; in all 7,312 died in the city, and another 2,977 in lazaretto—1,964 were men and 1,013 women. The outlying villages counted 2,099 plague deaths. More than 5,000 houses in the city were marked as 'suspect' and presumably locked up. The city spent 50,000 ducats on plague relief. Canobbio, the notary, ends his tract in the same fashion as the great majority of doctors' plague tracts, with remedies. His, however, were categorically different from the doctors', at least of those before 1575, whose cures pertained to the individual. Canobbio's were on the societal level of public health: 'The most valiant remedy against this plague is to send the afflicted and their belongings to lazaretti and those suspected of plague from the city to the huts [*caselle*] made of wood.'[121] His advice to individuals concerned hygiene and cleanliness: keeping clean and orderly (*mondi*), changing clothes and rooms frequently, using various perfumes and fires from sweet-smelling wood to purify houses and clothes, washing your face with rose water and a little vinegar and carrying a ball and a sponge soaked in vinegar.[122]

VENICE

In addition to Besta and Cannobio, another notary wrote a plague *successo*, this one centred on Venice. By contrast, despite the ubiquity of notaries in Italy in almost every form of literary expression and especially chronicling, I do not know of a single notary writing a plague tract before 1575.[123] Like Panizzano Sacco's lament, Rocco Benedetti's *successo* did not paint a picture of a steadfast,

---

[119] Canobbio, 30v.   [120] Ibid., 33r.

[121] Ibid., 34r. The canon Jacopo Strazzolini in his 'Avvertimenti' at the end of his 1598 plague diary said much the same: 'When a case [of plague] is discovered in a house, the best remedy for saving lives is to cordon off the street and the houses that had had contacts with the infected house and to impose a quarantine of forty days throughout the city or village . . . .' (*La peste a Cividale nel 1598*, 46).

[122] Canobbio, *Il successo*, 34v.

[123] During the plague of 1400 at Pistoia, Ser Luca Dominici, then head of Pistoia's hospitals, tallied plague deaths within his chronicle (*Cronache di Ser Luca Dominici*). However, his chronicle was neither a plague tract nor a plague chronicle; see Cohn, *The Black Death Transformed*, 111 and 120.

rational defence against the plague, even though Benedetti wrote his tract after the 'liberation' of Venice with the solemn and gay celebrations already in train.[124] Venice's experience during the 1575–7 plague was the worst of any major city in Italy as measured by the number and proportion of casualties. Of a population of around 190,000, over 50,000 died, more than a quarter, and some have pushed the mortalities higher to 60,000, its worst demographic calamity since 1348.[125] Like Canobbio, Bendetti placed the blame squarely on the Paduan academic physicians and their devotion to Galenic theory.

As with other *successi*, Benedetti's began with Trent, traced the contagion to Verona and thence to Venice. By Benedetti's account, the initial reactions of the city's health board were sound. Immediately it set in motion its time-tested procedures of placing the plague-afflicted in the Old Lazaretto, the suspected under quarantine at the New Lazaretto, and burning contaminated goods: 'With their diligence in utilizing these tools and other good ordinances, the governors soon gained so much success that the city appeared plague free.'[126] This happiness was, however, short-lived, and the governors responded to rising plague mortalities with stricter measures. For eleven days they prohibited neighbours visiting one another and banned women and children from venturing beyond their neighbourhoods (*contrade*). The city executed what Benedetti called 'a Sicilian Vespers' on Venice's cats and dogs, 'rounding them up and killing them, which caused great screeching and howling throughout the city'. The massacre created an intolerable stench with the dead beasts littering canals: servants had to be employed to clean up the mess.[127]

These measures caused the majority of Venetians to hate the governors, and with the plague's resurgence, 'a battle brewed among the doctors examining the disease-stricken corpses: some argued it was plague; others that it was *petecchie* or other curable diseases'.[128] The Venetian governors sided with the plague deniers, since the people (*popolo*) greatly despised the consequences that would ensue for families declared plague-stricken as well as further stringent ordinances on movement and commerce. For Benedetti this was shallow, short-term opportunism: 'none could have fooled themselves into believing that these glandular swelling, carbuncles, or other pestilential signs could have possibly been a "humour" of the French disease, a worm, a disease, a cough, a bruise, or an old spot.'[129] Despite their denials, neither physicians, nor surgeons, nor barbers could be found to treat the inflicted except at exorbitant prices. The government then invited the 'most famous doctors' Mercuriale and Capodivacca from the University of Padua to come before the doge and College of Physicians

---

[124] Benedetti, *Raguaglio*, 479r–94v (Vatican pagination). Benedetti's *successo* was published by two other presses, one under another title with a smaller font as *Noui auisi di Venetia*. On other works by Benedetti such as the celebration of Lepanto victory and Henry III's ceremonious visit to Venice, see Fenlon, *The Ceremonial City*, 176, 179, 183, 263, and 267–8.

[125] See Chapter 1, nn. 74–5.   [126] Benedetti, *Raguaglio*, 3r   [127] Ibid., 2v–3r.
[128] Ibid., 3r.   [129] Ibid., 3r–v.

to diagnose the disease; they judged it to be a malignant disease but not plague. Reassured, the people were allowed to mingle without regard for contagion: 'once again they ventured freely from place to place'. Consequently, the fury of the disease intensified. Many began to doubt the doctors' judgement and held them responsible for their city's impending doom. The doctors responded by presenting the doge with a long written statement defending their diagnosis.[130]

At the beginning of July, 'the princes of Italy' in growing numbers began to ban Venice and its commerce. Almost all foreigners, the nobility, and the well-off left the city for their country estates. These included cloth merchants, who provided livelihood for two-thirds of the city, putting many out of work. Notaries (*scrivani*), judges, and other ministers of the state also fled, leaving behind only the miserable. With the summer's heat, 'every hour brought a new massacre; every day a major terror'. As with other authors of the *successi*, but hardly seen in physicians' plague tracts before 1575, Benedetti turned to his own experiences, thoughts and nightmares: 'as he walked down streets and crossed canals', he heard 'the cries, laments, tearful sobbing, screams, and howling of the afflicted and those who had lost love ones to the disease'. With his heart ripped apart by scenes of misery, he imagined in front of the church of San Marco seeing the prophet Jeremiah dressed in a sack and hairshirt (*celicio*) predicting further gloom for Venice: 'all its gates destroyed, its priests wailing, its virgins corrupted; the city overwhelmed by bitterness with none to console him; his friends contemptuous of him'. Waking from the dream, he concluded that 'no one in living memory or among the city's historians had witnessed any disaster as great as the present one now oppressing Venice'.[131]

He described the progress of the plague, its increased terror of assaults: 'fathers and mothers carried to their doorsteps by their children' and vice versa; 'their bodies shamefully stripped nude in the public forum, examined to diagnose whether they had died of plague'. Benedetti experienced personally the same: 'I had to carry away three of mine, that is, a mother, a brother, and a nephew, none of whom showed any signs of plague in life or in death.'[132] As a result, Benedetti was sequestered in his home for forty days. He spoke generally of the misery and strain of being locked up alone, some dying a terrible death without any recourse of help, with no one appearing for two or three days to take account of the dead bodies. Then the gravediggers (*pizzicamorti*) would arrive, 'breaking down the

---

[130] Ibid., 4r. Before the arrival of the Paduan academics the government vigorously attempted to play down or deny the presence of plague in Venice. As the official historian of Venice, Andrea Morosini, wrote, 'If noised abroad that the city was in the grip of a pestilential disease, terror would arise in every estate, customs revenue would be diminished, traders of Europe and Asia would recoil from the city, and enemies of the Republic would be incited to revolt' (cited in Fenlon, *The Ceremonial City*, 220). There is no direct evidence, however, that Mercuriale and others were following dictates of the Venetian government.

[131] Benedetti, *Raguaglio*, 5r.   [132] Ibid., 5r–v [483r–v] (BAV).

door or crawling through a window to find the dead in bed or sprawled on the floor or in some other place where the madness of death might have transported them'.[133] As frightening was the view of thousands of houses throughout the city with crosses posted on them and 'the horrible spectacle of great numbers of boats that sailed continuously back and forth, some to the New Lazaretto, others to specified sites beyond the city, laden with their miserable cargos of unhappy plague-stricken and contaminated goods and returning with cargos of poor widows and sad orphans'.

For Benedetti, 'these painted a sad and mournful picture of the Triumph of Death'; the Old Lazaretto was Hell, 'every side oozing with stench and intolerable disgust, continuous sounds of groans and painful sighs, clouds of smoke languishing for long periods in the air from the burning plague corpses'. Inside the hospital were the 'great waves of the afflicted, stacked three or four per bed, left mostly unattended because of the great scarcity of nurses, who left them food at the door but did little else than dump the dead from their beds into ditches'. The New Lazaretto was purgatory. There, patients received some attention and medicine, although hardly all their needs were served. Yet only about 10 per cent of the inmates died here, 'about a hundred a day lying on those smoky, stinking beds'. Benedetti then described the wooden huts, about five hundred in all at Vignole, which resembled the blinds of bird hunters ('capanne da uccellatori'). In the world of plague, Paradiso did not exist.[134]

Benedetti turned to other dismal details of the plague's administration, a site called Cavanella on the Lido made into a burial ground (*campo santo*) with deep ditches laid in layers first with corpses, then lye, then dirt; the need for immense public spending by the doge; the chaos of services and confusion of not knowing how to supply these services on this unprecedented scale.[135] Noblemen and citizens were deputized as makeshift officers for every *contrada* with responsibilities of reporting 'everything' to the 'presidents' of each sixth of the city (*sestiero*), of setting up night guards, protecting the property of those sent to the lazaretti, and curfews established under threat of severe penalties. He described the problems the mounting deaths posed for the city, expenditures for temporary hospitals and the maintenance of 'so many people' and a shortage of gravediggers; the city's need to rely on the lowest and most despicable sorts for these necessary services. Those imprisoned were offered freedom if they served time carrying plague corpses from their homes. Still, because of the great scarcity of such employees, plague cadavers remained in houses for two, three, even four days, and 'with the summer's big heat an intolerable stench' wafted through neighbourhoods, 'killing by its nausea'.[136] Others died of starvation and every sort of hardship. To raise money, the city imposed taxes on rents ranging from one to three *grossi* on houses and shops receiving over 25 ducats a year. According to Benedetti this middle-class tax succeeded in impoverishing

---

[133] Ibid., 5r.   [134] Ibid., 5v.   [135] Ibid., 6r.   [136] Ibid., 6r–v.

the rest of the city, now filled with 'an infinite number of widows and orphans without care'. The multitude was forced to sell their belongings at negligible prices.[137]

Benedetti records the medical debates that followed during these desperate summer months, and, like the plague pamphlets themselves that soared in number across Italy, those presenting ideas to the Venetian senate and the *sestieri* were not confined to the medical elite of physicians.[138] With a sense of approval, Benedetti reports the opinions of a 'famous preacher from the order of charity [*dell'ordine della Carità*]', the most Reverend Padre Fiamma, who argued that the city had been misled by Galenic notions: 'this plague had not come from the air, which was as good as ever'. Instead, it had clearly spread from the interaction and intermingling of people (*per la pratica e conversatione delle genti*). He proposed the sequestration of the city for fifteen days to cleanse and purge it of the disease. According to Benedetti, the rulers of Venice took the preacher's advice seriously and considered evacuating 100,000 from the city.[139]

Benedetti mentions that many others presented ideas before the senate such as astrologers with great hopes for a quick turn in the stars that would ensure good tidings. He was as leery of these notions as of orthodox Galenic medicine. Instead, as a notary he relied on what he observed: 'almost all those afflicted had tumours of various sorts' ('qualche tumore, Parotide, Brusco, o ghianussa, o Carbone'), and he reasoned that many of these ones had not stepped outside their homes and so could not have been exposed to changes in the skies. He singled out, however, one astrologer, Annibale Raimondo, as worthy of careful consideration and described his recent published work ('un discorso publico in Stampa'),[140] that pointed to water supplies as the vital conduit of the plague's spread in Venice.[141] Raimondo was certainly not the first to see the mixing of salt and fresh water as inducing pestilence in Venice;[142] nor was he alone in 1575–7 in seeing the flood of sea water into the wells of working-class neighbourhoods during storms of 1574 as key to understanding Venice's plague.[143]

Benedetti was less approving of others who 'everyday appeared before the doge, offering their secrets for liberating the city'—'preservatives, purgatives

---

[137] Benedetti, 7r.

[138] The openness of the Venetian health board to outside ideas and discussion is illustrated by Crotto's *Memoriale delle provisioni generali*, 6r, which includes his written exchanges with health-board officials. He reports that he also communicated often with them orally (*Da parole dette in voce*).

[139] Ibid., 7v.

[140] See Raimondo, *Discorso*. Born in Verona in 1505, he was also a doctor, a mathematician, and author of nineteen publications.

[141] Benedetti, *Raguaglio*, 7v–8r.

[142] See Wheeler, 'Stench in sixteenth-century Venice', 32; and *I Diarii di Girolamo Priuli*, IV, 21. Priuli's explanation for the 1509 plague, however, differed from Raimondo's. According to Priuli, the mixing of fresh and salt water corrupted the air, which then led to the 'mala dispoicitione' for human bodies.

[143] See for instance, Crotto, *Memoriale delle provisioni generali*, 4r and 7r.

[*ellectuari*], and medicines that upset [*distempervano*] the stomach and ruined one's constitution'.[144] A Flemish merchant promised to free the city in eight days if the healthy fasted, drinking only three *sorsi* of their own urine and for dinner eating only a little bread dipped in vinegar with rue.[145] Similarly, the afflicted were also to drink their urine morning and night, to make a plaster of their warm excrement to be applied to their swellings, and to 'keep the sore clean with urine until it healed'. Another named Anibale Goroldini from a village outside Brescia went to the Old Lazaretto loaded with large barrels of liquid to cure the plague-stricken, but along the way plague afflicted him and his assistant: they died in a few days.[146]

Benedetti made no distinction between these foreigners, who may or may not have been licensed charlatans,[147] and Venice's recognized pharmacists. If anything, he found the latter more ridiculous with their broadsheets advertising 'in capital letters' their 'excellent such and such that could preserve with certainty against the plague'. Despite their confidence in advertising, he noticed they stayed locked behind their shop doors and washed their customers' money in vinegar as soon as they took it. 'Among other things that happened [at this time] worthy of memory in this city', one of those who sold these preservatives was rumoured to have been producing gold in his home and left money to the city to build a museum with a library (*libraria Regia*).[148]

Benedetti scorned equally certain spiritual attempts to liberate the city. An unknown man appeared three nights straight dressed in a habit of a confraternity, a large cross in his hand, singing the Litany in a plaintive voice, which drew a wide following from all the city's neighbourhoods. In imitation, they processed to the church of San Rocco. But, 'despite their intentions', Benedetti argued, they only succeeded in spreading the disease further. Official processions were limited to the piazza San Marco, where every morning long lines of senators, nobles, and others of the *popolo* processed with a cross and a painting of the Madonna of Grace. Despite these pious efforts, the plague worsened especially among the poor but began to hit the rich and nobles, creating great fear among Venice's ruling elite. Benedetti was not, however, sceptical of all spiritual remedies. He saw the turning point with the doge's promise of 10,000 ducats to build a votive

---

[144] Benedetti, *Raguaglio*, 8r.

[145] According to records of the Consiglio dei Dieci, the state accepted a secret antidote that prescribed drinking one's urine first thing in the morning as well as other remedies proposed by non-physicians; Laughran, 'The Body, Public Health and Social Control', 223–5.

[146] According to Benedetti, *Raguaglio*, 8v, fifty-nine doctors lost their lives fighting the plague in Venice.

[147] See Gentilcore, *Medical Charlatanism*.

[148] Benedetti, *Raguaglio*, 8v. Another author sceptical of plague secrets then being peddled to Venice's health board was Crotto, *Memoriale delle provisioni generali*. In an entry of 10 October 1576, he approved the health board's decision 'to put aside all these offers of particular and universal secrets [and] to attend to cleaning houses and diligently washing, perfuming, and purging contaminated goods . . . .' (12r).

church dedicated to Christ, Our Lord and Redeemer, with a yearly procession beseeching pardon for the city's sins.[149]

In September matters improved in three *sestieri* but worsened in the other three. The Senate did not neglect relying on all remedies, divine and human. They decided to sequester all residents in their houses of the first three *sestieri* for eight days beginning on 7 October and to help the poor with public finances, granting each six *soldi* a day. They divided the city in two at the Grand Canal with a barrier constructed in the middle of the Rialto bridge with guards posted there and in every *contrada*. City deputies and other officers patrolled the three worst hit *sestieri* to ensure that all were supplied with basic necessities. Benedetti again reflected on his personal experience as a notary called to redact the last wills of the afflicted. The horror of these tasks troubled him: 'walking through the abandoned and wild streets he could hardly hold back his tears, often these sights made his hair stand on end, to think that such a great city, celebrated throughout the world for its commerce, could have been brought to such a miserable state.'[150]

The plan of dividing the city in two proved ineffective; the Senate deliberated for two days and extended the period of quarantine, but they also turned to spiritual solutions with processions praying for God's intervention. 'All were armed' with perfumed gloves, a handful of rue on the neck, a small sack of aromatic herbs, and arsenic placed near the heart, and all took theriac and other purgatives as preventatives.[151] By 20 October the fury of the plague subsided for several days, but then returned as strong as ever. The government turned more attentively to the needs of plague victims in their homes and to purging infected property by various means—sand, salt water, soaps, and perfumes with different methods for different materials. Everyday fights and quarrels sparked among plague cleaners and gravediggers, who squabbled over the stolen goods of the dead. Benedetti reports a tragic-comic execution of four thieves including a voluptuous twenty-two-year-old woman placed between the men at the two columns of San Marco on 3 November. One of the men asked for a jug of wine and offered the assembled crowd a toast ('un brindise'), which was courteously accepted. He drank his cupful and then said to the executioner that he could now die in peace. The woman then turned piously to an image of the Saviour, bringing the crowd to silence. She addressed Christ, Redeemer of the World, who like her was innocent but had patiently endured his bitter and ignominious death. She then prayed to the Lord for her fellow thieves ('i suoi crucissori') and prepared herself as though Christ were present to receive her in His arms. 'And so it seemed to the crowd that on that day on the wood of the cross she had been delivered to Paradise.'[152]

---

[149] On the Redentore and its significance in Venetian history, see among other places Fenlon, *The Ceremonial City*, ch. 10.

[150] Benedetti, *Raguaglio*, 9v–10r.   [151] Ibid., 10r.   [152] Ibid., 11r.

By 22 November the plague began to wane and the government began its promised plans for the church on the island of Giudecca. By 5 December the city seemed liberated, and on the first of January (1577) for the first time since 1575 no urban plague death was recorded. The city proclaimed its liberation: a procession open to all marched through the streets 'with incredible joy', 'hearts now emptied of all the past horrors'; 'everyone rejoiced together, singing masses and giving thanks to God'. On the eighth the doge went with the entire government, sang the *Te Deum*, had a solemn mass performed, and arrived at the new church to set its foundation stone. Benedetti ended his account on 28 June 1577 observing with satisfaction that the Venetians, 'restored from the damage of their suffering, once again funnelled into the law courts to litigate and strolled through city streets and squares . . . as though the great mortality and overwhelming tragedy that had just swept through their lives had never happened.' He found incomprehensible this total and sudden change in behaviour along with the now past horror that such a city had almost perished.[153]

VERONA

As the brief *progresso* of the Jesuit Bisciola shows, treatises that traced the almost daily transmission of plague in 1575–8 were not limited to secular writers. For Verona, the writer of its plague story was probably its bishop and, later, cardinal Agostino Valier, an orator and philosopher, with sixty-four surviving publications on theological subjects, statutes and decrees, Church discipline, rhetoric, charity, women and marriage, a life of Carlo Borromeo, a life of Verona's martyred saint Zeno, letters to his congregation, *ricordi*, and more.[154] Some have attributed the text to Gabriel Chiocco, Cancelliere of the Veronese health office.[155] He signs as the author of this tract's dedication to the citizens of Verona, but for the body of the tract no author is explicit. The work, however, centres on the spiritual, charitable, and administrative contributions of the bishop (throughout, referred to in the third person)—his assistance to the poor, his spiritual and moral guidance to the people of Verona, his prayers, processions, and consolation, his efforts to persuade concubines to enter holy matrimony and calm the ire

[153] Ibid., 12v.

[154] By Hyacinthis Ponzetti's count assembled in 1795, Valier wrote over 600 treatises; see Pullapilly, 'Agostino Valier', 308. Valier studied at the University of Padua alongside the physicians Bernardino Tomitano and Bassiano Landi, who also wrote plague tracts. Unfortunately, Pullapilly's article does not mention the 1575-6 plague tract that concerns Valier's role during the plague. In fact, Pullapilly hardly mentions the plague except for Valier's pastoral letter of consolation and thanksgiving addressed to his congregation at the end of 1575 for the liberation of Verona (314).

[155] The Wellcome Library has catalogued this work under Chiocco, and Palmer, 'The Control of Plague', 240, has followed their assessment. A hand copy of this publication made in 1745 (conserved in ASVr, Sanità, no. 33) also attributes it to Chiocco. However, Edit 16, the Vatican Library, the Marciano in Venice, and other Italian libraries name Valier as its author.

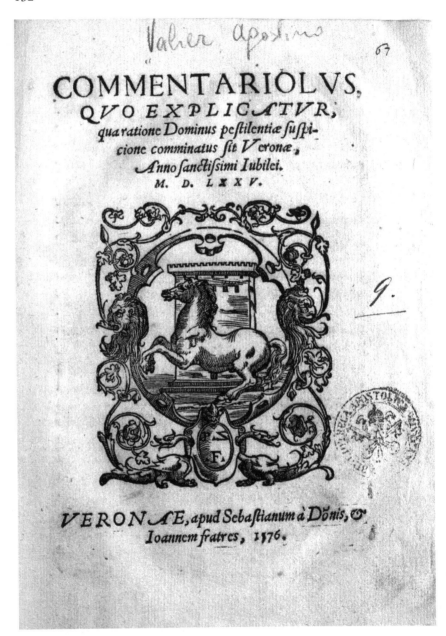

Valier Agostino

COMMENTARIOLVS,

QVO EXPLICATVR,

qua ratione Dominus pestilentiæ suspi-
cione comminatus sit Veronæ,
Anno sanctissimi Iubilei.
M. D. LXXV.

VERONÆ, apud Sebastianum à Dōnis, &
Ioannem fratres, 1576.

Illustration 2. Agostino Valier, *Commentariolus*.

of God, his building of plague huts ('quedam turguriola') in the parish of San Zeno beyond the city walls, his help sequestrating the ill from the healthy, his assistance at the city's lazaretto, and his love ('magno amore') and charity for the poor.[156] The text claims that 'in his opinion', the bishop was 'first in line' to encourage and console the dejected souls of the poor and fearful. Everyday he marched through the city and 'even visited the plague-stricken'.[157] The state archives testify to this service and public veneration of it: eight years after the plague, the city government of Verona, its health board, and the counsellors of the city's principal hospital, San Giacomo della Tomba, commemorated his charitable services during the plague for his governance of the city's hospitals, where the poor, both foreign and native, had been 'continuously' sheltered and feed.[158]

In addition, he called the city's monasteries for assistance to sing masses for the poor and afflicted and organized parish priests to say daily masses for their parishioners and deliver other spiritual services to the plague-stricken from the safety of the street and through windows.[159] He wrote to cardinals and to Pope Gregory XIII to gain their benediction for the people of Verona,[160] visited parishes and solicited charity for the poor, raising thousands of gold ducats. He even contributed the greater part of his own revenues to the poor during the plague.[161] In November (1575), he wrote again to cardinals and others seeking aid and to the Venetian senate beseeching it to lift its embargo on the city because of 'this terrible pestilence that should remain nameless' ('horribilissimo pestilentiae nomine non esse nominandam')—no doubt a barb aimed at the academic doctors of Verona and in anticipation of the bigger controversy stemming from Galenic logic to engulf Venice the following year. By contrast, Chiocco appears only once in the body of this tract, also in the third person, and there only as recording the number of plague dead in the winter months of 1575:[162] his authority and expertise—the workings of the health board and their reforms—are hardly mentioned.[163]

---

[156] Valier, *Commentariolus*, n.p., 67r–87v (BAV). I have used my own pagination beginning with Chiocco's dedication as 1r.

[157] Ibid., 9v. From the moment of his arrival as bishop of Verona, Valier reorganized the city's charitable organizations, beginning with the parish and its duties assisting the poor, sick, and aged; see Pullapilly, 'Agostino Valier', 313.

[158] ASVr, Sanità, no. 33, 202r.   [159] Valier, *Commentariolus*, 6r.

[160] Ibid., 7v. Ugo Buoncompagni, the future pope, had been Valier's friend and regular correspondent in the 1560s; both were members of the Accademia delle Notti Vaticane founded by Carlo Borromeo; see Pullapilly, 'Agostino Valier', 311–12.

[161] Palmer, 'The Control of Plague', 303.

[162] Valier, *Commentariolus*, 12v: 'Nulla die cadavera excesserunt numerum triginta sex . . . narrabat Gabriel Chiocus vir bonus, et scriba diligentissimus, qui eo in munere Cancellarii officio fungebatur.'

[163] In addition, this text recalls certain facts and themes Valier presented in his shorter *Lettera consolatoria* of 27 October 1575. In both works he cites the population of Verona as 70,000 or more and notes that, given such a large city and large diocese, few had died. In the letter, most likely from the health-office statistics, he also records that only 850 had died, or fifteen a day—fewer than in most years. Moreover, the character of the disease is described similarly in both texts as highly contagious and concentrated in the families of the poor, among which entire families were wiped out in a few days.

Like other authors of *successi*, this one (whom I will now assume was Valier) sought to trace the disease's transmission to his city and began with Trent.[164] For four months after its appearance there, Verona was able through God and administrative controls to keep the plague beyond its gates. But in July, despite the vigilance of city authorities, plague entered, transported, Valier maintained, down the Adige. According to him, 'the disease with swellings' began in the parish of San Zeno just inside Verona's city walls. He concluded the disease was plague not just because of the signs but also because of elementary epidemiological patterns of the plagues seen since the late Middle Ages and confirmed in early modern records.[165] In Valier's words: 'four, five, or more died in the same household with only a few days between them':[166] 'it was astonishing and horrendous to see the plague sweep so swiftly through these households, consuming the vast majority of them in a matter of days'.[167] Yet, despite these patterns some doctors in Verona, as in Padua, Venice, and Palermo, denied the disease was plague. 'With the great fear of contagion', the city convened a meeting of Verona's doctors (almost a year before a similar one occurred in Venice), where 'the talented doctor' Lodovico Lazisi argued with logic anticipating Mercuriale's and the Paduan professors' at Venice: because the disease infected only the *populos* and struck down only the poor, it could not be 'true plague' but must have been food poisoning. Moreover, the conditions of its rise did not conform to other antique theories: instead of a hot and humid summer, the previous summer (1574) had been temperate and dry.[168] Unlike the situation in Venice a year later, 'almost all the local doctors and surgeons of Verona rose up [*insurrexerunt*]' against Lazisi, affirming that the disease without doubt was plague ('pestilentissimum esse morbum').[169]

Yet, 'within a few weeks', opinions turned when, 'among other celebrated physicians', Alessandro Landi, Girolamo Giulari, and Lodovico Fumanelli supported Lazisi. Others then followed such as the later hero of numerous Veronese plague verses (as well as of Valier by the end of this tract), the town's podestà Niccolò Barbarigo,[170] and other city magistrates.[171] Several doctors, according to Valier, maintained that it was not a new epidemic but the acute disease that had struck Brescia in 1570. It had lingered on, they maintained, in the countryside and was contagious as evinced by the fact that it infected those within the same household but could not be plague because it struck down almost exclusively the poor. The disease was acute but not spread through corrupt air (afflicting

---

[164] Ibid., 4r.   [165] Cohn and Alfani, 'Households and Plague'.
[166] Valier, *Commentariolus*, 4v.   [167] Ibid., 5r.   [168] Ibid., 4v.   [169] Ibid., 4v.
[170] Although a civil servant, Barbarigo had been trained in the Arts Faculty at Padua by famous doctors such as Tomitano. See Palmer, 'The Control of Plague', 271–4; Rodenwaldt, *Pest in Venedig*, 98; Babinger, 'Barbarigo, Niccolò'; and Laughran, 'The Body, Public Health and Social Control', 211–12. Barbarigo had been the patron of Mercuriale and Capodivacca, had intervened on their behalf, was their intermediary with the doge, and condemned the Venetian health board during the controversy over plague in the summer of 1576.
[171] Valier, *Commentariolus*, 5r.

all) and for that reason too was not plague. Furthermore, it hit some villages but bypassed others; therefore, it could not be plague by definition since true plague was dependent on changes in air, afflicting all within vast regions.[172] Others went further, arguing that this supposed acute fever was hardly contagious, since it supposedly infected only those sharing the same bed ('ab illorum qui in lecto iacerent, familiaritate').[173]

Some said that the appearance of glandular swellings had been exaggerated. Thomas Bovius 'vir ingenio', author of a number of publications,[174] argued that the disease was not to be called plague because in the past four months the city's death books had recorded only twenty-nine bodies in which carbuncles were seen and attested by surgeons. Even though they also reported twenty-three other cases with glandular swellings ('aliis glandulas quasdam'), forty-four with the small bumps or spots, another thirty who died with various other tumours, and another thirty whose bodies had turned black and blue ('nigredine vero & livore confecta cadaver'). But mostly along with Lazisi these physicians turned to Galen arguing that the disease was not plague because it failed to fulfil his definition of a 'popular' disease (one that afflicted all classes): nobles remained unaffected, and only the lower plebs caught it. These arguments, however, did not convince the bishop, and, as he reported, the horrible plague gained momentum. Doctors, he tells us, also cited Marsilio Ficino's famous plague tract to substantiate their denials: the fact that the pestilential signs appeared was of no importance.[175] According to Valier, the disease was plague and also one that affected principally the poor, which had characterized this disease for at least a century. For those unfortunate few afflicted among the elites, he reported their sad stories, such as the plague death of the judge (*iuris consultus*) Petro Zaibanti, who 'with his most unhappy hands' buried his four children before meeting his own end.[176]

Valier reported the amounts raised in private charity from merchants and nobles spent on the lazaretto, plague huts, and charity to the poor, listing by name the major contributors as though a roll card of honour.[177] All was not, however, praise. At times, his tone recalls Panizzone Sacco's complaint. He detailed the crimes against the afflicted—theft of clothing and other property of the downtrodden and plague-stricken;[178] the insurrection of two strategic communities for communication and trade, Peschiera (on Lago di Garda) and Legnago, against their 'mother city',[179] the Venetians' decision to cut off all commerce with Verona and the consequences for Verona's labouring poor, the

---

[172] Ibid., 5r.   [173] Ibid., 5v.

[174] Tommaso Zefiriele Bovio, a doctor and astrologer, with six publications according to Edit 16, was born in Verona in 1521 and died there in 1609.

[175] Ibid., 9r.   [176] Ibid., 11v–12r.

[177] A decree passed by Verona's Council of Twelve beseeched citizens to assist the poor and those out of work because of the suspension of trade and industry, especially in silk production and other textiles; ASVr, Comune, no. 89, 109v, 10.x.1575.

[178] Valier, *Commentariolus*,

[179] Ibid., 6v. On these two towns, see Pasa, 'Quadri urbani', 144–5.

venality of pharmacists and surgeons who without pause profited from their portions and pills;[180] 'the many tumults, acts of fraudulence, theft, and sorcery [*aliqua veneficia*]'. Those from Vicenza and Padua refused to cross the territory of Verona. Illicit marriages increased. At first surgeons refused to inspect plague corpses, leaving commoners to make the crucial judgements on causes of death. Doctors did not grant even a minimum of assistance. The building of Verona's plague hospital of San Giacomo, for which funds had been allocated, languished, and, once built, was incapable of performing its services adequately: its ministers refused to fulfil their responsibilities. Even as the plague toll mounted to 3,000, Veronese doctors continued to call the disease a malignant fever that spread only within households with point-like bumps ('lenticulae & puncticula') and not by the corruption of air. Instead, the fevers arose from corruption of humours alone.[181]

The end of his treatise, however, turned to praise, commemorating (as with the later Veronese plague poetry) the podestà's adept handling of the crimes and threats to the city, his ability to obtain subventions for grain to feed the city and distribute it to the poor at low prices, saving them from utter misery.[182] Unlike other plague writers before 1575 who were clerics (and especially bishops or humanists such as Petrarch), Bishop Valier did not frame the tragedy of plague within clichés of *contemptus mundi*: a blessing in disguise that released mankind from its earthly chains.[183] Nor did he offer the usual justification for plague, as God's scourge and need to punish. Such justifications had been seen not only in religious plague tracts but also in the sophisticated writings of university-trained physicians, including the Palermitan *Protomedico* Ingrassia, as well as in the writings of lay observers, such as the *popolano* Giovanni Ambrogio of Milan.[184] Instead, Valier strove to help spiritually and corporeally the afflicted to survive, passing daily through the city to visit the stricken, seeking to console the dejected and those without resources, and to comfort the frightened. He called together Verona's parish priests, exhorting them not to abandon their flocks but to attend to their spiritual needs. Like Borromeo, he also had the priests' well-being and survival in mind, counselling them on various means for avoiding contagion such as consoling the afflicted from the street or speaking to them through windows. With the city's liberation from plague, over 30,000 gave their thanks and devotion. Like Benedetti and commentators elsewhere, the bishop was astonished to find that 'within the extremely short period of three months' the city had recovered and returned to its pristine beauty.

---

[180] Valier, *Commentariolus*, 6v–7r.

[181] On the concept of bodily humours and disease in Aristotle and Galen, see Temkin, *Galenism*, 17–18, and 103–4.

[182] Valier, *Commentariolus*, 16r.

[183] Such works certainly continued into the sixteenth century; see for instance *Il vero e santo rimedio*, 10v–11r.

[184] 'Le "Memorie" di Giovan Ambrogio', 13; see above 115–17.

OTHER FORMS OF *SUCCESSI*

Works attentive to the topographical details of the spread and development of the 1575–8 plague were also narrated from places where the plague threatened but did not arrive. In 1576, the Perugino historian Vincenzo Tranquilli charted plagues and prodigies over 2,311 years of Italian history with the remedies and laws used to confront them.[185] But he gave greatest attention to one plague, the one that stimulated his compilation and that threatened Italy top to toe in 1575. Tranquilli traced this plague from the Levant, where it had been 'grandissima' and recounted briefly the ordinances of the Venetian Senate to sequester goods and isolate the infected in the city's lazaretti. By his reckoning the plague spread from the 'hiding and secret selling' of infected goods. In Verona and Mantua, 'it was hoped that passing good laws' would contain it, but in both cities and especially Mantua, the plague entered despite such measures and began to rage by April 1575. Tranquilli reported that doctors in Mantua denied the pestilence was 'true plague', as would happen later in other northern cities. The disease, they argued, came from eating cheap fish caught or gathered from a part of the lake that had dried up and thus the plague attacked the poor alone. Tranquilli, however, never doubted that the disease was anything but 'true plague'. For Sicily, he reported less, but unlike many of the notaries and doctors who chronicled this plague's progress in northern cities, he showed greater awareness of its southern threat and transmission. By 1575, he noted, most places on the island except Catania had suffered. He then turned to his own city, which because of the threat from the north and south, elected twenty gentlemen as the priors of a health board to pass laws and measures to prevent the plague from entering. As far as the surviving printed sources reveal, they were successful.[186]

Although I have not yet found examples of physicians writing the new *successi* as such, the new concerns about contagion and detailed plotting of the plague's transmission in 1575–8 was not limited to those outside the medical profession. University-trained physicians such as the Mantuan doctor Giovanni Battista Susio,[187] a doctor of Salò, Andrea Gratiolo, a doctor of Pieve Santo Stefano, Jacopo Tronconi,[188] Tommaso Somenzi from Cremona,[189] and the Venetian physician and later professor at Padua, Alessandro Massaria, opened their plague tracts with new sections tracing the plague's transmission to and through Italy. For instance, Massaria began his tract by mapping the plague's transmission over the Alps to Trent in June 1575, estimated that 6,000 in Trent had died from the disease by November, that it reached Verona in July, Mantua in September, Milan, the following year, Venice in June 1576, and Padua in July.

---

[185] Tranquilli, *Pestilenze che sono state in Italia.*   [186] Ibid., 21–2.
[187] Susio, *Libro del conoscere la pestilenza*, non-paginated preface and 56.
[188] Tronconi, *De peste*, 1r.   [189] Somenzi, *De morbis*, 1r–3r.

Like the authors of *successi*, he charted the 'progress' of the plague from the health board records in his home town—Vicenza—where 1,098 died during the first year of plague.[190] As with the *successi*, Massaria structured his medical tract chronologically and drew on specific clinical cases or tales he had heard, such as a wife and all her children dying in the same household, all within two days, all with tumours and little black bumps (*papularium*) in various parts of the body. These stories were told, not so much to capture interest or to fascinate but to examine whether the disease was plague with its combination of epidemiological and symptomatic traits—quick death, household clustering of deaths, headaches, continuous fever, vomiting, glandular swelling, and bumps.[191] He then turned to the 'terrible disputes' that broke out in various cities, especially Mantua, over whether the disease was 'true' plague.[192]

Such chronological frames with specific stories grafted onto them also figured in verse, as with a poem by a translator from a prominent Umbrian medical family, from Florence, who had recently arrived in Venice. Borgaruccio Borgarucci celebrated Venice's liberation from the plague, but he began with the specific causes of this plague and continued chronologically with its spread, the 'heresy' that broke out between the Paduan and Venetian doctors on whether the disease was *petecchie* or 'true plague', the flight of the nobility, the closing of shops and barring of trade, the plying of 'secret medicines' by doctors, druggists, and charlatans,[193] the mounting of the dead, many of whom were thrown into ditches, 'the smell of the thick putrefaction of the air', increases in theft, the new administrative organization of the Venetian *contrade*, enforcement of law and order, increases in the numbers of 'the poor, naked, dirty, and mistreated', the eventual spread of plague to the nobility, the spending of 10,000 *zecchini* on the temple (the future Redentore), laws for cleaning clothes, burial, and care in homes, and finally the plague's decline, the 'white page' of the health board's register of deaths on 1 January, when for the first time in almost two years no plague-deaths were recorded. Jubilant but humble celebrations followed; the doge led processions in humility without his crown. Merchants once again engaged in 'big business', and now infused with great happiness, 'the people returned to play'.[194]

***

These tracts fail to substantiate a recent generalization about the 'paradox of plague literature': that 'the most detailed and realistic descriptions of plague' from Boccaccio to Defoe were written by authors who lacked personal knowledge of the disease.[195] All the authors described above not only witnessed the plague of

---

[190] Massaria, *De peste*, 3v.   [191] Ibid., 1r–2r.   [192] Ibid., 7r; also see Chapter 6.

[193] On plague drugs and charlatans in Italian medical life, see Gentilcore, *Medical Charlatanism*.

[194] Borgarucci, *L'afflition di Vinetia*. He came from a prominent medical family; his oldest brother, Giulio, migrated to London, where he became the physician of prominent aristocrats in Queen Elizabeth's court including William Cecil; Borgaruccio's other brother, Prospero, wrote a plague tract in Venice to be examined below; also see Firpo, 'Borgarucci', 567.

[195] Amelang, *A Journal of the Plague Year*, 26.

1575–8 first hand; they struggled passionately against it in daily acts of charity, in administrative roles on health boards, or with medical care to the afflicted. From these activities, as we have seen, they also became embroiled in disputes with governments and the medical establishment about the philosophy and theory of epidemics. In so doing, they broke from previous ways of presenting plague either of the physician's plague manual, the chronicler's static overview, or the theologian's silver-lining of *contemptus mundi*. Formed in the plague crisis of 1575–8 a new genre of plague writing was invented simultaneously across northern Italian cities. It was revived with Italy's next big plague wave in 1629,[196] and would later produce celebrated works of plague literature by Defoe, Manzoni, and Camus. Rigorous reporting of government statistics from plague burials to average sums governments spent on plague rations formed the backbone of these sixteenth-century narratives that then spilled into sentiment, illustrating sudden changes in the collective psychology as well as the daily trauma the authors themselves endured.

In their efforts to understand the disease and learn lessons to contain it, these writers also anticipated the discipline of epidemiology born in the nineteenth century that turned on detailed and precise tracking of diseases, such as yellow fever, and their modes of dissemination taken from rumours, stories, statistics, and direct observation.[197] The literary products of these sixteenth-century plague fighters went beyond telling stories; they arose from medical debates and opinions then swirling through Italy in 1575–8 that affected policy, commerce, and the lives of thousands. Through these narratives they argued from and for the observable, charting the disease's raging contagion and corresponding need for public health authority and policy, whose principal remedies focused on the separation of the plague-stricken from the healthy and decent care for the poor and afflicted.

[196] For the remainder of the sixteenth century, however, I know of only one plague *successo* of the sort seen from 1575 to 1579—that of Cividale's canon and curate Jacopo Strazzolini—but it was not published until the nineteenth century; Brozzi, *Peste, fede e sanità*.

[197] For disease tracking in the nineteenth century, see Coleman, *Yellow Fever in the North*, esp. 175, 182, and 194.

5

The 'Liberation' of the City and Plague Poetry

As with examples seen in the last chapter, the plague of 1575–8 gave birth to another literary form of plague writing, the *liberatione della città* or *liberatione della peste* in both prose and verse. The pope,[1] medical doctors,[2] and those who proclaimed to be 'crude and humble', lacking in literary talent as with an anonymous writer locked in solitude in Venice's Franciscan friary [Fratta] during the plague[3] or the Florentine exile Borgarucci, who apologized that his liberation poem was his first publication. Nonetheless, these new-born plague writers felt emboldened to write, and their efforts were published. Often these were songs, poems, prayers, or broadsheets of little more than a page but were grounded in the specific chronological developments of a city. I have found only one plague publication with liberation in its title before the 1575–8. Written during the previous plague in northern Italy of 1555–6, it was, however, strikingly different from those, spurred on by the next and more devastating plague of 1575–8. The place and time of *Il Vero e Santo Rimedio spirituale contra la peste . . . e così fu liberato dalla pestilenza*[4] reports nothing specific about the plague in Venice or Padua in 1555–6. Instead, the work is a consolation prayer, preaching the Christian virtues of death, portraying those who have died, not only in plagues but in wars, earthquakes, and famine, as the lucky ones, 'liberated from the prison of the world'. This anonymous author carried the implications of Christian *contemptus mundi* beyond that of the mendicant preachers or of Petrarch several centuries earlier: 'The dying children are liberated from the danger of aging, when it would have become easy for them to fall into sin; instead, they have died preserving the prize of their temperance and innocence.' 'Other beautiful fruits of this plague season' allowed the healthy to show charity towards the afflicted. Despite the 'liberation' in its title, little relief or praise was allowed for the living.

The fifteen 'liberations' I have found drafted at the end of the 1575–8 plague conveyed the opposite. They gave thanks for surviving the ghastly punishments of plague, not for perishing in it.[5] These liberation songs, prayers, and tracts were largely Venetian (ten of them); two were from Milan, one by

---

[1] [Gregorii PP], *Il sommario del Giubileo.*   [2] Glisenti, *Oratione divotissima.*
[3] *Canzone sopra la città di Venetia liberata da la peste.*   [4] See Chapter 4, n. 136.
[5] I found these principally in BAV, R.I.IV.1551; several have yet to be entered into Edit 16: for instance, Ionni, *Carmen. De urbe Veneta pestilentia liberata*, no. 39; and *Oratione al Signore Iddio per la liberatione del male contagioso*, no. 46.

Panizzone Sacco described earlier, another from Milan's inquisitor, the bishop of Cremona, a third from Verona, one for Palermo, and a fourth from the pope for Italy as a whole. To take one example: *La Liberatione di Vinegia* published in Venice in 1577 at the back of Rocco Benedetti's Venetian *Raguaglio* was penned by the little-known Muzio Lumina. Like Benedettii's *Raguaglio*, this work charts the Venetian experience chronologically: the arrival of plague in Venice dated precisely to 21 July 1575; its peak in September 1576, and the Senate's declaration of the plague's end on 21 July 1577. The author then describes in minute detail the processions: visits to various churches, votive offerings, and artistic embellishments constructed for that day of liberation. In contrast to the *contemptus mundi* literature, Muzio celebrated the material world and the collective exhilaration of survival. He described the construction of a new door for the Venetian church of the Capuchins, 'covered masterfully with minute leaves that climbed an image of a tree trunk'. From the door 'fine and very expensive cloth covered a long passageway that led to the spacious choir, beautifully decorated and adorned with gold.' Fine rays emanated from its centre on the high altar with an image of Our Lord 'painted by a masterful hand', and a back ('spalliere') made of gold and a frame ('seda') of silver.[6] He described other streets and palaces covered in cloth and with 'innumerable banners, standards, tapestries, and shields decorated with the arms of the health board of Venice' and other paintings created for the event. In one 'by an excellent Master doctors were treating the plague sores as a bearded man looked on filled with great amazement as if to say such a horrible sign has never before been seen'; in it the Lord was 'flanked on one side by the genuflexing Donzella, her hands tightly grabbing the cross, and on the other by San Rocco, one hand on his breast, the other blessing the afflicted flock crushed by the present misery'. Sixteen further paintings of popes were placed above it and unveiled with a fanfare of trumpets, tambourines, and other musical instruments: while 'the skies opened with a comforting ray of sunshine; a soft west wind [*Zefito*] blew in a new air of happiness'.[7]

After God, Lumina praised the Venetian government: 'under its fortunate rule and wise ordinances the city had been cleaned of the contagion'. He described the rulers' wish to display their happiness through works of art and a procession of liberation that went to the Scuola of Santa Maria della Carità, where 'an infinite number of candles were lit to honour God'. They then marched to numerous other *scuole* and shrines, the clergy and laity in tow. Lumina carefully counted their standards and described the jewelled-encased relics they carried, detailing the clothing worn for the occasion by the doge, ambassadors, and senators as 'the sound of artillery fire, trumpets, tambourines, and the songs of the *popolo* gloriously and instantaneously struck the air'.[8] He ended his happy account in astonishment: 'Lord, having witnessed the plague in Venice, I would have

6 Lumina, *La liberatione di Vinegia*, 476v (BAV).   7 Ibid., 477r–v.

8 Ibid., 477v–8r.

never believed that so many could have survived. Now, it seemed the population suddenly doubled. With such a great throng of people, it was difficult to imagine how they all could be contained even within the spacious square [*campo*] and on the balconies and sun roofs of the palaces.' According to Lumina, the crowd covered the entire length of the Grand Canal. 'Such was the crown of this liberation, dated at Venice, 22 July 1577.'[9]

We have already seen how Olivero Panizzone Sacco's 'Gubileo' for the 'liberatione della contagiosa infermità pestilentiale', celebrated on Saint Sebastian's day, 1578, suddenly shifted the perception of his plague experience from one of governmental corruption and inadequacy and wickedness on the part of the populace to praise and rejoicing. After God, Panizzone Sacco, like Lumina, praised the city's secular forces for liberating Milan, singling out individual governors, doctors, and health workers for their valiant and courageous service. Ultimately, his praise redounded on the citizens of Milan as a whole. This tract, too, was a celebration of human survival. The longest 'liberatione' and praise of a city's plague leaders, however, comes from Sicily and from a doctor. Dedicated to the health board of Palermo, it celebrated every member ('illustri Heroi') for freeing Sicily from this 'frightful monster': 'the fierce and untamed beast' that had converted the author's 'dear and sweet homeland from happiness to misery, from laughter to tears'.[10] Girolamo Branchi (Branci)—cavaliere, doctor, poet, and a magistrate of Palermo—praised these health officials and other rulers—from 'wise senators' to fathers of households for 'their heroic and immortal deeds' as administrators and counsellors, 'expediting all that needed to be done': 'you are the new founders of the city' and, at the same time, 'the true conservators of the greatness of this city'. With liberation from plague on 22 July 1576 'a new life and spirit' was celebrated, 'the city now dressed in happiness'.[11]

PLAGUE POETRY

These 'liberation' tracts were not the only literary forms invented during the 1575–8 plague to celebrate the deeds of individual bureaucrats and rulers and to express collective relief in surviving plague. This plague stimulated a rush of a new form of plague poetry, many yet to be entered into the Edit 16 database, and others, no doubt, awaiting discovery. One collection from Verona written in the late stages of their plague in 1576 contains as many as thirty-five poems.[12] Other than prayers and Baravalle's 'History of the plague in Padua in 1555', to

---

[9] Lumina, 478v.   [10] Branchi, *Oratione . . . fatta per la liberatione*, 3r (in text).

[11] Ibid., n.p. (13r–18v).

[12] The count may be higher; it is difficult to distinguish when one anonymous poem ends and another begins in this collection: *Raccolta delli componimenti*. Still other poems on the 1576–7 plague in Verona are found in the Vatican's miscellanea R.I.IV.1551, several in manuscript such as no. 26, *Canzone di M. Girolamo Verota*.

be discussed shortly, I know of only two publications of plague poetry in the sixteenth-century Italy before 1575. For earlier plagues, not even short songs or liberation pieces celebrated their end in 1511, 1523, or 1528, and certainly nothing of the character of the Latin and vernacular poems produced in Milan, Mantua, Venice, and Verona with allusions to Herculean deeds, honouring their health-board directors, podestà, judges, and citizens.

Furthermore, the 1575–8 plague verse shows great variety, from published prayers[13] to epic poems on combating the plague.[14] There was a compilation of poems by Venetians who had left the city because of the plague and a selection of 'the most beautiful and bizarre rimes and sayings [*motti*] found scribbled on the walls of locked shops' by the plague victims inside.[15] One poem, an ode to Apollo, even appears within the plague legislation of Milan in 1577.[16] In addition to these free-standing publications of plague poems, often verses penned either by the authors or by others introduced plague tracts in prose published during the 1575–8 epidemic. For instance, Branchi's *Oration presented for the liberation of his country from plague* led off with three sonnets by three gentlemen in praise of the author, followed by the author's 'protest' in verse against their flattery, and his oration finished with four further poems of his own plus two more, one by a Sicilian gentleman, the other by a Greek doctor and canon, again in praise of the author.[17]

Of course, the Black Death and its successive strikes of the later fourteenth century produced its plague poems, but they were remarkably few in number. One of the earliest was by the Montpellier-trained doctor Simon de Couvin, who, in Paris in 1350, wrote a long poem, *Libellus de judicio Solis in conviviis Saturni*, on the Black Death.[18] Another by the French poet Guillaume de Machaut lamented the terrible slaughter of 1349 along with its disruption to economic life and agricultural production.[19] In addition, a striking Welsh poem,

---

[13] RI.IV.1551 contains a number of short plague prayers in verse, *c.*1575–6, in which the press is often not indicated, and many of which have yet to be entered into Edit 16, such as no. 44: *Oratione alla Vergine Maria contra la peste*; no. 45: *Orationi devotissime contra la peste*; no. 47: *Oratione devoto da dirsi ogni giorno da tutti li fideli Christiani massime in questi tempi calamitosi*; no. 48: *Tempore pestis oratio*; no. 58: *Oratione alla Vergine Maria contra la peste*; no. 59: *Una devota supplicatione della citta di Venetia al Signore Iddio . . . con farci liberi del presente contagio*; no. 60: *Supplicatione divotissima sopra queste due parole, Ave Maria, in otto stanze*; no 72: *Preghi . . . per la liberatione del popolo di Vinegia*.

[14] Celebration in verse over the victory of Lepanto in 1571 prefigured the 1576–7 outpouring of popular verse on plague; see Fenlon, *The Ceremonial City*, 263–7.

[15] Neither *Rime di diverso a gli habitani di Venetia* nor *Scelta de i piu belli e bizari motti* is found in Edit 16; BAV, RI.IV.1551, no. 67 and 69. The success of Fracastoro's *Sphylis sive morbus gallicus*, published in 1530, may have set the vogue for disease and verse but, if so, its effect was delayed by more than a generation.

[16] *Gride diverse*, no. 62: 'Ad Deum Opt. Max. Precatio L. Annibalis Cruceii'. It also appeared separately.

[17] Branchi, *Oratione . . . fatta per la liberatione*. Another example, Complani, *Pestilentis morbi*, began with two poems in praise of the chief physician of his town, Brescia, Franciscum Modegnanum, Archiater.

[18] 'Opuscule relatif à la peste de 1348'. See Coville, 'Écrits contemporains sur la peste', 372–82.

[19] See Herlihy, *The Black Death*, 40–1.

first thought to have been written by Jeuan Gethin, who flourished in the early fifteenth century,[20] now believed to have been by Llywelyn Fychan, written during Wales's second plague in 1363,[21] lamented the deaths of his daughters. It was, however, little known until the twentieth century. Others were orations such as those penned in 1349 by the abbot-chronicler Gilles le Muisit to God, Jesus, the Virgin Mary, the Holy Ghost, All Saints, and Saint Sebastian, characterized by Alfred Coville as 'banal and without personality'.[22] Another longer one in le Muisit's chronicle said little about the disease but did reveal facts particular to Tournai's experience, such as a conflict between the magistrates and populace over burying plague victims in new plague pits placed outside their parishes and away from their ancestors.[23] Perhaps a handful of others can be cited within verse chronicles and across Europe such as the section on plague within the universal chronicle of Scotland by Andrew Wyntoun.[24] But after Francesco Petrarch's *Ad seipsum*[25] and Antonio Pucci's few verses on 1348,[26] I know of no other plague poems from Italy until the sixteenth century.

Furthermore, the late medieval verses did not narrate the developments of the plague or celebrate a community's liberation or conquest of it. Quite the opposite, they grovelled in the horrors and carnage of mass mortality, bemoaning lost ones and describing the disease's horrific scars and remote causes. Simon de Couvin's poem, for instance, describes the configuration of planets, the plague's signs and symptoms, and doctors' inability to cure or prevent it: Hippocrates' art had failed. Llywelyn's moving poem on the black scales and pustules that deformed the fair skin of his young daughters likewise shows no development of the disease from its initial infection within a town or region until the moment of a community's liberation. Scholars are not even certain when or exactly where this plague may have struck. Petrach's *Ad seipsum* begins by surveying the grim funerary and ruined landscape wrecked by plague,[27] churches filled with abandoned coffins of nobles and plebs, cemeteries overflowing with cadavers, threatening all human kind with a terrible end: 'death conquers all'. The poem continues with Petrarch's mental conflict between fear and an Augustinian *contemptus mundi*, longing for liberation from his earthly sentence, the chains

[20] Rees, 'The Black Death in England and Wales', 33.

[21] 'Pestilence', in *Galar y Beirdd*, 50–8.

[22] Coville, 'Écrits contemporains sur la peste', 382–4. On his poetry also see Guenée, *Between Church and State*, 74–6, who is less harsh and judgemental.

[23] Coville, 'Écrits contemporains sur la peste', 384–5.

[24] Cook, 'The Influence of the Black Death on Medieval Literature', cites an English Black Death poem by an unknown author, 'The Catell did ye men devoure'. For Wyntoun's Black Death verse, see *Andrew of Wyntoun's Orygnale Cronykil of Scotland*, 483.

[25] Petrarca, *Opere*, 433–41. [26] Pucci, 'Delle crudeltà della pestilenza', 413.

[27] A manuscript in the Biblioteca Laurenziana in Boccaccio's hand has the date 1340. Literary scholars such as Wilkins, 'On Petrarch's *Ad Seipsum*', and the editors of this edition of *Ad Seipsum* have strongly contested this date and attribute it to 1348.

that bound his borrowed body.[28] Antonio Pucci's eighteen lines repeat the common refrain seen in chronicles across Europe in 1348: brothers abandoning brothers; fathers abandoning sons, wives abandoning husbands; and vice versa, and points to the fear and selfishness of the clergy and the uselessness and greed of doctors. [29]

The first freestanding publication of plague verse in sixteenth-century Italy that I have spotted does not appear until 1549 and differed from the plague poetry that gushed forth from 1575 to 1578 in several respects. First, it was not an edition in cheap print (the usual sort for most of the plague literature during the sixteenth century) but a luxurious one. *Elegiae de peste* by the French doctor and poet Jean Ursin[30] comprised sixteen poems printed with gold-leaf-edged pages, dedicated to Cosimo I de' Medici. Unlike other plague poems, the arrival, presence, or recent departure of a particular plague did not prompt it. In fact, it was an elegy on disaster in general, 'Pestis, bella, fames, nos mala cuncta prement'/ 'Plague, war, and famine, all of which oppress us'. Diseases other than 'contagious plague' were also invoked, such as 'phthisis' (now thought to be tuberculosis), which the poem describes as 'infecting the lungs through breathing foul air [*vitiant Pulmones Aera tetris Flatibus*]'. Again, unlike the celebratory plague verses sparked by 1576, this poem did not turn to a secular ruler—not even to its dedicatee, Florence's Grand Duke—or to doctors, cardinals, citizens, or other 'heroic' individuals whose wisdom and courage helped liberate a city from hydra-headed plague. Although it honoured the great men of philosophy and medicine such as Albert the Great, and especially Galen, and provided some of the standard remedies and preventatives including Galen's six 'non-naturals' about sleep, exercise, diet, etc., and other recipes of aromatics and perfumes, its central message was spiritual: no medicine or medical skill could alone conquer plague:

> Hoc sine nil artes, nil medicina valet.
> Ergo salutifero solum fidamus in IESU.[31]
> [Without Christ, no skill or medicine is worthwhile
> To be healed we can rely only on Jesus.]

For the next important plague that spread through parts of northern Italy, confined mostly to Padua and Venice in 1555–6, two plague publications appear in verse. One focused on Venice; the other on Padua. 'Carmen of the pestilence that shook Venice' by the Latin poet Giacomo Ruffini from the Marche was an ornate portrayal of the horrible misery wrought by plague that transformed 'that most beautiful throne of the city of Venice' in 1556.[32] To stir up dread and visions of death, it entered the underworld of Greek mythology,

[28] *Francesco Petrarca Poesia Latine*, 128–37. Also, see Bergdolt, *La Pesta Nera*, 348.
[29] *Storia letteraria d'Italia*, 413.   [30] Orsini [Jean Ursin], *Elegiae de peste*.
[31] Ibid., 9.   [32] Rufini, *Carmen de pestilentia Venetam urbem*.

of threatening and dangerous places in northern Europe, the Mediterranean, and Asia: the rivers of the icy-cold Styx and Phegethon, whose waters were fire, Sarmatia, Istria, and Rhodanusia (Lyon), the Rhine, the Dardanelles, the land of the Seres (Eastern Asia), and Erthyreo, an island in the bay of Cadiz where the giant Geryon dwelt.

Like Petrarch's *Ad Seipsum* or the final verses of Lucretius' *De rerurm natura* (which Ruffini probably had read), it conveyed the horrors of plague's mass destruction, the funerary landscape of 'earth-strewn cadavers', 'deserted homes', 'temples of God where no one dares to enter', and the psychological torments of a city 'pressed down by black plague [*atra lues*], the monster of blackness [*Monstra nigrantis*]'. The citizens of Venice fled their homes, loved ones, blood relations; wives abandoned husbands in their final hours; 'children fled from the dangerous embrace of motherly love', 'the repulsion of dear ones reigned'; 'fathers and mothers stood alone tearless at their children's graves': 'where has piety gone?'. 'Funerary incantation' filled the *calles* of Venice. This was hardly an uplifting poem of hope and triumph over plague, celebrating survival with secular or ecclesiastical heroes placed on pedestals of civic action and pride.

The other poem of that plague, *L'Historia della Peste di Padoa del'Anno MDLV* by the Piedmontese doctor and professor of medicine Baravalle, broke with this lugubrious imagery and efforts to stir fear and depression so engrained in the fabric of previous plague verse. His poem of over four hundred verses anticipates much of the form, style, content, and key metaphors of what became common with the poetic outpouring in 1576–7.[33] First, unlike earlier sixteenth-century Italian tracts, in prose or verse, it narrated chronologically the events of a plague, in this case the one in Padua of 1555: the outbreak lasted six months, was carried to the city in March from Venice, and spread as though 'made by ants carrying food'. Baravalle described the signs and symptoms of the disease—swellings 'pur giacea' behind ears, in the groin, and the armpits; 'often they lay under the skin'; some were 'large tumours; some white, others black, some flat, others raised'. Larger and smaller spots, the *carboni* and *petecchie*, also formed. In June the plague reached the 'monstrous proportions of a wild animal' ('Hebbe gran strage l'animal feroce'). Until then, it had been 'a war'; now its 'enormity' was such that that metaphor was superseded ('Enorme veramente, non più guerra'). In July the scourge became still more 'atrocious'; all who could, fled, leaving the city abandoned. In August the plague remained as severe, if not more so. For September, Baravalle described the effects of poverty and famine on those who remained, the horrors and fears of the lazaretto, the streets, where only dogs, cats, and chickens now prowled, of increased criminality and

---

[33] For instance, the BAV has a volume with twenty-seven works on plague, mostly published during the 1555–6 plague in northern Italy or immediately thereafter (R.I. V.487): Baravallo's is the only work in verse. Compare this to R.I.IV.1551, which contains over fifty plague poems written exclusively in 1575–7.

its punishments. Finally, in October the plague declined, and the city was liberated. Anticipating the verses of 1576–7, Baravalle's poem did not turn to God but remained within the secular realm: it was a heroic epic. The plague now was dubbed the seven-headed monster Hydra, and the city's salvation relied on the strength and wisdom of a Hercules. Hercules here, however, was not a single figure: first he was the Piacentine physician then practising in Padua 'the excellent' Bassiano Landi, author of a plague tract on this plague's origins; then, he was the city magistrate Messer Antonio Brusco, who 'shot the arrows that dismembered the seven-headed monster'. The poet-physician ended with the city's celebrations, the ringing of bells and processions, new 'signs of happiness and infinite gratitude', feasts and games: 'Padua had never before been so embellished' ('Cui mai piu Padoa [credo] non ornorno').[34] But Baravalle's poem was a lone survivor as far as I can find. Plague verse of 1576–7 was different, quantitatively and qualitatively. It moved sharply from the moaning of the Middle Ages, when its rare examples of plague verse turned to God with dark hues of death and doom, streets of corpses, destruction, and human misery; the world bereft of human care or love, all celebrating the triumph of death.[35]

The new epic plague poems clustered in Verona, but it was not alone in producing such odes to plague. In Venice and elsewhere the new plague stimulated publications of various types of verse—songs, madrigals, laments, and religious prayers. Most were produced in cheap print and survive in few numbers.[36] Not all, however, were classical epics celebrating secular triumph over plague. Several, such as one from Padua in 1576, beseeched God to keep the four horsemen of the apocalypse of war, plague, famine, and fire far away.[37] Another poem by the Veronese Francesco Cieco composed in 1576 while the plague still raged began with all Venice crying: the poem's content and spirit were much in the vein of plague poetry from the mid-fourteenth century to 1575. For Cieco, Venice had never been so sad, sorrowful, or deserted; few were left to clean it, since so many

---

[34] Baravalle, *L'historia della peste di Padoa*. Another early reference to Hercules in plague tracts appears in the dedication by a physician of Modena to the duke of Ferrara of a translation from Greek into Latin of Al-Razi's plague manual, *Libellus de peste*.

[35] Given the flourishing of publications by women in mid-sixteenth-century Italy and their salons that sponsored new anthologies of verse, perhaps it is surprising that all of the plague poets I can presently identify were men. On the sudden rocketing in women's writing and poetry in mid-sixteenth-century Italy, see Robin, *Publishing Women*.

[36] See for instance *Preghi . . . per la liberatione del popolo di Vinegia* (only two copies according to Edit 16, one at the Vatican, the other at the Marciana, Venice); *Canzone nel calamitoso stato di Venetia*; *Canzone alla gloriossima Vergine* (two copies: BAV and the Biblioteca Civica Bertiliana in Vicenza); *Scelta de i piu belli e bizari motti* and *Rime di diverso a gli habitani di Venetia* (both published in Venice in 1576, neither has been included in Edit 16); *Lamento della città di Vicenza*; *Il pianto della sconsolata città di Vicenza* (located in three Italian libraries); and *Madrigali spirituali nel tempo della peste nella città di Vicenza* (found in the BAV alone). In addition, the 1575–8 plague stimulated poems that remain in manuscript; twelve are found in R.I.IV.1551, and see the Venetian one, 'Di alcuni versi inediti sulla peste del 1575', and its analysis in Laughran, 'The Body, Public Health and Social Control', 242–4, 253–4, and 274.

[37] Montecchio, *Carmen epicum*.

had fled its filth. His refrains recall the clichés of the Black Death: 'the father fled his dear child; mothers went in exile; matrimony and kinship no longer counted':

> Piangan tutti amaramente
> Son Venetia poverina
> Pianti e stridi, urli, e dolori
> Cresce mia doglia infinita.
> [All cry bitterly
> I am Venice the poor little one
> Cries and screams, yells and pain
> My grief increases beyond all bounds]

And the poem's tone fails to brighten:

> Altro piú non so che fare
> Se non pianger e suspirare
> Il Signor del ciel pregare
> Che mi voglia aiuto dare
> E con la sua santa mano
> Far che'l popolo sia sano.
> [I know nothing more that can be done
> If not to cry and sigh
> And pray to the Lord of Heaven
> That he should wish to help me and
> With his holy hand
> Make his people healthy.]

Furthermore, the poem showed no more confidence in the medical profession or curing plague than the Black Death verses of Simon de Couvin:

> Ogni medico eccellente
> Ch'era dotto e sufficiente
> L'arte sua non li val niente
> Ma chi scampa è assai valente
> Perch'il ciel n'ha destinati
> Forse per nostri peccati.[38]
> [Every excellent doctor
> Who was learned and well trained
> His craft was now worthless
> He who ran was valiant enough,
> Because the heavens had its own ways
> Perhaps because of our sins.]

Yet unlike the Black Death verses this poem had a firmer sense of place. It was not plague anywhere but in Venice as the Veronese poet recalled the transmogrification of pre-plague Venice with its balls and musicals along canals and *calles*; few now promenaded through city streets cracking jokes:

---

[38] Cieco, *Barceletta sopra il lamento di Venetia* (not inventoried in Edit 16; BAV, R.I.IV.1551, no. 40).

Piú non se usa suoni e balli
Per le cale, e ne' canali
. . .
Pochi van scherzando intorno.

A short collection of five poems completed on 25 September 1576 by Lodovico Ronconi and Cesare Campana[39] also written before the city's 'liberation',
expressed the misery and pessimism of this, Italy's worst-hit place in 1575–8.
As with Petrarch's *Ad Seipsum*, these poems depicted the desperate pestilential
conditions as Venetian death counts peaked in early autumn: 'of a punishment
beyond contemplation, of death, which is always hard to bear'. But plague death,
Campana explained, was much worse still because with this death, 'the father
rejected his son, the son, the father', leaving survivors 'bathed in so many tears
their eyes could not shut'.

In punire ch'l suo fin mai non contempla;
Duro è sempre il morir, ma il morir quando
Nega il padre al figliuolo, e 'l figlio al padre
. . . Di lagrime bagnarli . . .
Et non può chiuder gli occhi.[40]

Unlike Petrarch and others of Black Death days, these two poets, even during
their worst days, saw some hope at least in the celestial realm with the 'king of
heavens', but they expressed little if any confidence in the labours of men:

Ma s'egli è ver, Signor verace & giusto
. . .
Seco & si lagna & pregate, che mostri
Limpido, puro, sacro, eterno fonte,
Entro'l cui picciol seno il Re del cielo
. . .
Accio 'l buon gregge tuo, che langue & erra
Ne l'acqua sante ssue salubri & belle,
Lavi & risandi i membri egri, & piagati.[41]

Another Venetian poem, *De foeda pestis rabie in Venetam ciuitatem saevius*,
also written in 1576 before signs of relief, invoked the horrors of pestilence as
expressed earlier, but in these darkest days this Venetian poem gave a rousing
call for hope urging courageous actions in the struggle against plague:

Ipsa lues, urbem populans, gliscitque medendo,
Hosteque ab occulto patimur miserabile bellum.
Urbe tamen morbo attrita magis ipsa virescunt

---

[39] Campana was a historian, poet, and orator, born in L'Aquila in 1540 and died in Vicenza in
1606 with twenty-six publications (Edit 16); Ronconi is identified by Edit 16 only as a Vicentino of the
sixteenth century with one publication.
[40] Campana, *Alcune compositioni volgari et latine.*   [41] Ibid., 2r–v.

Consilia, & pietas Patrum, qui ad proelia magnis
Invitant pretiis animos, & numera dignae
Grandia virtuti ponunt, auroq. lacessunt
Illustrem ad pugnam. Haec pietatas gratissima fulsit
Ipsius ante oculos Genitoris cuncta videntis;[42]
[Ravaging the city, this plague caused fear to blaze through it.
And we suffered miserably from the war waged by our invisible enemy.
Although the city became greatly worn down by the disease,
Counsel and love of country summoned its resources to battle
And numerous worthy ones came forward with great bravery
to challenge this illustrious one to battle.
And this most gracious love of country propped up
The rest before our parents' eyes for all to see.]

Still other poems from other places were simply plague remedy books in verse. Five such published sonnets that now survive only at the Vatican Library give advice on pills, plasters, and syrups, different herbs to carry by hand during the plague, and the like. But unlike the usual plague recipe books of cherished (and expensive secrets), these 1576–7 poets were often more sceptical:

Le lor virtú, non sai, che son mancate,
Per li peccati horrendi:
[As for their virtues, you never know if they are enough
To cure our horrendous sins.]

In the end, some recommended the old lessons: flee as far as possible and fear God.[43] The poem of the Sienese biographer of Gregory XIII, Marcantonio Ciappi, published in 1576, was much longer than the sonnets above. Beginning with his credentials—ancients and moderns he had studied—he charted the plague's spread to Venice, the accompanying circumstances of war and famine, the laws and provisions of the Venetian state, the infection centred principally among the poor, the abandonment of family members, and then a long series of cures, remedies, and drugs interspersed with jokes exposing the contradictions from one famous physician to the next:

Mangia pan bianco, e bevi del bon vino
Parmi Galeno prohibisca il pesce;
Cardano non lo vuole prohibire
. . . .
Che'l pover corpo mai lo digerisce
Il simile vo far delle cipolle.
Et altri mali da empirne un volume;

---

[42] BAV, RI.IV.1551, no. 95. No place, press, or date are indicated. According to Edit 16 it was not published before 1576 and probably in Venice.

[43] *Sonetto sopra tutti gli rimedii che si usano contra la peste*, R.I.IV.1551 (six sonetti, no. 98a–f). This publication has not been listed in Edit 16.

E sopra tutto fan puzzar il fiato,
Che chi ti sente gli pari ammorbato.

. . . .

Perche Mercato nel suo scriver tocca,
Che tutti i mali vengon per la bocca.[44]
[Eat white bread and drink good wine
Those who adhere to Galen prohibit fish

. . .

Cardano[45] wishes not to ban it.

. . . .

Even if the poor body never digests it.
And similar things are said of onions
And other bad things could fill a book;
And above all else they make you fart
And whoever smells you also gets it.
As Mercato[46] wrote
All things bad come through the throat.]

Ciappi continued in this jocular vein with other standard concerns of the typical plague tract—dress, sleep, exercise, attitudes and behaviour, perfumes, bathing, cleanliness, remedies, and other preservatives. But he also included matters that had not been part of the traditional plague tract—that is, until 1576. These concerned public health and politics—ordinances against leaving waste and the issuing of *bollettini*, the government's passport control: 'without one you'd be thrown out even if you were king of the Tartars'.[47]

Milan, so important in the production of the new plague narratives in 1576–8, also published plague verse for this plague. One described pestilential symptoms, where buboes formed, and the nature of contagion, providing information similar to those found in medical tracts.[48] Another, *Componimenti Christiani in materia de la peste*, a compilation of six songs and sonnets by the nobleman poet, historian, and court secretary to Ferrante Gonzaga, Giuliano Goselini, went beyond the grist of previous plague poetry. The first one was black humour addressed to 'Mr. Plague', 'the voracious one and his perverse sons', but ending with a hopeful plea for the afflicted to 'repent, hope, and live'. In the spirit of other 1576 plague verses, Goselini's poems charted the plague's origin in the Levant, its spread and pincer movement against Italy, 'devouring Sicily and the north simultaneously'. In the poem's long dedication and its verses it praised Milan's ruler, Don Antonio de Guzman, for sustaining the people of Milan,

---

[44] Ciappi, *Regola da preseruarsi*, 467v (BAV).

[45] Girolamo Cardano: famous doctor, mathematician, and philosopher, born at Pavia in 1501, died in Rome in 1576, author of thirteen texts on Hippocrates, medicine, and arithmetic; also see Belloni, 'Carlo Borromeo e la storia della medicina', 167–8.

[46] Michele Mercati (1541–93), doctor and naturalist of San Miniato, was called by Pius V to direct the Vatican's botanical gardens and was the doctor of Pope Clement VIII.

[47] Ibid., 470r.   [48] Della Croce, *Ad Deum Opt. Max. Precatio*, [155r-8v] (BAV).

visiting and consoling the afflicted, providing them with an abundance of doctors and medicines, nourishing the poor, supporting artisans thrown out of work, and ensuring that the masses did not perish from famine. Goselini then celebrated the prefects of the health board and 'a hundred other ministers of the lazaretto, the huts, the city gates, and the parishes', 'who enforced ancient and recent laws with Christian zeal, maintained the quarantines, and administered precisely [*esattamente*] the supplies of foodstuff, charity, and medicine'. He finally turned to Cardinal Carlo Borromeo, 'Our Pastor' in thanks for 'his prayers, communal fasts, devotions, frequent processions, and role in organizing the Holy Jubilee'.[49]

Another by the doctor and mathematician Bernardino Baldini, who taught at the universities of Pavia and Milan, was an epic in line with numerous other verses from Verona in 1576 to be examined shortly. The first and principal poem of his collection of seven, *In pestilentiam libellus*, is a 136-line *Elegiae* describing the horror of plague—'the kingdom of the black' ('qui nigra regna tenet')—physical pain and deformity, heart failure, overpowering headaches, fiery fever, burning of the throat, great thirst coupled with an inability to drink, and then the ugly many-coloured tumours that swell behind ears, on the femur, and other parts of the body, accompanied by a multiplicity of spots ('papulas') of various sorts and colours, while nausea and bile pour from the stomach. Baldini then turned to the social and economic desolation wrought by plague: separation and fear of friends and family, absence of surgeons to administer medicines and gravediggers to carry away the dead, the end of commerce, the paucity of food that trickled into the city, and with winter, the freezing of the poor, especially those locked in the wooden huts with only straw for warmth, tormented by ice, pouring rain, and snow.

From these grim conditions and threats to humankind, the poem, however, shifts gears to the human struggle against the invisible enemy, enlisting hope and ending in triumph. Here, as in Verona, plague's metaphor suddenly becomes the seven-headed Hydra of Hercules' labours. As a result of human intervention, the plague lifted by the following winter, shops reopened, craftsmen returned to work, and goods were no longer wanting; tears dried, and joy, jokes, fun, and games returned to Milan, even if sorrow for recent losses was not wholly forgotten. The poem ends with the survivors' ultimate revenge on plague—human fertility—life springing from its seeds. Ultimately the victor was the city itself.

Baldini followed this elegy with six shorter poems, two dedicated to the citizens of Milan, another to Cardinal Borromeo, two to the two presidents of Milan's health board during the 1576–7 plague—Galeazzo Brugora and Girolamo Montio—another to one of its judges—Giovanni Gasparo Barchini—and

---

[49] Goselini, *Componimenti Christiani in materia de la peste*. As these and other poems attest, Carlo Borromeo was not the only or even principal one singled out for praise during this plague in Milan as is sometimes assumed; see for example Wallis, 'Plagues, Morality and the Place of Medicine', 2 and 23. Carlo's dominance over this plague came after his canonization (1610) with works such as those by Etienne Binet; see Worcester, 'Plague as Spiritual Medicine'.

finally an obituary in verse praising the plague service of the priest and musician Niccolò, the city's *protomusicus*, conductor of the cathedral choir. Plebs and Milan's rulers alike—Don Antonio de Guzman and his lieutenant in charge of the city, Gabrio Serbelloni—were also celebrated as local 'heroes', for their deeds, hardships, courage, decrees, and fortitude, which had vanquished the plague with its multiple threats. The choral master Niccolò with his 'ancient songs, Doric harmonies and gamely and elegant witticisms helped the afflicted banish from their minds 'the horrors and monstrous destruction of the plague'.[50]

Nor were these 1576–7 examples of plague poetry limited to principal cities or to northern Italy. The Bresciano doctor Bartolomeo Theani (or Tiani) published a Latin poem of over 2,000 lines decrying the horrors of plague—the loss of friends, abandonment of the city by the rich, social and economic disruption, the sudden widespread domination of fear—along with the most detailed descriptions in verse of the signs and symptoms of the plague. Within this lugubrious setting, Tiani, however, pointed to one shining light that gave his city hope: Magnificus Dominus Honophrus Madium, 'the illustrious knight and lawyer' then governor of the town's lazaretto to whom his long poem was dedicated; as Moses leading the Israelites, he kept the lazaretto stocked with medicines and other necessities and watched over the ill day and night.[51]

The professor of medicine at the University of Salerno, Francesco Alfani, began his plague tract of 1577 with five poems, mostly academic in praise of the philosophy and medicine of Homer, Hippocrates, Aristotle, Galen, Alexander the Great, and others of the classical past. But, like Baldini, Alfani also celebrated local heroes—the monk Filippo Rennanti, the magistrates Gabriele Quaranta and Giovanni Francesco Lombardi from Naples, and the canon and musician Gaspare for steadfast services during the plague just ended.[52] A sonnet by the Palermitan doctor and statesman Branchi also praised musicians during the 1575–6 plague for their 'impassioned harmonies'.[53]

Verona, however, emerges from the surviving publications as the centre of a new form of plague verse penned as the 1575–8 plague began to decline. A collection of thirty-five poems broke profoundly with previous plague verse. Written mostly by Veronese citizens in Latin, Italian, Venetian, and one in Spanish, and arranged according to language, these did not dwell on the horror and dread of death-threatening buboes, vomit-sputtering, abandonment of loved ones, and the hopelessness of the physician's craft; nor did they explain plague as the consequence of man's sins, or rely on God as the sole remedy. Although they

---

[50] Baldini, *In pestilentiam libellus*. Also, see the long lament in verse on the plague in Milan by Civelli, *Carmina*.

[51] Tiani, *De singulari pestilentiae magnitudine*, 6v.

[52] Alfani, *Opus, de peste*. Other plague poetry from southern Italy includes an anonymous one on the 1575 plague in Palermo, *Le lagrime di Palermo*, known only from the typographical evidence.

[53] Branchi, *Oratione*, n.p.

154

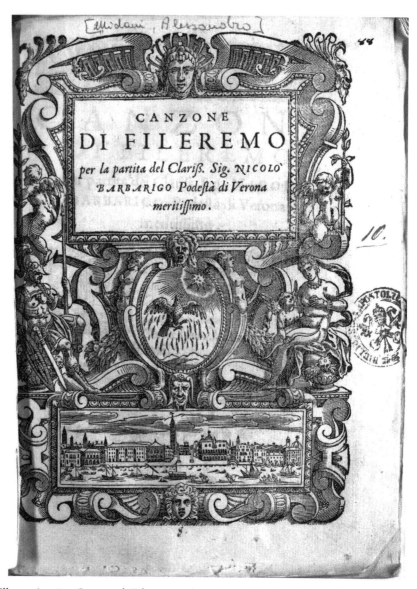

Illustration 3. *Canzone di Fileremo per la partita del Cl. Sig, Nicolò Barbarigo Podestà di Verona meritissimo.*

began with the plague's threats to survival, they rapidly passed to extol the earthly means by which local heroes such as Michelo da San Zen, the sub-prior of the Battigelfi, and especially Verona's podestà from 1575 to 1576, Niccolò Barbarigo, confronted these threats and triumphed over them.[54] The prose preface, part in Latin, part in Italian, by Cesare Nichesola (another writer who finds no trace in Edit 16) did not invoke God as an explanation of Verona's liberation from the plague but instead placed the credit squarely on the city's plague-time podestà for his 'deeds, advice, generosity, and diligence'. Barbarigo masterfully preserved law and order, while he showed charity toward prisoners. As a result, homicides fell sharply, and although 'innumerable conflicts (*pretersioni*)' arose between city and countryside, through wise laws Barbarigo dampened factional strife initially fanned by the social ills of plague.[55]

Nichesola then further magnified Barbarigo's achievements and glory comparing him to Hercules and his labours in slaying the many-headed Hydra. In the verses that followed Hercules' labours became the overriding metaphor unifying the collection. Nichesola along with the collection's poets pointed not only to the disease itself that ravaged the population but also to its social and economic consequences. Conditions worsened with the end of commerce, not only between Verona and other cities, which refused to trade with Verona, but within Verona itself with one household refusing or forbidden to deal with the next. As a result, merchants no longer had the means to sustain their workers.[56] 'Under pretence of fearing the plague', peasants worsened conditions further, 'stubbornly refusing' to provide the city with its sustenance. They 'even rebelled' against public authority, showing utter disdain, disobeying every order to feed the city, selfishly 'attending to their own health'. Their refusal to transport food brought immediate hardship especially to those who had lost their livelihoods. But the podestà stepped in, swiftly confronting the 'horrible progress of the *contagio*': he cut deals with city bakers and relieved the healthy poor with an abundance of bread. By appealing to noblemen and merchants for charity, 'he procured new and fitting ways to provide housing, medicine, food,

---

[54] *Raccolta delli componimenti*. Other contemporaries also praised the deeds of this podestà during the 1575–7 plague—the Venetian notary Benedetti, *Raguaglio*, 2v (for valour in defending the passages and gates of Verona); and Valier, although he noted critically that Barbarigo was among those in Verona who initially resisted calling the disease plague; see Chapter 4. Curiously, I find no praise or even mention of Marcantonio Cordino, Verona's representative at Venice, who persuaded the government to lift its ban, which had so damaged the Veronese economy. On Cordino, see Palmer, 'The Control of Plague', 276. Also, see *Canzone di fileremo*, a collection of five poems in praise of Barbarigo; a single-sheet published poem to him by Bartolomeo da San Zeno, *Sorano so chi poeti desgirlande*; and several other single-sheet poems or ones of several folios by anonymous poets, R.IV.1551, no. 15–19.

[55] For the Black Death, historians have argued that crime and civil law suits increased: see Bowsky, 'The Medieval Commune and Internal Violence', 16; Carpentier, *Une ville devant la peste*, 178: Smail, 'Telling Tales in Angevin Courts', 186–7; and Falsini, 'Firenze dopo il 1348', 457–66; for the early modern period, see Pastore, 'Note su criminalita e giustizia in tempo di peste', 31–43; and *Crimine e giustizia in tempo di peste*.

[56] Nichelosa in *Raccolta delli componimenti*, 3r.

clothing, and other necessities'; as Hercules he triumphed over all the plague's monsters'.[57]

For the most part, the poems that follow were by authors without other literary traces and unmentioned in Edit 16's comprehensive survey. Only eight (twenty-two were named and three wrote two poems apiece) are found in Edit 16, had another publication, or can be identified by an occupation. Most prolific was Federigo Ceruti (1532–1611), a Veronese *letterato* and doctor with thirty-five published works.[58] Antonio Pasini was professor of medicine from Brescia with four publications;[59] Angelo Maria Maggi, a noble lawyer and notary with six legal publications; Giovanni Pietro Moretti, a literary figure with two other short treatises in 1598 on triumphal entries; Tommaso Becelli, a lawyer, humanist, and magistrate of Verona with only one other publication; Adam Fumani, a Veronese canon, poet, translator of Saint Basil, secretary to Cardinal Navagero at the Council of Trent and author of two further works;[60] Bartolomeo Vitali, a judge and knight from Desenzano with three publications;[61] and Garbinel de Fruffa de Berton, a dialect poet with one other brief poem, 'Saonetto de Garbinel. . .', again extolling Barbarigo's plague-time deeds.[62]

The poets praised the podestà's leadership that tamed the social and economic dangers unleashed by plague. A poem by Antonio Pasini described how death suddenly seized the city, the foul plague brought down the people ('Foeda contages, humilem popellum'); furiously, afflicting the plebs ('Plebe grassatur furibunda tabes'), it caused crafts to languish and left the city deserted, shaking in fear ('Urbe deserta, trepidans pavore') and embroiled in social unrest. But Barbarigo reversed the tide of this monster, restoring the city to its former glory.[63] Others, such as Giovanni Battista Dondonini, pointed to famine and exile, which accompanied the illness and brought Verona to ruin:

> fame plebem, morboque cadentem
> Exilia & patriae crudeli peste ruentis.[64]

For Giovanni Pietro Moretti hunger redoubled the blow of disease, and its misery crushed the people:

> Fame raddoppia il colpo, e di moleste
> Miserie, il popolo preme.[65]

[57] Nichelosa, 3v–4r. [58] Also, see Ceruti, *Prosopopeia amphitheatri*, 149r–54r (BAV).

[59] He was born at Calvasesio (Brescia) and lived at Salò in 1574–5. He must have moved to Verona before or soon after the plague flared. Two works are listed for him, one on air, water, and place in Hippocrates, and another, published in three editions, on the famous pharmacist Pietro Andrea Mattioli. His plague poetry, however, is not listed.

[60] Edit 16: one on Saint Basil; the other, a much shorter work, on Pope Sixtus V.

[61] Edit 16: one was a short chronicle of Brescia; the other two, saints' lives of the Brescian bishop Hercoliano; neither is found in more than two Italian libraries.

[62] Edit 16: the only known copy is at BAV.

[63] *Prosopopeia amphitheatri*, n.p.; also included in *Raccolta delli componimenti*, 118r–v (BAV).

[64] *Raccolata delli componimenti*, 15v–16r. [65] Moretti, 'L'horrido mostro', in ibid., 20v–21r.

In Bernardino Cavadoro's poem, the Herculean 'Barnadici' before conquering plague, first had to banish the wicked threat of hunger; 'Il rio timor di fame fu sbandito'. And as in Moretti's poem and Nichelosa's introduction, Barbarigo countered the threat of social unrest:

> . . . Egli à romori
> Corre provede, da mille ristori.

Leonardo Riardi, another local poet (unknown to Edit 16), enumerated how Barbarigo, this Hercules, expelled the wild and horrible beast from Verona:

> Herculis egregios inter numeratur honores. . .
> Atque feram horribilem Verona, expellis, egestas.[66]

In Girolamo Brenzoni's poem, Barbarigo bravely confronted and surmounted the plague's multiple challenges by embodying the unconquerable and immeasurable courage of Hercules:

> Si tulit & tantos potuit superasse labores
> Invictos animos Herculis instar habens.

In Moretti's poem, 'Barnardici' was the great champion, who came to Verona to declare war on plague and confronted and overcame all its horrors, giving new vigour to the people:

> Move a Verona guerra un'aspra peste
> Trafitto aspetta ogn'un gli estremi horrori
> S'opponi il gran Campion queta i furori,
> Vince, predon vigor le genti meste.

Instead of the usual religious language and iconography of God's wrath, these poems depicted the disease as serpent-like (as in Tommaso Becelli's poem, 'Serpebant passim contagia dira per urbem' ['the terrible contagion snaked through the city']), or, as in Bernadino Cavodori's, 'Il pestifer Dragon, c'ha tanti ucciso' ['the plague dragon, which slaughtered so many']). In Moretti's poem, as in others, this 'cruel serpent' was more than plague or any specific disease; it encompassed the tangle of epidemiological, social, and economic conditions that engendered theft and evil: 'L'empio serpe coi furti accresce il male'.

The poems further named Barbarigo as 'Apollo',[67] 'the New Apollo',[68] compared him to Moses bringing manna down from heaven to his starving people,[69] and called his 'valour the equal of the famous Theban'.[70] Still others, such as Leonardo Riardi in a second poem—this one in Italian—praised the city, its physical surroundings, and especially its river: the Adige, 'the envy of the

---

[66] A poem by Giovanni Jacopo Todeschi, in ibid., 14v.
[67] A poem by Aurelio Prandino, in ibid., 27r.   [68] Another poem by Prandino, in ibid., 20r.
[69] A Latin poem by Giovanni Iacobi Todeschi, in ibid., 14r.
[70] A poem by Bernardino Cavodoro, in ibid., 20v.

Arno, Ganges, and Rhine', which washed away the fog brought down from the hills, opening the city to an everlasting and beautiful day' (perhaps implying that the plague had derived from climatic conditions of dense humid air).[71] And in this poem, as with others, the hydra-headed monster plague was a complex of social, economic, political, and psychological trials and tribulations engendered by the disease—the end of trade and commerce, the absence of provisioning from the countryside, famine, theft, fear, and social disorder: 'plague, famine and a thousand, thousand other threatening and monstrous horrors', as Aurelio Prandino's poem put it.[72] Finally, another collection, this one of four poems signed by initials only, celebrated Verona's plague podestà at the moment of his departure from office. Again, recalling Hercules' labours in praise of the podestà's valour and love of virtue ('Il Philarete') during the plague, they also praised Verona's citizens and the restorative power of its river Adige.[73]

Such eulogy of a local podestà was not unique to Verona. A similar collection of verse composed by Giovanni Battista Maganza, Sandron de Magagno, and other, anonymous poets is found at Vicenza, lauding its local chief administrators—Nicolò Michele, the town's *capitano*, Geronimo Schio, who presided over the town's Lazaretto (*Proveditor di Campo Marzo*), and members of its health board. These, they instructed, were 'to be sung by excellent musicians to the lords of the health board ('Versi recitati da molti eccellentissimi musici alli Magnifici Signori alla Sanità').[74] Other poems extolled the podestà of Venice and its plague-time doge, Alvise Mocenigo, similarly as Herculean conquerors of plague.[75] Such symbolism and praise extended, moreover, beyond verse. A painting by Jacopo Bassano (now in the Museo Civico of Bassano del Grappa) executed in 1576 for the chapel of the town hall (Palazzo Pretorio), portrays Saint Roch presenting the town's plague-time podestà, Sante Moro, to the Virgin during this plague's early stages. It was a public offering of thanks to his wise governance, in which only eighty perished of plague in Bassano. After his eighteen-month stint of office, however, the plague struck the town again, in 1577 to 1578, with much greater casualties.[76] Other paintings executed during the 1575–8 plague or soon afterwards praised other local leaders such as Venice's Doge Alvise Mocenigo, and, most significantly, Cardinal Borromeo, who shortly thereafter became a major plague saint across Western and Central Europe and was of especial iconographical significance during the plagues of the seventeenth century.[77] Not

---

[71] Ibid., 18r. The Adige is also praised in poems by someone signed as Al. M., 27v–28r, and Aurelio Prandino, 25r–27r.

[72] Ibid., 19v.   [73] *Canzone di fileremo.*

[74] *Lamento della città di Vicenza*, and *Alcuni sonetti al clarissimo sig. Nicolò Michiele*, esp. 50r (BAV), which also praised the lords of Vicenza's health board.

[75] See the Venetian dialect poem, *Picegaton di memorosi Beretaro de la contra di San Lazaro al clarissimo podestà*, and *Carmen. De urbe Veneta pestilentia liberata.*

[76] 'Catalogo: le immagini della peste', 247.

[77] Ibid., 253–64 on Alvise Mocenigo. For paintings of Carlo Borromeo and the plague, see among other places *Hope and Healing*.

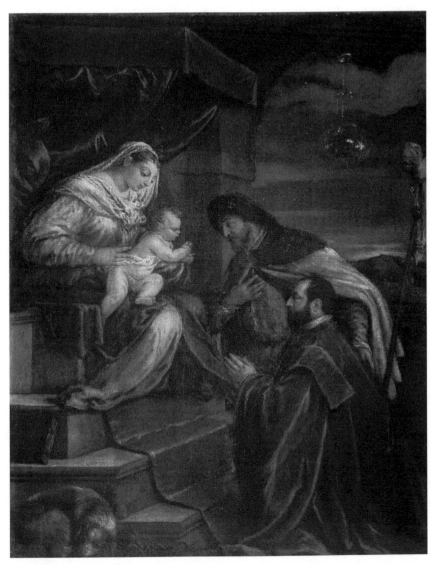

Illustration 4. Jacopo Bassano, *Il podestà Sante Moro presentato da San Rocco alla Vergine col Bambino.*

only is this wider social and political complex of the plague wholly missing from earlier plague verse in Italy (with the exception of Baravalle's 1556 poem), it is also absent from plague literature across Europe before the seventeenth century and perhaps later. The 1576–7 outpouring of plague verse constitutes another strand of this plague's creative force, bringing to publication those from professions who earlier had not written on plague in prose or verse. In contrast to plague poetry from Lucretius to Petrarch to Ruffini, their verses centred on the wider world of plague, its social and economic consequences, and its political and administrative remedies. Instead of celebrating death, these hailed local heroes, from health board directors to choir masters, who delivered their cities from a misery worse than war or any other form of death. We now turn to physicians to see how the 1575–8 plague affected their writing and thinking as seen in supposedly the most conservative form of medical writing before the eighteenth century—the physician's plague treatise.[78]

[78] For this assessment in the recent historiography, see the Introduction.

6

Plague Disputes, Challenges of the 'Universals'

Every plague no doubt created controversy over its causes and nature. For instance, probably not all doctors agreed with the highly astrological bent of the University of Paris plague report of 1348,[1] but no manuscripts survive of any who might have refuted it. Indeed, its rich manuscript tradition shows that it continued to curry favour well into the fifteenth century.[2] During successive plagues in the late fourteenth and fifteenth centuries, when with sharply falling rates of mortalities doctors became more confident of their plague cures, tracts such as that by Saladino Ferro, cited through the sixteenth century, translated and published for the first time in 1565,[3] challenged earlier generalizations of astrologers, philosophers, and physicians. Yet before the plague of 1575–8, plague publications rarely show debates aired among doctors. Only two doctors produced public pronouncements or exchanges within the sixteenth-century published tracts before 1575. Both publications surfaced in the non-plague years of the early 1570s. Neither involved big clashes of ideas or challenged systems such as those of Galen or variations of it by Ficino towards the end of the fifteenth century. The first, in 1569–72, was a polemic between two doctors where ego, honour, reputation, and treatment of individual plague patients were more at stake than ideas. It involved, however, all the doctors of Rimini, and certain barbers and pharmacists who adjudicated whether Bartolomeo Traffichetti's diagnosis and treatment of plague patients had been correct against charges levied by Marcantonio Cappelletti. The dispute brought even the pope into the fray and threatened to strip Traffichetti of his doctorate, licence to practice, and to excommunicate him.[4]

In 1570, a second controversy brewed among three doctors in Brescia over the use of strong purgatives called theriacs for treating plague.[5] A younger doctor, Vincenzo Calzaveglia, challenged Giuseppe Valdagno's claim that theriac was

---

[1] See Introduction, n. 5. For instance, the first French plague tract by Pierre de Damouzy, *Cum autem pestilencia jam regnet. . .*', drafted two months before the *Compendium*, paid much less attention to the astrological; see Coville, 'Écrits contemporains sur la peste', 330. According to Barkai, 'Jewish Treatises on the Black Death', 12–13, the Hebrew tract of the southern French Jew Issac ben Todoros criticized one point of the *Compendium* 'that the plague resulted from a loss of balance of dryness'.

[2] Coville, 'Écrits contemporains sur la peste', 336–58.   [3] Ferro, *Trattato della peste*.

[4] Cappelletti, *Apologia . . . aduersus Bartholomeum Traffichettum*; Traffichetti, *Antidosis . . . aduersus Marcum Antonium Capellettum*.

[5] On the theriac, see Chapter 1, n. 45.

an appropriate remedy for pestilential fevers. In two pamphlets, the well-known Paduan-trained physician Girolamo Donzellini (c.1513–87), who had been both the pope's and emperor's doctor, rallied in support of Valdagno, launching a stinging *ad hominem* attack against the younger doctor with a scholastic defence of theriacs for treating pestilential fevers.[6] Perhaps reflecting the change in medical treatment and suspicion of fighting poison with poison especially against plague, the two better-known physicians lost the debate, and the city's College of Physicians banished them from town.[7] A Milanese surgeon writing in 1577 showed similar doubts. He began his discussion of plague cures by attacking two well-engrained methods of plague treatment that would endure to the eighteenth century: purging the patient with a wide variety of strong drugs and prescribing specific diets.[8] The creative energies unleashed by the 1575–8 plague, however, turned on another issue that went beyond recipes and treatments of the individual patient; instead, it deeply affected health policy and the survival of thousands.

'TRUE PLAGUE'

No plague in Italy sparked as much debate, controversy, and bitter antagonisms both within the medical community and between it and outsiders as that of 1575–8. The 1576 disputes that arose from the pronouncements about plague made by Girolamo Mercuriale, Girolamo Capodivacca, and their colleagues at the University of Padua are best known. Invited by the Venetian senate to diagnose the disease then afflicting Venice, they judged that the current disease did not satisfy Hippocratic or Galenic criteria of 'popular' or 'an epidemic' and thus was not true plague: to qualify it had to spread over a vast region, killing all or most in that region regardless of age, social class, or other characteristics of a population. They held fast to their position despite the appearance of the historic tell-tale signs and symptoms and against the vigorous counter-arguments of Venice's health board and most of its doctors.[9] Yet during this plague, the dispute was not isolated to Venice; nor was Venice the first place to see this question divide medical and public opinion.

---

[6] Donzellini, *De natura*, 6r. Yet, while defending these strong purgatives, Donzellini also advised doctors to abstain from phlebotomy in most cases of plague.

[7] Calzaveglia, *De theriacae abusu*; Donzellini, *De natura*; idem, *Eudoxi Philalethis*; Valdagni, *De theriacae usu*. See Palmer, 'Physicians and the Inquisition', 124–5; and Redmond, 'Girolamo Donzellino', 59–123. According to Gentilcore, *Medical Charlatanism*, 213, 'only by the eighteenth century did doctors voice strong doubts about the efficacy of the theriac; until then, it was the most potent cure—all the medical establishment had to offer'. Evidence from the plague tracts tells another story.

[8] Grassi, *Diario empirico*, 26r.

[9] Numerous descriptions of these debates can be found in the literature as far back as Corradi, *Annali*, I, 603ff. See Rodenwaldt, *Pest in Venedig*; Preto, *Peste e società a Venezia nel 1576*; largely from the records of the secret archive of Venice, Laughran, 'The Body, Public Health and Social Control', 204–20; and most recently Palmer, 'Girolamo Mercuriale'.

Already in 1575, the Sicilian physician Giovanni Filippo Ingrassia had argued that Palermo and other towns and villages in Sicily were not experiencing plague, despite buboes and carbuncles in lymph nodes, black and purple pustules across bodies, headaches, vomiting, and an epidemiology that for over a century had been the criteria for doctors and health boards in Italy in diagnosing plague. Moreover, he maintained that the doctors of Palermo in 1575 held the same opinion.[10] In the same year Veronese physicians denied that the epidemic was plague ('vera peste'), splitting the medical community roughly between physicians and surgeons; the surgeons diagnosed the disease of quick death with the bumps, buboes, carbuncles, and other signs and symptoms as plague; while the physicians denied it. As can be seen in the works of Agostino Valier, Alessandro Canobbio, and Vicenzio Tranquilli, this debate flared also in Mantua and Padua. It penetrated beyond learned medical circles and engaged a wide literate public. They came before city chambers to debate these medical issues and protested against decisions such as that taken by the Venetian senate in 1576 when, endorsing the diagnosis of the Paduan physicians, the Senate rescinded Venice's long-tested procedures for plague protection.[11] Not only were notaries, gentlemen administrators, and religious leaders aware of doctors' arguments about plague in 1575–8, they vigorously challenged them, despite their lack of medical training.

In addition to Valier, Benedetti, and Conobbio, whose arguments have been touched on in previous chapters, the poet and proofreader Borgaruccio Borgarucci was another outsider to publish his doubts about the 'dotti' during the 1575–8 plague. His was in verse:

> A certain heresy sprung up among many
> Between the doctors of Padua and Venice;
> Some were said to be plague-stricken.
> Others were said not to be taken,
> But wished to maintain that they were spot-ridden,
> which often reigned here in Venice.
> So friends and family were in trouble
> Not knowing whether they should be dead.
> Once these learned and prudent ones had left,
> the plague was then found to be real.[12]

Pastarino, a druggist in Venice, also expressed doubts about 'rumours' spreading among native Venetians (before the arrival of the Paduan professors) that 'this pestilence' was not 'really plague', since the corruption of air was held not to

---

[10] Ingrassia, *Informatione*, 47.

[11] For evidence of members of the public writing letters to and discussing their notions with health-board officials, see Crotto, *Memoriale delle provisioni generali*.

[12] *L'afflition di Vinetia*, 4–5. His name appears as a translator or editor of thirty-seven works during the later part of the sixteenth century. He was the author of only one published work, the poem above.

have been the cause. He challenged learned opinion 'based on experience and with previous histories [of plagues]', concluding: 'this plague, beyond any doubt, is plague'.[13] The Udinese author Gioseppe Viscanio was equally empirical. In April, 1576 before the Paduan professors had been called to Venice, the 'Vulgo' of Venice were already denying the plague because, they claimed, only a few women, children, and the poor were dying from it. But because of the tell-tale pestilential signs and symptoms, he supported the health board of Venice and their stringent implementation of quarantine and sequestering.[14]

This controversy was not, however, a conflict between two distinct groups: on the one hand physicians supposedly bound by bookish and ancient authority; on the other, practical men outside the academy—surgeons, notaries, administrators and the like—who treated the disease and its consequences. Academic physicians led the chorus that found the opinions of Mercuriale, Lazisi, and others who denied the plague to be unsupportable and dangerous. The attack of the Veronese doctor (and secret Protestant) Donzellini was written in a Venetian prison, where he had been condemned for life by the Inquisition. But because of the plague, he was freed to treat the infected in 1576.[15] Perhaps, because of his political circumstances, he was more guarded in his criticisms than the non-medical critics. In his tract of 1577 he named no one and, without any sense of irony, couched his critique in praise of the Venetian state as though it had not followed the opinions of Mercuriale and the Paduan physicians.[16] Yet, as Richard Palmer has shown, despite Protestant works on medicine and science being put on the Index of Prohibited Books, a republic of letters among physicians continued to flourish through the sixteenth century. Staunch Catholics such as Mercuriale acquired and read such works without penalties so long as they did not read or at least acquire banned theological works, a line that Donzellini began to cross in his years at Rome during the early 1540s.[17] Furthermore, as Donzellini's repeat bouts with the Inquisition attest, his Protestant belief in predestination may have given him a protective psychological shell; he was fearless in pursuit of scientific knowledge and his bibliomaniac craving to acquire new printed titles, regardless of their origins.[18]

---

[13] Pastarino, *Preparamento*, 4v. The humanist historian Tranquilli said that such debates also split the medical profession in Mantua in 1575; see Chapter 5, 137.

[14] Viscanio, *Regimento del viver*. This discussion appears in his second dedication, written first and signed on 11 April 1576. The first was dated 13 July 1576, at the height of the dispute in Venice on the character of the disease, but Viscanio did not mention the arrival or opinions of the Paduan physicians.

[15] Schutte, 'Donzellini, Girolamo'. He was freed temporarily in 1576 to treat plague victims and definitively in 1577 by an intervention from Rome.

[16] Others such as the *scrivan* of the Venetian health office during these years, Cornelio Morello, were not as circumspect; however, he never published his account of the Venetian plague.

[17] Palmer, 'Physicians and the Inquisition', esp. 128. Also, see Ongaro and Forin, 'Girolamo Mercuriale e lo studio di Padova'; on Mercuriale's relations with the 'German nation' of students at the University of Padua, see esp. 47–9.

[18] Palmer, 'Physicians and the Inquisition', 126–7.

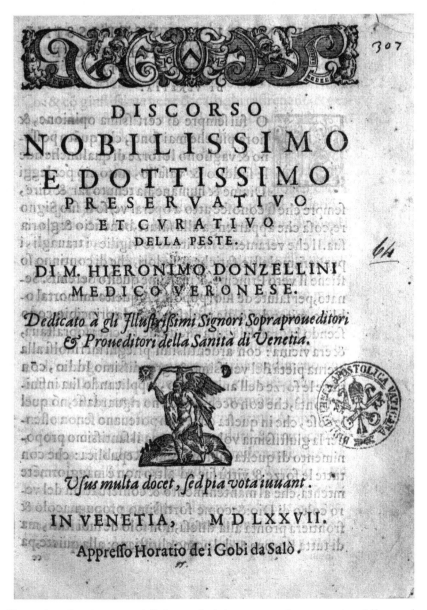

Illustration 5. *Discorso nobilissimo e dottissimo preservativo et curativo della peste* by Girolamo Donzellini medico Veronese, 1577.

On the other hand, his refusal to name Mercuriale or other doctors may not have come from fear of personal or professional reprisals. Donzellini graduated from the Medical School of the University of Padua in 1541, taught there before going to Rome, and was a friend of Mercuriale, supplying him with scientific books, some of which were on the Index.[19] As for his praise of the Venetian government, one arm of it, the Venetian health board, had in fact challenged Mercuriale and his colleagues as soon as they made their pronouncements. The health board had even broken the law: it ignored governmental orders and continued to separate the inflicted, the suspected, and the healthy when transporting them to hospitals and plague huts.[20] Donzellini dedicated his jail-house tract to these magistrates.[21]

Yet, despite his circumspection, his attack against those denying the plague was scathing. First, without citing Fracastoro, he held that plague in his day was most frequently generated and spread by mechanisms which ancient writers knew nothing about or at least never mentioned. This was contagion by clothing and other goods—'ad esser fomite' (Fracastoro's second mode of contagion).[22] Donzellini did not then describe the third means—*ad distans*—so crucial to Ingrassia's argument against calling Sicily's 'morbo contagioso' 'vera peste'. Instead, Donzellini praised the Venetian magistrates for passing decrees prohibiting the free circulation of inhabitants and thus impeding the spread of plague. Their actions, he maintained, cut against the common judgements of doctors and others that this *peste* was not an 'Epidemia' based on Galen's definition:

I say that everywhere one finds the same sets of characteristics, that is, the effects, signs, and accidents of the plague, and [if these are present] it is right to call it by its name, even if only one man is found with them. To the opposition which retorts that such is not an epidemic, I say that this is not pertinent . . .

Donzellini maintained that the Venetian magistrates had been effective in impeding the spread ('il progresso') of plague by not listening to the Paduan physicians. In support of the government, he alleged that they had passed decrees that sent the infected beyond the city's gates, locked up those already in the city who were infected or suspected, and prohibited commerce and the movement of people. By these means they had blocked the plague from 'snaking through the city'. Although the government had in fact supported and may have even influenced the opinions of the Paduan physicians out of commercial interests, Donzellini, perhaps considering only the health board as the 'government', concluded that because of its actions (but against the facts), the plague had not become 'an epidemic' in Galen's sense.

---

[19] Ibid., 128.   [20] Palmer, 'The Control of Plague', 249.

[21] He was tried several times for heresy and eventually executed by drowning in Venice in 1587. Perhaps brushes with the Inquisition caused him to be guarded in his criticisms and account for his attempts to ingratiate himself with the Venetian government.

[22] Donzellini, *Discorso nobilissimo*.

At the time of his dedication to the health board, the city had already suffered from the major force of the plague with at least 50,000 or more than a quarter of its population felled by the disease. Donzellini's praise may have been for the city's abrupt change of policy by the end of the summer and return to its original decrees. As a result of the suspension of their traditional quarantine and other defences against plague, Venice's mortalities had soared beyond those of any other city. The notary of the Venetian health board, Cornelio Morello, declared that Mercuriale and Capodivacca had been 'the number one cause of Venice's mortality and ruin'.[23] Even Mercuriale had implicitly realized his errors and changed his mind. By late summer the disease (by the Galenic criteria) had become 'vera peste'. But for Donzellini it had been so from the start, not because of any Hippocratic or Galenic definitions of 'epidemic', but because it 'possessed the nature, effects, and signs of true plague' and thus was to be treated as plague by doctors and governors. To prevent the spread of contagion, the plague-stricken, 'dead and alive' had to be separated from the healthy.[24]

With still stronger words two other doctors condemned physicians then denying that the 1575–8 disease was true plague. These tracts, moreover, were written in Latin and in the academic style current in medical schools across Italy. Their arguments turned heavily on copious citations of antique sources—Hippocrates, Galen, Aristotle, Thucydides—as well as of medieval and modern philosophers and physicians—Averröes, Albert the Great, Aquinas, Ficino, and Fracastoro. Like Donzellini, the Cremonese physician Tommaso Somenzi, who practised medicine in Milan,[25] never named Mercuriale, Capodivacca, Lodovico Lazisi, or other physicians, then arguing against calling the current pestilence true plague. Unlike most academic physicians whose tracts often proceeded from ancient and modern authority and definitions to 'experience',[26] Somenzi established his authority by citing first his experience. At the time he was assisting the Milanese doctor Agostino Terzagi, probably on the Milanese health board. The two had been employed to treat the new wave of illness then threatening the city.[27] Unlike Ingrassia, Mercuriale, and others, Somenzi did not begin with Galenic premises on what constituted an epidemic and therefore plague. Instead, his arguments focused on the epidemic patterns and symptoms he and his fellow doctors had been observing in Milan. Like the non-physicians Bisciola, Cannobio, and others then describing the daily 'progress' of plague in their cities, Somenzi began with a narrative of the disease's transmission from Trent to Mantua, Verona, and Venice, and the measures these cities employed to prevent plague from entering

---

[23] Palmer, 'The Control of Plague', 277; and Laughran, 'The Body, Public Health and Social Control', 220.

[24] Donzellini, *Discorso nobilissimo*, 310v.   [25] Somenzi, *De morbis*.

[26] See Nutton, 'Books, Printing and Medicine'.

[27] Somenzi, *De morbis*, 1r: 'Ego & Augustinus Terzagus Medicus Mediolanen. vir insigni morum probitate . . . in quibus vagari nova Morborum clades ferebatur, ut num quidpiam in illis pestilens, contagiosumue appareret diligenter inquireremus.'

their gates. In fact, according to Somenzi, Venice had initially been the most successful in preventing the plague's entry, but eventually the disease penetrated all these cities. By Somenzi's account (like those of the notaries and others), it spread through contagion either by contaminated goods or infected individuals. By contrast, Mantua was one of the first to be infected, he charged, because early on its city authorities had 'neglected' to call the plague a plague.[28]

Somenzi then considered the symptoms, not in any theoretical sense or ones compiled from ancient authority in Hippocrates or Galen of what constituted epidemics in general but 'as they appeared in Mantua'—acute fever, headaches, delirium, sleeplessness, painful vomiting, intense thirst, excrement corrupted by stomach convulsions ('excrementa per aluum corrupta'), turbid urine, stench, a change in facial expression and colour, eyes that assumed a look of horror, and especially the high lethality of the disease. Somenzi's diagnosis combined these symptoms observed at present as well as in previous bouts of plague with the tell-tale signs: the swellings in many parts of the body, but especially in the glands (*adenes*) of the armpits, the groin, and behind the ears. According to Somenzi, these swellings were mainly buboes, but they also appeared in various other forms—bumps around the ears (*parotides*) and tumours (*tubercula*), carbuncles and various types of spots and *pettechiae*, also called *morbilli* and *variolae*.[29] If by the seventh day these swellings suppurated, Somenzi claimed the patient could survive. But mostly the boils did not erupt and 'most of the afflicted died in three days, some in four, some in two, and some on the same day [as the first signs of illness] or even within a few hours.'[30] In other words, the criteria were roughly those observed by Milan's health board doctors going back to the beginning of its necrologies in 1452.

Having established similarities between the present affliction and the signs and symptoms of previous plagues, Somenzi then concentrated on epidemiological traits: 'the first thing to be noticed about plague is its contagion, as can be gathered from the historical sources ('ex praenarrata historia colligamus')'.[31] Once plague had infected a place, it quickly afflicted many others in that place, spreading from family to family. But, most importantly, as doctors since 1348 had noted, the plague spread within households, 'afflicting one after another within a very short space of time' ('cumque in iisdem domibus, unus post alium, plures modicissimo tempore').[32] For Somenzi, 'there was no doubt' the disease currently infecting Milan was contagious, had spread to places nearby and further afield, and possessed the same terrible symptoms seen in the history of other plagues'.[33]

He then reported on the current disease in Trent, Mantua, and Milan, and historical experiences of plague to engage in a more academic discussion

---

[28] Ibid., 2r.   [29] Ibid, 2r–v.   [30] Ibid., 2v.   [31] Ibid., 3r.
[32] Ibid., 3v. On these epidemiological patterns, see Cohn and Alfani, 'Households and Plague'.
[33] Somenzi, *De morbis*, 4r.

of contagion. He narrowed his focus to classical and modern definitions, distinctions, and disputes. Instead of relying on Fracastoro, he cited Aristotle to discuss how the disease spread *ad fomitem* or by objects and *ad distans*, or by the putrefaction of the air (but despite his footnotes, he surely was relying on the new terms and ideas of Fracastoro). Somenzi rejected the Epicurean notion of atoms and attacked Fracastoro for supposedly adopting this position and for attacking Galen on issues such as putrefaction of the humours.[34] Suddenly, in contrast to his opening pages, Somenzi shifted to a conservative and academic defence of Galen but grounded it in specific historical examples: Italian plagues in 1528, a sixteenth-century plague in Tripoli, the 1555 plague in Padua, and the plagues then raging in Mantua, Milan, Venice, and elsewhere in northern Italy.[35] He also continued to emphasize the importance of signs, symptoms, and epidemiology such as plague's historic tendency to spread predominantly among the poor. This criterion, so essential to Mercuriale and others for ruling out plague (because it supposedly failed to satisfy Galen's definition of 'epidemic'), was for Somenzi the historic evidence that the current disease must be 'true plague'. He then tried to explain this social-epidemiological pattern, a subject to which we will return in the next chapter.

The physician Francesco Stabile, from the southern town of Potenza but who practised in northern Italy, was another to attack vigorously the physicians' denial of plague in 1575–8.[36] Like Somenzi, Stabile began not with theory or authority found in ancient texts but with empirical observations and reports from the spread of the present plague in 1576. First, he reported for Venice that many died from the disease in three days or less and few survived as long as a week[37] and that many were afflicted with 'large swellings the size of nuts in the groin, armpits or behind the ears'. In addition, carbuncles appeared on many under the chin, on thighs, shins, the back, and nape of the neck. Further, often spots ('macules') like black lentils appeared in various parts of the body. He then described in detail the symptoms: weakness of the entire body, headaches, delirium, a tendency to lie in bed without sleeping, pale complexion, a wild look in the eyes ('occuli horridi'), failure to notice light, loss of appetite, vomiting bile, intense thirst, dry tongue, slurred speech, stomach convulsions with corrupt and smelly excrement sometimes filled with worms, turbid urine for most, but for some it was thin or weak ('tenues'), for others bilious or with a sickly sediment. Stabile confessed to not taking his plague patients' pulse but reported from doctors who had that it

---

[34] On the atomistic theory of nature and Galen's rejection of it, see Temkin, *Galenism*, 17. The theory was introduced into medicine by Asclepiades, a contemporary of Cicero. Somenzi was mistaken: Fracastoro criticized the atomism of Democritus, Epicurus, and Lucretius as 'crude and silly' (*rudis et ineptus*); *De sympathia et antipathia*, 32; also see Pennuto, *Simpatia, fantasia e contagio*, 17–18, 167, 214–18, and 417–52.

[35] On the importance of history for doctors' analysis and diagnoses during the sixteenth century, see Siraisi, *History, Medicine, and the Traditions.*

[36] Stabile, *Breuis quaedam defensio.* Curiously, he dedicated his tract to Girolamo Capodivacca.

[37] Stabile, *Breuis quaedam defensio*, 1r–v.

was weak and rapid. He reported at length on aspects of plague corpses, their colour, contortions, stench, puss erupting from the spots, eyes wide open, and blackened nails.[38] As for Somenzi, these observable signs and symptoms were the crucial criteria, not antique definitions.

Like Somenzi, Stabile did not name names but made it clear that in Venice a major dispute ('lis magna') had erupted among 'our honourable College of Most Excellent Doctors' (suggesting that Stabile had become a member).[39] He then outlined more thoroughly than Somenzi the arguments of the physicians who denied the plague. In short, by Hippocratic and Galenic doctrine, to qualify as true plague a disease had to be common ('communis'), meaning spreading to most living in a region and thus having been caused by pestilential air. These doctors argued that no such air had afflicted Venice that year, and although the disease had afflicted men, women, the old, and young, it had failed to affect them equally. Rather, it had been confined almost exclusively to the *ignobiles* with nobles and the wealthy left largely untouched. Given these class differences, they argued, the disease could not have originated from the air; otherwise, the majority would have perished.[40] True to the physicians' academic credentials, Stabile loaded his treatise with citations to Galen and with Greek terms for 'epidemic', 'common', 'popular', 'vulgar', and more.

Thus armed, he then refuted the Paduan doctors' claims on their own terms, utilizing Galenic definitions to maintain that the disease 'was in fact *vulgaris*: many in the city of both sexes and of all ages were afflicted and many of these had died; therefore, the disease must have been spread by air'. To demonstrate this theoretical point he then turned to empirical evidence—detailed disease tracking, in fact, at a more microscopic level than that seen in the notaries' tracts or in any other plague tract I know for the sixteenth century. He reconstituted the lines of contagion within specific households in Venice as well as from one household and one street to another. His analysis began with a sixty-year-old pauper, Iacobus Cadorinus, who lived with his second wife and a daughter from his first marriage. Stabile alleged that Iacobus carried the disease from Trent to Venice.[41] In a short time, all these family members caught the disease and died but before dying passed the disease to their neighbours and in particular to two households that Stabile maintained had had contacts with these first Venetian victims. Through these and similar interconnections Stabile argued that the disease disseminated through touch, clothing, 'but especially by breathing venomous air',[42] and concluded (slightly changing definitions seen in Mercuriale and others) that the disease had

---

[38] Stabile, *Breuis quaedam defensio*, 2r.

[39] Another doctor not to name names but to support the Venetian health board and oppose vigorously the opinions of the Paduan doctors was Crotto, *Memoriale delle provisioni generali*, 6r–v. He alleged that the Paduan doctors had been advised by charlatans (*ceretani*).

[40] Stabile, *Breuis quaedam defensio*, 2v–3r.

[41] On the geography of contagion, also see Preto, *Peste e società a Venezia nel 1576*, 13–14.

[42] Stabile, *Breuis quaedam defensio*, 5r–6r.

to be called plague because it was 'common' ('vulgaris'), 'deadly' ('perniciosus'), and spread by air. Again turning to case studies from the Venetian registers and his own inspection of the plague corpses (probably as a member of the health board), he addressed another pillar of the Paduan denial: that the current disease could not be plague because it infected only certain neighbourhoods and not the entire city. Instead, to maintain that the disease was plague, Stabile pointed to the clustering of deaths within households and the quickness of death.[43]

How this proved his case against Mercuriale and other doctors who denied the presence of plague based on strict Hippocratic and Galenic definitions of 'common' and 'epidemic' is not clear. Like Somenzi's tract, the later parts of Stabile's drifted from empirical analysis (in his case the Venice's plague registers) and his own clinical observations to present classical texts heavily laden with references to Thucydides, Galen, and many others. But also like Somenzi, he continued to rely on recent histories of plague, such as the description of the Paduan plague of 1555–6 by the 'celebrated' doctor Francesco Frigimelica, to argue that the present plague resembled this previous one (which had been seen by Paduan physicians as 'true plague'). Both were highly contagious, and both displayed the 'well-known signs' on the bodies of the living and dead.[44]

Still other doctors further removed from the most severe outbreaks of the 1575–8 plague and distant from major seats of medical learning adopted new notions of plague and 'epidemic' that had been filtering through Italian academic medicine over the past decade, if not longer. For instance, the communal doctor of Camaiore Giovanni Battista Giudici began by defining plague. He 'restricted its name' to a disease that was common in Galen's sense, that is, infecting lethally the great majority of a region ('nihil aliud est, nisi morbus vulgaris et communis'). Yet, unlike Mercuriale and others in the north who began their arguments with Galenic definitions, Giudici did not employ them to deny the presence of plague now threatening Italy top to toe. Instead, he turned the words to make a new argument: because plague was 'vulgar', or 'common' to a large proportion of a population, physicians' plague tracts should now be written in the vernacular, not in Latin.[45] He then quickly departed from the Galenic strictures to define plague according to his own criteria that relied on signs and symptoms alone. The doctor and poet Sebastiano Ajello, writing at the end of 1576 in Naples, also began his tract by defining plague according to Galenic principles as 'popular' and deadly. His definition, however, incorporated Fracastoro's new definitions of contagion, and, like Giudici's, stressed the presence of the plague's

---

[43] Ibid., 8r–10v. He cites the records of Morello, notary of Venice's health board; see Chapter 4, 115.

[44] Ibid., 11r. Another doctor to begin with classical definitions of plague, mutation of air, and bodily humours was Crotto, *Memoriale delle provisioni generali*; however, he rejected the opinions of 'the two Paduan doctors'. Crotto based his argument on the appearance of 'carbonchi' and other plague signs, raging mortality and ideas of contagion largely digested from Fracastoro (6r–v).

[45] Giudici, *Il trattato della Peste*, 6.

historic and well-known signs and symptoms—swellings behind the ears, in the armpits, in the groin, 'and more often there than in the other two places'. Like Somenzi, Ajello challenged the plague deniers and even Galen by turning to contemporary historical examples and attacked from an altogether new angle: not all diseases that were in fact 'popular' and 'mortal' were plague. He cited the example of a coughing disease ('i catarri'), perhaps akin to bronchitis, that broke out in Naples in 1562. 'Precisely because it was not contagious, it should never be called Peste.'[46] Ajello then examined the question, 'what is contagion or infection?'[47]

During the 1575–8 outbreak not all doctors in Venice or elsewhere adopted Hippocratic or Galenic definitions of plague that depended on definitions of epidemic or made distinctions between plague-like 'morbo contigoso' and 'true plague'. Most remarkable of these was the Venetian David de Pomi, the first Jewish doctor in Italy to publish a plague tract and one of the few to leave a manuscript on plague in Italy since the Black Death.[48] Because de Pomi's 'discussions and memoirs' ('discorsi e ricordi') were dated letters presented to the health board of Venice, they give the earliest precisely dated reactions to the plague in Venice of 1575–7. From his first report of 15 February 1576, he never questioned that this disease was plague. Nor was he an armchair physician who stayed safe from it; instead, he 'visited a great number of the afflicted from their front door'. At the plague's height he continued to treat the plague-stricken in the three worst-afflicted neighbourhoods (*contrade*) of Venice. Despite the initial low levels of plague mortality, he used criteria similar to those employed by health boards: if victims died suddenly with tumours in the groin, under the arms, or behind the ears, they had died of plague. He did not refrain from the dreaded words 'segno pestifero', 'luoghi pestiferi', and 'peste' or attempt to mince words with the less precise *morbo contagioso* used in Sicily as well as in the north. In his last report presented on 27 and 28 February 1577, with the disease in steep decline, he continued to use terms for plague despite the fact (as seen in previous Italian plagues) that the disease was no longer as lethal as it had been during its height in summer: 'at this time in the splendid city of Venice there was again plague [*peste*], even if cases were seen that were not very dangerous [*non molto perniciosa*]'. By Hippocratic-Galenic definitions, the disease would no longer have qualified as plague. Instead, de Pomi accounted for the disease's change in lethality (probably mistakenly) by speculating (perhaps with Fracastoro as his guide) that these cases had been transmitted by clothing with a weak residue of

---

[46] Ajello, *Breue discorso*, 7r–8v. In later chapters, he discussed in detail the symptoms of plague ('Segni per conoscere un'huomo appestato'), headaches, condition of the eyes, tiredness, etc., 29r–v.

[47] Ibid., 8v–12r.

[48] De Pomi, *Brevi discorsi*. He also wrote on Jewish-Christian relations and published a Hebrew dictionary in three languages. No Jewish plague tracts appear in Karl Sudhoff's survey from 1348 to 1500. Barkai, 'Jewish Treatises on the Black Death', claims that Jewish physicians produced a great quantity of plague treatises for the late Middle Ages but names only five, and none of these was by an Italian.

the plague poison.[49] In effect, Donzellini, Somenzi, Stabile, and de Pomi had returned to the trusted means of diagnosis as seen in the day-to-day operations of northern Italian health boards. Symptoms of continuous fever, headaches, and vomiting, together with signs of buboes and other pustules and quick death, were paramount in their rules for recognizing plague, and not academic definitions adopted from Galen.[50]

Curiously, before 1575, physicians' plague tracts contained little discussion distinguishing 'true plague' and other lesser categories of pestilential fevers or the use of new terms *morbo contagioso* to avoid the terrorizing realities of *peste*. During the previous plague of 1555–6 in Padua and Venice, Lodovico Pasini distinguished between 'true plague' and that which was not. But his analysis did not deny the presence of the plague then striking these cities. Its point was instead to rule out an accompanying disease occasionally mistaken for plague. This disease was in Pasini's terms 'both a pestilential fever and one with spots, commonly called "petecchia"'. It was not plague because it was not as contagious or unavoidable as 'true plague' ('non esse contagiosas, nec fugiendas').[51] Indeed, members of health boards in places such as Milan had diagnosed this disease of bumps or red *morbilli* as early as 1477 as one 'without suspicion' of being plague because of the consistent epidemiological differences that Pasini highlighted.[52] A doctor from the Veneto, practising medicine in Venice during the plague of 1555–6, also distinguished plague from *petecchie* on epidemiological grounds that did not rely on Galen's definition of 'epidemic'. Instead, although Fracastoro was not mentioned, his notions of contagion lay behind this doctor's diagnosis: 'The said "petecchie" are contagious but not in the manner of plague'. With *petecchie*, the contagion is spread only by direct contact with the ill, while plague is transmitted not only directly by handling ('maneggiandolo') the inflicted, but also by coming near without touching the patient, or by touching his clothes and similar things. The contagion of plague is much quicker and lethal than that of *petecchie* because the poison of plague is more intense.[53] He then cautioned that because of plague's swift contagion and the intensity of its poison it had to be treated rapidly.[54]

Another professor of medicine at Padua, Bernardino Tomitano (1517–76) writing during the 1555–6 plague, defined 'true plague' also to distinguish it from *petecchie*. His definition, however, relied more on Galen than his colleagues and may have anticipated the controversies of the next plague wave. Neither the signs and symptoms nor epidemiological traits such as the speed of contagion or quickness of death were crucial for him. Instead, he distinguished 'the variety

---

[49] De Pomi, *Brevi discorsi*, 305r.   [50] Daciano, *Trattato della peste*.

[51] Pasini, *De pestilentia, Patavina anno 1555*, 13v.

[52] See the diagnoses of the Milanese doctors during an epidemic principally of red *morbilli* in 1477 and 1478; Popolazione, no. 75. On average patients took two weeks and not two to three days to die from this disease.

[53] da Marostica, *Copia d' vna lettera*, 309v (BAV).   [54] Ibid., 312r.

of *petecchie*' from plague 'in this manner': if it kills many, it is to be labelled 'petecchie'; if it kills the majority, it is plague.[55] Still he had no doubts, the 1555–6 plague in Padua and Venice was true plague.

The 1575–7 plague in Venice had not been the first occasion a city council had assembled doctors to decide whether a disease in their midst was plague or something less acute and malignant. In 1555 the Venetian government summoned Niccolò Massa before the College of Physicians 'to determine by common opinion or true science if the disease was plague [*Peste*], glandular swellings, Giandussa as it was commonly called, or some other disease'.[56] Massa reports that until he had examined the corpses and patients still alive with the disease, he had refused to make a diagnosis.[57] Once he had, however, there were no doubts; the disease was plague, despite the fact that in Padua it was afflicting almost exclusively the poor ('queste infirmità morivano questi dì, sono stati poveri, & non ricchi, nè nobili').[58] Rather than denying plague, he instead attempted to explain why the poor caught and harboured it, concluding that 'the condition of their bad bodies filled with bad humours', the variety of the bad and cheap food they ate, their sexual appetites, and their cramped housing filled with too many children made them 'less resistant to the corruption'.[59] Although his explanation may strike us as unconvincing, Massa's reasoning did not derive from antique logic or definitions but was lodged in clinical observation and in housing and living conditions:

the poor lived in tiny and wretched houses [*casupule strette*], without sunlight or air, and were made ill by being locked up with their stench. Moreover, in such a small space few possessed the means for removing their filth, and what was even sadder, in these conditions, the ill easily infected the healthy.[60]

He further argued that the rich fared better than the poor during plague time, because they had much greater access to medical care.[61]

For Massa, 'peste' was hardly a catch-all term for any epidemic as current historians sometimes claim was generally the case with medicine before the Enlightenment.[62] Instead, like many other sixteenth-century authors of plague tracts, Massa took pains to distinguish plague by its specific 'accidents' of buboes and carbuncles from other epidemic diseases, such as those with sneezing ('delle distillationi') and coughs, heart disorder ('sqinantie'), smallpox ('ponte') and other pains and illnesses'.[63] Nor did he consider illnesses of 'many smallpox'

---

[55] Tomitano, *Il consiglio sopra la peste*, 11v.   [56] Massa, *Ragionamento*.

[57] Ibid., 2v–3r.   [58] Ibid. 20r and 21r.   [59] Ibid. 20v

[60] Ibid., 17r–18v. In his first work on syphilis (*Il liber del mal francese*, first published in 1527), he was also pragmatic and not ruled by antique doctrines. He encouraged physicians 'to try everything provided that one proceeds reasonably . . . for I am not of the opinion that nothing can be added to the discoveries of the learned . . . ' Cited and translated in Palmer, 'Nicolò Massa', 393. He made similar proclamations in other works (ibid., 395).

[61] Massa, *Ragionamento*, 21r.

[62] See for instance Cosmacini, *Storia della medicina*, 101. Many others can be cited.

[63] Massa, *Ragionamento*, 22v.

('variole') or bumps ('morbili') or other such marks ('espilsioni') that afflicted children to be 'plague'. He also recognized that other diseases could produce apostemes in various parts of the body, and that 'not every *antrace* or *carbone* was necessarily pestilential'.[64] Rather, for him as with doctors on health boards since the mid-fifteenth century, rapid contagion, household clustering of cases, and sudden death were the plague's hallmarks: 'The first and most trustworthy principle is if one dies in a household, most of the others living there along with those serving it, suddenly become ill from the same disease, and most of them die.'[65] Massa's manual written in the midst of the 1555–6 plague was no academic exercise. Its intent was to instruct individuals and governments on how to recognize the 'true signs' of plague and to separate and sequester the plague-stricken from the healthy as soon as possible and 'without any error'.[66]

Francesco Frigimelica (1490–1558) was another authority of the 1555–6 plague cited by other doctors through the second half of the sixteenth century, and who also was a professor of medicine at Padua. He devoted the first part of his plague treatise to distinguishing pestilential fevers from plague (which he simply called 'peste' and not 'vera peste'). By Frigimelega's definition, as with Massa's, pestilential fevers did not have 'the terrible accidents, *apostemi*, *carboncoli*, and *pruni*'. Frigimelega placed even greater emphasis than Massa on one epidemiological aspect of plague and was more precise—the speed of death from the onset of the first signs of illness. With the fevers patients took two weeks or more to die; for plague it usually happened by the fourth day. He used this criterion (as Milanese doctors had done during an epidemic of 'petecchie' in 1477–8) to diagnose a contagious epidemic with spots ('con macchie o parotide') that had erupted in 1528 alongside plague. The disease, he argued, had not been plague, not only because carbuncles and *pruni* had not formed, but because the victims took from eleven to fourteen days to die.[67] Similarly, a decade earlier Fracastoro had distinguished *pestilentes verae* or *vere pestilentes vocatae* from other diseases such as one called 'lenticulae' or 'puncticulas'. At

---

[64] Ibid., 5v.   [65] Ibid., 15v.

[66] Ibid., 13r. On changes in Massa's analysis of plague from his first tract published in 1540 (but probably written in the aftermath of the plagues of the 1520s), his *Ragiomento*, written in 1555 and his third work on plague, *De essentia causis*, see Palmer, 'Nicolò Massa', 396–8. On the traditional character of plague as miasmic and dependent on the stars in this earlier text, see Pennuto, *Simpatia, fantasia e contagio*, 397–400, but she does not comment on Massa's later tracts.

[67] Frigimelega, *Consiglio sopra la pestilentia*, n.p. Still others during the 1555–6 plague made distinctions in their definitions of plague without drawing a dichotomy between pestilential fevers and plague or 'true' plague. For instance, the Venetian doctor and astrologist De Forte (*Il trattato de la peste*, n.p.) distinguished four categories of plague based on skin disorders but did not relegate or advance any of them as criteria for rejecting 'true plague'. Around the same time, Georg Agricola, best known for his work on mining and metallurgy (*De Re Metallica*), published a plague tract distinguishing plague from other diseases by signs and symptoms, beginning with the glandular swellings and carbuncles, then supplying a long list of familiar symptoms—headaches, nausea, vomiting, etc.; Agricola, *De peste libri tres*, 24–6. The plague tract of the English doctor Thomas Moulton, *Myrour or glasse of healthe*, also called 'A treatise of What is ment or signifyca by thys worde pestylence', defined plague by its signs and symptoms.

first his definition approached that of Mercuriale and the Paduan Athenaeum thirty years on. This disease was not true plague because it killed principally (in this case) the nobility and not 'the greater part of the people'. However, when he came to his chapter on 'true pestilential fevers', his criteria like those writing in 1555–6 depended on the formation of buboes, speed of contagion, and quickness of death, and not on Hippocratic-Galenic notions of 'popular', 'vulgar', and 'epidemic'.[68]

***

As claimed above, it would be incorrect to conclude that those outside the medical profession such as Valier or the notaries, gate-guards, and gentlemen administrators were the ones, even the leaders, of the attack on the plague deniers. Of the printed sources, in fact it was physicians who overwhelmingly led this assault, and they often did so by becoming more attentive to defining the crucial characteristics that separated true plague ('peste vera') from pestilential fevers or other diseases. With these criteria, they argued that their current plague was plague and that time-tested public health measures were not to be abandoned. In 1576, Gioseffo Daciano employed by the commune of Udine, published a tract on plague and the spots ('delle petecchie') in which he devoted three chapters to various forms of plague and what constituted the difference between true plague and pestilential fevers.[69] Despite his copious references to Hippocrates, Galen, and Avicenna, Daciano's judgements replicated the diagnoses and actions of doctors on health boards and writers of earlier plague manuals such as Niccolò Massa. Daciano's three forms of plague were distinguished by visible signs: first, *petecchie* or black marks and bumps like lentils 'or like the bites or stings [*beccature*] of fleas';[70] secondly, the *posteme* or *buboni*, which formed in the glands, behind ears, under the arms, or in the groin and were accompanied by great pain; and thirdly, the *carboni* or *antraci*, which formed indiscriminately over the entire body. All three were highly contagious and were accompanied by malignant fever. Although plague and pestilential fevers all had their origins in the putrefaction of the air, plague was the most contagious and could be distinguished by the speed of death, 'killing within two, three, or four days with victims rarely surviving to the seventh day'.[71] Further chapters returned to the problem: 'on the signs for recognising the plague'. He repeated his earlier

---

[68] Fracastoro, *De contagione*, ch. 6–7, 46–53. As with later plague writers, he also pointed out that not all diseases 'common' or 'popular' in a district were necessarily contagious (54–5).

[69] Daciano, *Trattato della peste*, 1–9.

[70] Similarly, Fracastoro, *De contagione*, 103, described the purplish-red spots that appeared on the arms, back, and chest. Modern historians have assumed that this disease (which Fracastoro and other contemporaries called by names such as *lenticulae*, as 'looking like flea bites, though they were often larger') was typhus. No sixteenth-century author said that these spots were flea bites or came from stings of lice or other insects. Nor were medieval or sixteenth-century doctors so oblivious to insects as modern historians sometimes assert. See for example Albert the Great's careful distinctions in the appearance and habits of lice and fleas idem, *Man and the Beasts*, 437–9.

[71] Daciano, *Trattato della peste*, 9.

descriptions of the skin disorders and the quickness of death, but added what he considered as the most important criterion—contagion: 'if one in a household caught it, within two, three or four days, most of the others died, even if they showed no pestilential signs'.[72] But, along with doctors on Milan's health board who diagnosed causes of death, he believed that the combination of epidemiological and symptomatic traits was crucial. In 1552, at the beginning of his career, he tells us, he went against the opinions of older colleagues on Udine's health board concerning an epidemic of *petecchie* or spots, in which the victims, as in plague, died rapidly but where none of the corpses showed swellings in the usual lymph nodes.[73]

A doctor Marino Massucci of Jesi,[74] also distinguished *petecchi* from plague, maintaining that many of his colleagues had confused the two. In contrast to plague, *petecchie* did not always kill the majority of those it infected, it was not as malignant, nor always as contagious as plague. He then turned to history, recalling his experiences practising in Padua when he diagnosed a fever of *petecchie* in 1560 and 1561 not to have been plague: it was not 'popular' or 'regional' but confined only to a few families in Lombardy and especially to the city of Padua. He contrasted that experience with the disease of the past year (1576) in the Marche, which he called plague: it was truly 'epidemic', spreading over a vast terrain in 'Venice, Padua, Mantua, Milan, Trent, and many other regions [*paesi*]', inflicting death on the majority who were infected.[75] Perhaps Massucci was unaware that he was now in conflict with his former colleagues. He further elaborated that many epidemic diseases—coughs ('catarri'), dysentery ('dissenterie'), scurvy ('schelentie'), and other fevers—spread beyond households and occupied cities, provinces, and even regions but were not plague, even when these diseases killed the majority they infected as they had done in 1527 and 1528.[76]

***

On his return to Padua and after plague had declined in Venice during the winter of 1576, Mercuriale delivered lectures on plague, collected by a former student (Girolano Zacco) and published in January 1577. These represent a defence of the Paduan position during the disastrous summer of 1576 along with a thinly veiled concession that his earlier advice might have been mistaken. Although he continued to ridicule the position of the Venetian health office, that their policies of isolation of the sick had not been correct, he now diagnosed

---

[72] Ibid., 40.   [73] Ibid., 25.

[74] He informs us in this tract (his only publication) that he had been a student of the famous professor of Anatomy at Padua, Gabriele Falloppio (1523–62).

[75] Massucci, *La preseruatione dalla pestilenza*, 24–5 and 66.

[76] Ibid., 25. Later he described other diseases that were contagious, covered vast regions, and had to be called 'mali Epidemiali' but were not plague. Such was a 'very contagious disease of coughs' that had struck Marcerata in 1562 'along with the cities of Perugia, Rome, Naples, Venice, Padua, Milano, Ferrara, Bologna, and in many parts of Europe' (43).

that the Venetian disease had become 'true plague'.[77] His definition had in fact shifted: its overriding criterion was now contagion—'there was no plague without contagion, and plague is the most contagious of all diseases'.[78] In addition, the accidents specific to plague—swellings in various parts of the body, especially in the groin, underarms, and behind the ears, along with carbuncles in all parts of the body, often numerous—had become essential to his diagnosis.[79] His tract continued with long lists of the other signs and symptoms of plague that would enable doctors to recognize the disease, including characteristics of urine, excrement, eyes, vomiting, and the colour, number, positions, and forms of various smaller bumps and spots ('macule'). These characteristics were essentially those that had determined thousands of diagnoses of plague found in Milanese necrologies from the mid-fifteenth century on. As in other physicians' plague tracts and with practising doctors' diagnoses, he also turned to the standard epidemiological criteria of 'true plague': 'this disease most frequently wiped out entire families and the afflicted rarely survived to day five'.[80]

With the next major plague outbreak in northern Italy after 1575–8, one in 1584 that struck Turin and Piedmont, where the 1575–8 plague had failed to penetrate,[81] the University of Turin physician Bucci, also without naming names, looked back critically over physicians' judgements during the previous plague in 'Padua, Venice, Palermo, and other Italian cities':

On whether the disease was true plague or not, some affirmed that it was not, because not enough died of the same illness on the same day, transmitting the disease from one to another, to be true plague. Others denied it because the air was not corrupt. Thus by praising such opinions, governments returned to commerce as usual, and, as a consequence, the disease spread with incredible mortality.[82]

Bucci's experience came from his practice in Ivrea, where he charted his current plague as having begun in Piedmont. From his practice, he compared plague with others diseases, which were contagious by contact—scabies, leprosy, inflammation of the eyes, and venereal diseases—and rejected the definitions and models of epidemics formulated in Hippocrates and Galen. For Bucci, neither mortality counts nor the social or geographic dimensions of a plague were relevant; rather, if victims died immediately and those infected spread it much more readily than with other diseases of contact, the disease was plague. If

---

[77] Mercuriale, *De Pestilentia*: quidem Tridentinus circa m. Iulii, quo tempore Tridenti grassabatur pestis, appulit Venetias . . . usque ad totum Decembrem 1575 duravit (4)'; and 'ostenditur, Venetam & Patavinam fuisse veram pestem' (10); also see, 2. This tract was published at Venice and Basel in the same year. They were his lecturers at the University of Padua in January 1577. See Durling, *A Catalogue of Sixteenth Century Printed Books*, 396; and Palmer, 'Girolamo Merucriale', 64.

[78] Mercuriale, *De pestilentia*, 11.   [79] Ibid. 3, 102–03, and 110.   [80] Ibid., 3.

[81] According to Corradi, *Annali*, I, 593, the 1575–7 plague struck only a few villages on the eastern borders of Piedmont.

[82] Bucci *Modo di conoscere*, 7r–v. As early as July 1576 in Venice, others outside the medical profession without published works had concluded much the same and placed the blame squarely on the shoulders of Mercuriale and Capodivacca; see above, 167–8.

these conditions were observed, immediately, individuals and governments were to enact the necessary preventative measures.[83] In a latter chapter, 'Concerning the pernicious error of those doctors who denied that the disease was plague', Bucci's condemnations became harsher still as he speculated on the government's motives:

Notwithstanding that many doctors saw the afflicted dying so suddenly and quickly, that the disease was transmitted from one to another within the same household, that the exterior and well-known signs were staring them in the face, and that the disease progressed in the usual manner, they were deceived by the opinion that this disease could not be plague or true contagion. The people willingly latched on to this opinion, partly to hold on to what they had, partly from abhorrence of the disease and fear of sequestration and privation of commerce. But he who examined well the beginnings of the past plagues in Trent, Padua, Venice, Mantua, Milan, and other places can show that these doctors had been deceived; there was no question but that these cities suffered from plague.[84]

Ultimately, whether a disease was 'true plague' was not so complex. Bucci applied Occam's razor to the perplexities created by the new and refined readings of Galen and Hippocrates during 1575–8: it is enough to affirm that plague is 'true plague' if many die of these symptoms on the same day, and the disease is passed from one to another.[85] Later in his tract, he would take great pains specifying the exact signs and symptoms of plague to assist laymen, physicians, and health boards.[86]

After 1575–8, other plague writers would also characterize diseases that they did not call plague or 'true plague' as an 'Epidemia o, volemo dire, morbo populare' in the Galenic sense. This was how the Augustinian friar Evangelista Quattrami from Gubbio described a disease that began in Flanders and France in 1580 and soon reached Rome, infecting the lungs, and which modern historians have called influenza.[87] It met the Galenic conditions for an epidemic but was certainly not plague. For the next plague in Sicily, Pietro Parisi accepted the Galenic definition that an epidemic had to be popular, 'that is, common and dangerous to all or most', but he did not stop there. Instead, he specified five signs of plague beginning with the bubo, but warned: 'To recognize plague, it is not only necessary to recognize its signs from medical texts; one needs to recognize it through experience.'[88]

Despite Mercuriale's loss of face and semi-retraction, those in the medical academy continued to cite him with respect and pride.[89] Even in 1577, the doctor Andreas Gabrielli of Senigallia, then practising in Genoa, praised 'the

---

[83] Ibid., 7v.   [84] Ibid., 12v.   [85] Ibid., 7r.   [86] Ibid., 57v–58r.

[87] Quattrami, *Breve trattato intorno alla preservatione*, 4r. For this epidemic, see Cavini, *L'influenza*; Pyle, *The Diffusion of Influenza*, 23–5; and Cohn and Alfani, 'Households and Plague', 184–5.

[88] Parisi, *Trattato della peste et febre pestifera*, in *Auuertimenti*, 15–17 and 20.

[89] When he and Capodivacca arrived before the Venetian Senate, they were praised as 'two Gods of medicine . . . sent by God to rid Venice from plague', but with the steep climb in plague deaths in July the Senate abruptly dismissed them. According to Venice's official historian, Andrea Morosini, this 'ugly

celebratissimo Gymnasio' of Padua and their advice (presumably to the Venetian Senate) on the importance of air in plague time: Mercuriale and Capodivacca were noted in the margins.[90] In later plagues of the sixteenth-century, their scandalous advice seems to have been mostly forgotten. Alessandro Massaria of the medical school of Padua, writing in 1591,[91] and the Sicilian doctor Pietro Parisi, writing in 1593, despite implicit criticisms of Mercuriale's position in 1576, cited approvingly the opinions of 'the renowned Mercuriale'.[92] By then (1587), Mercuriale had been persuaded to move to Bologna 'with a contract more flattering than any previously offered to a professor of medicine at Bologna (an annual salary of 1,200 *scudi* in gold), honorary Bolognese citizenship, and an exemption from all taxes', and in 1592 the Grand Duke of Tuscany offered him even more to accept a professorship at Pisa.[93] Yet, at least in Padua, the 1576 debacle may not have been completely forgotten or forgiven: in 1598 Mercuriale applied for the chair following Massaria's death and was refused.[94]

By the time of the next big plague in Italy, that of 1629–33, the Florentine doctor Alessandro Righi (who also denied that Florence was experiencing true plague as late as 1630[95]) heralded Mercuriale as the 'summa cum laude medicum' and called his plague manual 'the most beautiful work on plague' ('pulcherrimo suo libello de peste').[96] Tragically, Venice seemed destined in 1629–31 to repeat its errors of 1576. The dispute over 'true plague' erupted again; denial of plague came again from professors from Padua. This time, however, Venetian doctors who argued that the disease was 'true plague' and for swift implementation of quarantine were few, and the life of one of them, Venice's *Protomedico* Giambattista Fuoli, was threatened.[97] Further, the College of Physicians demanded that he use greater discretion in expressing his views that prejudiced Venetian commerce, thus 'threatening the liberty of the country'.[98] History repeated itself. The consequences in terms of the absolute number of death counts was almost exactly the same as in 1575–7, from 46,721

separation' engendered a loss of faith in the medical profession by the Venetian populace'; see Preto, 'Catalogo: Le Pesti dell'età moderna', 127–8; and Palmer, 'The Control of Plague', ch. 9.

[90] Gabrielli, *De Peste*, 35v–6r   [91] Massaria, *De abusu medicamentorum*, 3.

[92] Parisi, *Trattato della Peste et febre pestifera*, 46, who praises Mercuriale for his identification of twenty-six signs of plague in Mercuriale's tract of 1577.

[93] Gnudi and Webster, *The Life and Times of Gaspare Tagliacozzi*, 135.

[94] Ongaro and Forin, 'Girolamo Mercuriale e lo studio di Padova', 50, point to several reasons for his failed application, but one may have been the 'grossolano errore' of 1575–6.

[95] On Righi's denial of plague in Florence, see Henderson, 'Public Health'.

[96] Righi, *Historia contagiosi morbi*, 13r. Others during this plague, however, made no mention of Mercuriale, 'true plague', or Galenic distinctions on what constituted an epidemic, see Baccei, *Della peste e suoi rimedii*, 4; and Rondinelli, *Relazione del contagio*; Mocca, *Discorsi preservativi e curativi*; Mugino, *Trattato breve sopra la preservatione*; *Raccolta di avvertimenti et raccordi per conoscer la peste*, esp. 17–19.

[97] Palmer, 'The Control of Plague', 278; and idem, 'Girolamo Mercuriale and the Plague of Venice', 65.

[98] Preto, 'Le grandi pesti', 125. Alexandra Bamji, currently researching plague, medicine, and religion in early modern Venice, contends that Venetian doctors defending 'true plague' in 1630 were not in the minority; rather the medical community was split more or less evenly.

to 51,000 as compared with 46,490 in 1630–1; the second time, however, this number represented a higher proportion: now 30 per cent of the city perished.[99]

Yet for the remainder of the sixteenth century, I have found only three stalwarts who continued to support the initial reactions of the 1575–8 plague denial—Massaria mentioned above, Giovanni Marinelli, a Modense doctor who had practised 'for a long time' in Venice before the plague, and a doctor from Mantua, Giovanni Battista Susio, trained briefly at Padua but who graduated at Bologna.[100] Marinelli devoted his entire plague tract of 1577 to the plague controversy of 1576 in Venice. While he described the Senate's request for doctors' diagnoses of the disease, he did not mention the physicians from Padua or those on the opposition from Venice.[101] He presented four arguments, which Venetian doctors supposedly used to argue that 'true plague' was then invading their city. Steeped in methods of scholastic logic, he refuted them one by one with counter-arguments grounded narrowly in the Hippocratic-Galenic definition of epidemic. As with the arguments of Mercuriale and Capodivacca, the disease in Venice was not 'dangerous enough': almost all who caught it, did not die; nor was it 'popular', because not all classes and sections of the population were afflicted. He also argued that the seasonal and atmospheric conditions required for plague purported by Aristotle, Galen, and Avicenna were not observed: there had been no change of the air ('mutatio aeris') putrefaction, poisonous vapours, or other 'universal causes', such as a hot and humid summer followed by a hot and dry autumn.[102] While the absence of such conditions would lead other doctors in 1575–8 to question the framework of antique medicine and its 'universal causes' (as we will see), Marinelli stuck with the system and rejected the plague. Nonetheless, even this scholastic thinker bent on upholding antique notions at

---

[99] Preto, 'Peste e demografia'; Pullan, *Rich and Poor in Renaissance Venice*, 322, continues to claim that the initial advice of the Paduan academics to Venice was correct: 'the government did depart from the rigid and mistaken policy of confining plague contacts in the houses whose vermin had caused the sickness'. Such a judgement misinterprets the character of rats and *Yersinia pestis*, even if the early modern plagues were a rat disease (despite evidence to the contrary). Furthermore, it disregards the comparative context of Venice's disastrous experience in 1576; beyond any other city during this plague, Venice suffered the highest plague mortalities anywhere, and the surge in mortalities erupted when the Venetian Senate forced its health board to rescind its cautious measures of sequestration and quarantine. Pullan attributes the change to the incidental coincidence between the Senate's decisions and the summer plague season. However, the change came after mid-July and into August, when the plague season was often on the decline. As we have seen, moreover, plague in early modern cities in the north of Italy could peak as late as November as happened with Venice's next disastrous plague in 1630.

The comparative data of early modern plague strikes in Italy versus the north of Europe, where plague controls were weaker, also lends credence to the effectiveness of quarantine, plague passports, and other measures reviewed in the book. Between 1540 and 1666 devastating plagues struck London, for example, nine times (Slack, *The Impact of Plague*, 151) and, between 1550 and 1660, Denmark (which did not institute state-wide plague regulations until 1625) eleven times (Christensen, 'Appearance and Disappearance of the Plague', 17 and 19). For a vigorous and comparative argument for the effectiveness of the Italian system of plague control, see ibid. and earlier Slack, 'The Disappearance of Plague'.

[100] I thank Vivian Nutton for this information.   [101] Marinelli, *De peste*, 1r.

[102] Ibid., 5v and 10v.

the expense of contemporary judgements cannot be accused of failing to observe events around him. He described the buboes and spots that covered victims' bodies and the passage of plague from Trent to Venice. Unfortunately, Marinelli leaves no date at the end of his dedication (as many did) or elsewhere in his tract indicating when he completed it: was it during the summer of 1576 before plague mortalities began to soar and before Mercuriale subtly shifted positions?

The dating of the second case is, however, clear. Susio wrote two plague treatises during the 1575–8 plague. The trajectory of his opinions was the opposite of the Paduan authorities sent to Venice in 1576. In the first (1576) he maintained that the disease afflicting his city, Mantua, was plague, but in the second (1577) he held that the disease with the same symptoms and accidents could no longer be called plague because its death counts had fallen. His use of health board statistics on 'plague' mortalities to demonstrate these changes in mortality is hardly convincing. His emphasis, however, fell on the citing of authorities. He began his argument against the common hordes ('il vulgo', who had apparently savagely attacked his first book), by citing those who he claimed were the two most excellent doctors of his time, Ingrassia and Mercuriale, both of whom (at least initially) had argued that the plague had been a 'contagious illness' but not 'true plague'.[103] As with the earlier arguments of Mercuriale and others, the Galenic definitions came to the forefront: not enough people were then dying in Mantua in 1577; it was not sufficiently widespread ('comune'); and it was no longer killing the majority of those who became ill from it.[104] Moreover, the disease by 1577 was confined exclusively to the poor; noblemen were no longer victims. According to Susio, not even doctors, surgeons, and barbers who treated the afflicted, parish priests who gave them last rites, or the gravediggers were now dying: thus the disease failed to meet the Galenic standard of 'comune'.[105] As with others who began challenging Galen and Renaissance models of plague in 1575–8, Susio maintained that the causes of plague were absent—conjunctures of the stars and mutation of the air.[106] But like Marinelli, Susio chose to challenge the plague's reality rather than Galen or Ficino. Unlike his first work, which stimulated heated debate, the second seems to have fallen on deaf ears, at least in press. No rebuttals appeared; nor did Susio feel compelled to publish a third tract against further recriminations of the 'vulgo'.[107]

Finally, the first of Massaria's two-book plague tract of 1579 was devoted entirely to the controversy over the nature of the 1575–8 disease. Yet he was much more equivocal than the others mentioned above, despite his support of his beloved colleague, 'meus nobilissimus Mercuriales'.[108] Massaria presented dispassionately both sides of the argument—that based on the signs, symptoms,

---

[103] Susio, *Libro secondo del conoscere la pestilenza*, 4r (pagination of introduction) and 8v bis (text).
[104] Ibid, 5r (pagination of introduction).   [105] Ibid., 8r–9v (text)
[106] Ibid., 4v (pagination of introduction), 42v and 68v (text).
[107] The text is riddled with internal inconsistencies and contradictions.
[108] Massaria, *De peste*, 13v, 20r, and 27r.

and epidemiological aspects of the disease such as the quickness of death, contagion, and household clustering, and that on the Galenic definitions. Throughout, his refrain was 'nescio' ['I do not know']. He concluded his first book saying he would embrace the best opinion from all doctors.[109] However, by the end of his second book on the signs, causes, and treatment of plague, he was calling the 1575–8 disease 'peste'.[110]

On the other hand, doctors during the last years of the sixteenth century continued to use Galen's principles to distinguish pestilential fevers and other diseases from 'true plague'. But as with the 1555–6 plague, these definitions did not lead physicians such as Asti's Pietro Francesco Arellani to deny the disease with the historic signs and symptoms then afflicting Piedmont at the end of the century as plague. [111] Similarly, the Bolognese physician Georgio Rivetti began his tract of 1592 in the traditional manner of definitions—'Che cosa sia pestilenza?'—and referred to the controversies of the 'learned' over definitions during the previous plague. He rehearsed Galen's definitions of epidemic and endemic diseases and agreed that plague must be epidemic, but unlike the Paduan professors in the summer of 1576, he did not end his definitions here. Instead, he saw signs and symptoms as the distinguishing characteristics of different epidemic diseases: 'some gave birth to carbuncles, others to dysentery, others to glandular swellings [*ghiandole*], and some to smallpox [*varuoli*]'.[112]

Other doctors such as the *Protomedico* of Rome and physician from Fermo Antonio Porto in 1589, [113] Gerardo Columba of Messina, describing plague in Sicily in 1596,[114] and the Roman doctor Giulio Durante for the plague of 1600,[115] also continued to cite Galenic definitions of 'pandemic, endemic, and epidemic', but these definitions did not lead any of them to deny the bubonic plagues then invading their territories even though these killed far fewer and spread over much less territory than had the plague of 1575–8. For them, if the disease killed quickly and was accompanied by buboes and other historic signs and symptoms now well known from historical descriptions or experience, it was to be diagnosed as plague and health boards were to impose stringent controls. These physicians instead rejected the Renaissance model of disease. After Galen's definitions, Porto, for instance, turned to his own observations, historical comparisons, and to Fracastoro's notions of contagion to argue that the disease in 1575–8 as in his own day (1599) had been 'true plague'. He then had the confidence to break the Galenic mould: these plagues had not originated from polluted air but instead from 'pure and simple contagion'.[116]

---

[109] Ibid., 18r, 22r, and 38v.   [110] Ibid., 81v.   [111] Arellani, *Trattato di Peste*, 1.

[112] Rivetti, *Trattato sopra il mal delle pettechie è gianduissa*, 10. Edit 16 attributes this collection of several authors to Oratio Campioni; the Wellcome to Rivetti.

[113] Porto, *De peste libri tres*.

[114] Columba, *Disputationum de Febris pestilentis*, Liber 1: Disputatio I.

[115] Durante, *Trattato della peste*, 1r.

[116] Porto, *De peste libri tres*, 5; also see Massaria, *De abusu medicamentorum*, 2–3.

As we have seen, similar debates on whether the disease was 'true plague' were already in circulation in various parts of Italy before the Venetian Senate invited Mercuriale and his colleagues to diagnose their disease in the early summer of 1576. The arguments and consequences, however, were not everywhere the same. In Sicily, disputes within the medical community and outside it—what Ingrassia called the popular rumours—were present in 1575. Ingrassia's decision to deny plague also turned on Galenic and Hippocratic notions of an epidemic. But, as we have seen, Ingrassia was not trapped by erudite definitions and changed his mind several times based on clinical observation and his health board statistics about the character of the disease in Palermo, its severity, and the proper measures to confront it. He argued for and instituted strict quarantine and sequestration, because the disease was *morbo contagioso* and not 'true plague'. His logic was the very opposite of that used by physicians then denying plague in northern Italy: since 'true plague' was so omnipresent in the air, separating the ill from the healthy would be senseless; in 1348 no political action could have been effective.

***

Before 1575 I know of only one doctor, the Sicilian *Protomedico* Giovanni Filippo Ingrassia, who employed strictly the Galenic definition of epidemic to deny that a contagious disease was 'true plague'.[117] However, in this case (the epidemic of 1558) there is no evidence that the disease possessed the usual swellings and spots; it was probably influenza. Others, such as Donzellini, who later in 1577 attacked the claims of the Paduan physicians, seemed to rely on the Galenic definitions of epidemic but in the abstract. In his earlier tract of 1571, pestilential fevers, unlike true plague, did not derive from the air but came from bad food and drink. Against those who saw the plague's distinguishing feature to be its contagiousness, he further stressed that many diseases were contagious.[118]

Why did the Hippocratic-Galenic distinction of 'popular' epidemic suddenly become an overriding principle for diagnosing plague, leading Italy's most renowned doctors—Ingrassia in the south and Mercuriale in the north—to deny it? We find no evidence of one doctor influencing another. Less significant doctors without any publications to their names, such as Lodovico Lazisi, anticipated Mercuriale's denial of plague based on Galenic notion of 'popular' and 'epidemic'. Richard Palmer has suggested that this new questioning of plague depended on the Renaissance zeal to return to the sources, which in medicine led to the recovery of an unadulterated Galen available in its original Greek, no longer corrupted by Arabic commentators. To be sure, the sixteenth century had witnessed an upsurge in interest in classical medicine.[119] But this was not a sudden development of the 1570s; in fact the plague years 1575–8 initiated a reverse swing at least as regards language: from a predominance of tracts in

---

[117] Ingrassia, *Trattato assai bello*, 19v. On the distinction between 'De caussis superioribus' and 'inferioribus', see for instance Gabrielli, *De Peste*, 17v and 34v.

[118] Donzellini, *De natura*, 23v–25v.   [119] Palmer, 'The Control of Plague', 254 and 266.

Latin, now 87 per cent were in the vernacular. Moreover, the interest and return to Galen preceded the change in 1575–8 by almost a century.[120]

As early as 1505, humanists such as Filippo Beroaldo, the elder, had read Galen in Greek and had grounded their understanding of plague solidly in the Galenic tradition of humours and corrupt air.[121] In 1507 the Turin doctor Pietro Bairo defined plague and epidemic citing Galen and other classical sources, pinning both to mutation of the air but maintained that various diseases could be epidemics such as those with coughing and *catarrah* and, in Naples, gout (*podagra*) because of the humidity of the ground.[122] As we have seen, the testimony of Massucci reveals that Galenic notions of 'epidemic' had been already rife in Padua by 1560 and probably before without leading any to deny plague if the historical signs and extraordinary contagion of the disease were present. In Sicily these Galenic terms were also well entrenched in medical discourse when Ingrassia published his first plague tract in 1558.[123] Finally, the first genuine Greek texts of Galen were published in Venice in 1500, and editions of Galen's complete works in Greek became more widespread (although limited to readers who knew Greek) with the Aldine Venetian printing in 1525. The most significant spurt in Galen publishing in Italy was between 1525 and 1560; afterwards the number of editions dropped sharply.[124] Yet fixation on Galen's epidemiological definition and its effect to deny plague against historically known 'accidents' did not provoke controversy until 1575. Nor did these Galenic definitions of plague based on what constituted an epidemic have the same consequences in other countries, leading academic physicians to deny plague or influence governments to disband quarantine and other plague policies.[125] Something else

---

[120] For a brief overview of the translation and publishing of Galen's work from the end of the fifteenth century, see Porter, *The Greatest Benefit to Mankind*, 168–76; and Maclean, *Logic, Signs and Nature*, 37–8. Diomedes Bonardo, a physican of Brescia, published at Venice works of Galen in Latin in 1490; see Castiglioni, *A History of Medicine*, 220 and 376–78. Galen's *Ars parva* was published as early as 1478. In addition, early writers such as Guy de Chauliac (1300–68) had shown a keen awareness of the works of Galen, citing thirty-one of his books 890 times in his *Chirurgia magna* of 1363; Durling, 'A Chronological Census of Renaissance Editions', 236.

[121] Beroaldo 'il vecchio', *Opusculum de Terraemotu et pestilentia*.

[122] Bairo, *Nouum ac perutile opusculum de pestilentia*, n.p. Bairo also wrote medical books of secrets; see Eamon, *Science and the Secrets of Nature*, 162.

[123] Ingrassia, *Trattato assai bello*, 19v. However, by his definitions (and presumably by Galen's) it was not an 'epidemio', because it did not derive from 'cause superiori'. He rejected the current plague as plague: although it struck most, most recovered, and the reason most died was because they had not been treated properly (22r–v). For the Galenic interconnection between plague and epidemic in 1570, again coming from the University of Padua, see Oddi, *De pestis*, 6v–8r and 33v.

[124] Durling, 'A Chronological Census of Renaissance Editions', 236 and 242; Palmer, 'The Control of Plague', 254; Temkin, *Galenism*, 125–7. Also, see the many editions of Galen's *Opera omnia* published in the sixteenth century and the numerous libraries where they survive (Edit 16). This trend was not unique to Italy. Between 1526 and 1560, translations of Galen across Europe jumped to over twelve a year, reaching a peak of thirty-one in 1549; after 1560, the number dropped to three a year until the end of the century; Nutton, 'The Fortunes of Galen', 371.

[125] See the tract by the Montpellier doctor, Sovirolius, *Brevis & accurata de peste*, ch. 4: 'Popularium morborum pesti affinium & eam saepe concomitantium distinctio', 9v–10r.

was in the air: the threat of plague attacking the peninsula simultaneously at both ends suddenly produced this academic act of denial as well as a creative and impassioned counter-attack from physicians and others. For the first time in print a wide spectrum of intellectuals, government officials, and others outside the medical profession suddenly felt compelled to enter a medical fray and to voice their judgements about contagion, diagnosis of diseases, causes of plague, and the proper public health policies to be implemented.

VENICE AND POLLUTION OF WELLS

Another dispute sparked by the 1575–8 plague, this one centred entirely on Venice, caused almost as much controversy, at least in print, as 'true plague'. Set off by the astrologist Annibale Raimondo in a tract published in Padua in 1576, reissued in Venice, and presented to Venice's health board the following year, it concerned flooding, wells, and the mixing of sea and fresh water.[126] These arguments were hardly abstract academic ones lodged in theory and 'superior causes'. Instead, like the *successi della peste*, they were grounded in specific localities with minute attention to the chronological unravelling of the plague's momentum during 1575 and 1576. Already in 1576 Raimondo had issued a defence of his treatise addressing his critics and trying to resolve their doubts.[127] He dated the origins of the plague in Venice precisely to the night of 11 October 1574, a half year or more before any cases were discovered. A storm and violent winds had broken over the Lido, sweeping in volumes of sea water that flooded the city, washing waste and rubbish through the canals and squares (*campi*), polluting wells and fountains with rubbish and salt water. By March, the wells in the *campi* remained a mix of fresh and salt water and smelly mud. Raimondo 'judged' that those continuing to drink from these wells became sick, and ten died from 'a strange infirmity'. The health board became concerned and ordered the *Sestieri* of the *campi* to clean the wells. But still the poor, who could not leave the city or afford wine, were forced to drink and wash their vegetables in these sources. They continued to become ill, turning roan and yellow with bloated bellies and '*pettecchie*, and worse', while those who could fetch their water elsewhere and who had large and clean housing were unaffected. According to Raimondo, the combination of drinking this water, eating poorly, and living in hot, cramped, smelly hovels 'weakened the complexion and humours', making the poor susceptible to the disease. Poor women were most prone because of their weaker constitutions ('assai piu deboli di complessione'), having less access to medicine and medical services, and living in even more squalid conditions than poor men.

---

[126] Raimondo, *Discorso*.   [127] Raimondo, *Apologia*.

DISCORSO
DE ANNIBALE
RAIMONDO VERONESE,

NEL QVALE CHIARAMENTE SI CONOSCE LA VIVA ET
nera cagione, che ha generato le fiere infermità, che tanto hanno molestato l'anno 1575, & tanto il 76 acerbamente mole-
stano il Popolo de l'inuittissima Città di
VINETIA.

Indirizzato à tutti quelli che non sono idioti delle cose Naturali, de gli Acci-
denti, & che molto intendono la prattica della Città di VINETIA.

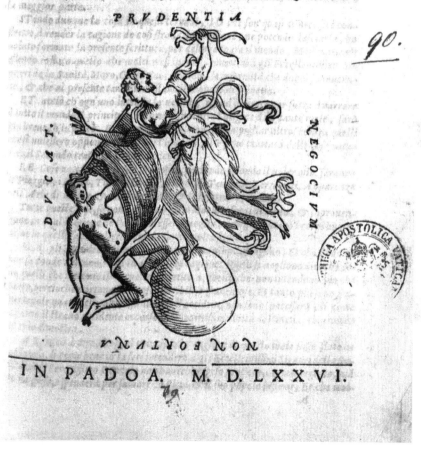

IN PADOA. M. D. LXXVI.

Illustration 6. *Discoro de Annibale Raimondo Veronese,* 1576.

According to Raimondo, this strange disease began in 1575 and continued for several months 'not without giving considerable trouble to the poor but ended as if having made a truce with the people'.[128] Yet it returned in 1576 with greater rage and higher levels of mortality than previously, hitting those who had been living off the 'fatal water' for the previous fifteen or sixteen months. Moreover, merchants, wishing to avoid endangering themselves, stopped work in these quarters, leaving the poor penniless and unemployed, worsening matters. Until May 1576, Raimondo considered the disease treatable, since it was *petecchie* and not so malignant. He claimed that of every ten patients attended, eight were cured, but of those not treated 'nine and a half of ten died'. He cited a case of one house where ten were stricken with the *petecchie*, all of whom were cured through medical assistance.

At this time, others 'appeared to have the *pestilenza* with headaches, swellings under arms, behind ears, or on thighs [*cosce*]'. In one household ten were afflicted and sent to the Old Lazaretto. 'Perhaps it was because of the quality of the air during May', the disease was not so lethal and many could be cured. Despite the change in the disease's signs, Raimondo thought it was still the milder *petecchie* and might be connected to an abundance of worms and caterpillars ('pinocchie bruschi').[129]

The Venetian government ordered all the city's doctors to meet in a room of the Grand Consiglio to discuss the character and causes of the disease, compare it with previous epidemics, and issue decrees. There, Raimondo refuted the standard causes of the rise of epidemics and plague in particular—mutation of the air and humidity—by making the common-sense argument: 'every year the summer brings on hot, even intolerable weather and then the summer changes to cold; yet such mutations do not produce pestilence. Others made arguments about the corrupt air of 1574 and 1575 and a bad crop of wheat, and 'worse still' that the plague was born from dead fish in the sea. Going back to 1348 and earlier, Raimondo dismissed older explanations of plagues: 'certainly this time no one could point to earthquakes to explain it'.[130] Perhaps less convincingly, he also refuted the notion that the disease had invaded the city by boats coming down the Adige from Trent and unloading at the Lido.[131] He returned to his hypothesis: 'The birth, growth, and nourishment of these illnesses within the most splendid city of Venice comes from the mixing of fresh and salt water in its wells.'[132]

In the meantime, 'terrible rioting' erupted in the city over rumours that the pestilence had killed everyone in Trent; fear spread through the city and many doctors left. According to Raimondo, all the major cities became depopulated.

---

[128] Raimondo, *Apologia*, 392r.   [129] Ibid., 392v.   [130] Ibid., 395v.
[131] Ibid., 393r–4v.

[132] Ibid., 395r. At the same time other physicians in Venice, such as Tiberio Superchio, prior of the College of physicians, and Vincenzo Negrono (whose remarks are found in the records of Venice's secret archives and not in published treatises) expressed similar scepticism about corruption of the air being the cause of the present plague; Laughran, 'The Body, Public Health and Social Control', 228.

He reported 'seven or eight unfortunate ones' ('poverini') dying in the same household. Those who survived were sent at first to the lazaretto, but increasingly many of the poor were left in their homes and allowed to walk about, infecting the rest of their households and others through the city. These factors along with the mounting numbers of human and animal corpses in May, Raimondo admitted, could have caused the putrefaction of the air and contributed to the plague's spread. Matters worsened also because the poor did not receive medical care or other basic needs. 'Terror and fear' spread through the districts of the poor (which were without clean sources of water), making, 'the disease dance there more wildly and to become more malignant'.[133]

As is clear from his refutations and theories, Raimondo questioned parts of the old astrological and miasmic causes of plague but still held to notions of the putrefaction of air. While the mix of fresh and salt water was Raimondo's prime mover of the Venetian plague, it was not its sole determinant. As with others, especially during the plague of 1575–8 (as we shall see), social factors—poverty, bad food, lack of medicine, filth, poor housing, and stench—increasingly played an essential role for those like Raimondo trying to understand the plague's spread and severity. Clearly, critics must have hammered Raimondo immediately on his lack of a comparative perspective. His explanation for the 1575-6 plague was based on an occurrence unique to Venice, the storm of 1574, the flooding of the city, and the contamination of wells in the *campi* that served principally the poor. Why had the plague spread within inland cities, in fact, before it reached the Venetians? That these questions were raised is apparent from his published 'Apologia', which begins: 'They have said that the *pestilenza* is certainly present at Padua, Mantua, and Milan; yet these cities have no mixing of salt and fresh water.'[134] Citing the earlier astrologer and professor of medicine at Padua, Pietro d'Abano (*c*.1250–*c*.1316),[135] Raimondo defended his position by emphasizing that plague could develop from many causes and, in an Aristotelian-Hippocratic vein, from earth, air, or water.[136] He did not explain, however, why plague happened to spring up in these various places with different causes and origins at roughly the same moment.

The doctor Antonio Glisenti (1513–76), called Bresciano but actually from Vestone in Valsabbia, published four works on the 1576 plague—a tract on proper living during plague time, a summary of the causes that put humans at risk of catching the plague in 1576, an oration thanking God for liberating Venice from the 'male contagioso', and a response to Raimondo on the causes of the current plague. The text of this last short 'apologia' or defence, suggests that Glisenti may first have lodged an attack on Raimondo's water theory, which

---

[133] Ibid., 395r   [134] Raimondo, *Apologia*, 396v (BAV).
[135] On the significance of d'Abano for sixteenth-century medical thought, see Siraisi, 'The *Expositio Problematum Aristotelis* of Peter of Abano'; and Pennuto, *Simpatia, fantasia econtagio*, 59–60.
[136] Raimondo, *Apologia*.

either was delivered orally or, if published, has not survived or been found in the typographical sources. Nor is there any trace of a counter-attack by Raimondo that occasioned Glisenti's response. Without Raimondo's text or what may well have been his oral criticisms delivered at the medical meeting of the Gran Consiglio, it is difficult to know Raimondo's objections to Glisenti's *Summario*; perhaps, he thought his own theory had not received the weight it deserved in explaining Venice's plague.

Glisenti's summary of the causes of the 1576 plague in Venice vigorously eschewed any mono-causation and was more traditionally cast within a Galenic model, certainly much more so than Raimondo's original and heterodox text on the 'active and true' cause of the 1575 plague. Glisenti's multiplicity of causes did not refute any hypothesis, including Raimondo's theory of bad water. First, Glisenti argued that the plague had entered Venice through the transport of clothing and goods from Trent, and, as other contemporary doctors had argued, such goods could transmit the plague *ad fomitem*. He alleged that a single leather jacket that had been passed from one infected victim to another had killed twenty-five in Venice. A precondition of this transmission had been 'aspects of the skies', the position of the stars, and putrid vapours. He also pointed to the mounting of plague corpses and their production of putrid vapours, first at Trent, then Venice. Moreover, the seasons played their role: recent climate had predisposed humans to suffer corruption.[137] That is, the summer of 1575 had been particularly hot and was followed by a hot and dry autumn, followed by a dry and not cold spring in 1576. Without explaining why these combinations would make the human body more susceptible to plague, Glisenti went on to incorporate Raimondo's theory of salt water running off into wells as another component of his multiplex argument: 'I would not dare deny that the salt water that poured over this city on 11 October 1574, according to Master Annibal Raimondo Veronese, would have had some effect causing inhabitants to be disposed to catching the putrid plague nourished by the wells in the *campi* that had taken in the salt water.'[138] Economic conditions, behaviour, and social class (cast in a Galenic mould) then entered Glisenti's equation: plague struck principally the poor (*persone basse*) because they ate bad food and had other bad habits such as their inability to control their sexual appetites, their 'disorderly exercise, which heated them up and made their humours alternate', and their tendency to get drunk in their taverns.

In Glisenti's argument, the weather was pivotal, but against earlier doctrinal arguments based vaguely on notions of humidity and dryness, derived from ancient sources, Glisenti turned to health-board statistics in an attempt to discover new climatic correlations. Rain after 14 May had slowed the pace of plague mortality to less than eight a day; after 13 July the weather turned humid and hot, resulting in plague mortality climbing to forty-seven a day, not

---

[137] Glisenti, *Il summario delle cause*, n.p.   [138] Ibid.

including those dying at the Lazaretto vecchio and 'other such places'. Rain returned and plague deaths correspondingly fell; then on 29 July 'the sun's rays brought extreme heat and humidity' and plague deaths soared to 143. With the health board's numbers, Glisenti continued to sketch a rough trend between rainy periods and a decline in mortality, rises in temperatures and humidity and a climb of mortality, which reached its peak on 4 August with 219 plague fatalities.

Another mild critique of Raimondo came from a Brescian doctor Faustino Bucelleni, who in fact dedicated his pamphlet to Raimondo, calling him his patron.[139] Accordingly, it began with praise of 'the astrologer' and his 'elegant and learned *discorso*'. He pointed to the problem of explaining why the less malignant epidemic of *petecchie* suddenly exploded into the disease with carbuncles and glandular swellings in May 1576 and suggested that there may have been errors with the initial diagnosis.[140] Secondly, Bucelleni pointed to the obvious: at this time, plague had not been unique to Venice but was raging in Trent, Verona, Messina, Constantinople, and Padua. Then he suggested other long-term determinants of the disease—war and famine that scarred the region in 1571 and 1572, and the drying up of Venice's canals during the autumn of 1575.

Except for Raimondo's lack of a comparative perspective, curiously, no one challenged further his logic. Although the pollution of wells with sewage and other filth may well have led to the disease of *petecchie*, which troubled the poor immediately after the flooding in 1574 and may have made them more susceptible to plague a year later, why would the mix of salt and fresh water have caused plague? By the time of the 1575–8 plague doctors and health boards recognized that salt water made a good disinfectant for purging clothing and other goods. At least two different broadsheets published by the health board of Venice on 9 November 1576, to be displayed on the city's street corners, sensibly instructed Venetians to purge their infected belongings in salt water ('Modo di nettar le robbe con l'acqua salsa').[141]

Even if some may not have agreed with Raimondo's formulation of the pollution of water supplies, many looked to water sources as a cause of the plague's spread in 1575–8. The plague doctor Massucci advised his readers in 1577 that fresh springs were the best sources of water during plague, followed by rain water, and lastly, water from wells, which was by far the worst. If water had to be taken from the last two sources, it should be boiled and filtered ('cuocerle & colarle').[142] Before 1575, admonitions about public wells, fountains, and drinking water had been rare, and when they appeared, as in a tract written during the plague of 1523 by Luca Alberto Podiani (1474–*c*.1552), who taught 'theoretical medicine' at the gymnasio of Perugia, they were generic, couched in ancient or Arabic

---

[139] Bucelleni, *Faustino Bucelleni*. Little is known of this doctor, not even his dates of birth and death.

[140] There could have been two diseases in Venice in 1575–6, with the less fatal *petecchie* weakening the population and making the poor more vulnerable to the more lethal *peste*.

[141] *Col nome d'Iddio modi, et ordini che s'hanno da tener in sborar . . . .*

[142] Massucci, *La preseruatione dalla pestilenza*, 87.

authorities, and placed under the dietary chapters on food and drink. These were matters of personal hygiene, not public policy. Citing Avicenna's personal health manual, *De regimine sanitatis*, chapter one, the Perugino doctor advised drinking clear water from recently cleaned cisterns and good wells, where the specks had been filtered ('bone levis subtilis'), or better yet from sources that are opened ('bene discooperti').[143] He then proceeded to the vices of gourds, melons, and other fruits and vegetables.[144]

CHALLENGES TO THE GALENIC MODEL
AND RENAISSANCE MEDICINE

Despite problems in Raimondo's logic, he appears even among his critics to have been a respected doctor and astrologer whose opinions were seen neither as short-sighted nor heretical. Clearly, the Venetian notary Rocco Benedetti had been influenced by 'the excellent astrologer' to break with the Galenic orthodoxy and declare that 'disease was not born from spoilt air' ('contagio non nasceva dall'aere quasto'),[145] and that the present plague was not caused by malignant influences of celestial bodies or a malign constitution of the air. Instead, he insisted his ideas derived 'from experience', 'from all that he had seen'.[146] As seen in Chapter 4, another creative impulse of the 1575–8 plague was a departure from the old plague-tract divisions—definitions, followed by causes, Galen's six non-naturals, then preventative remedies and finally cures. But ideas, too, were at stake. Writers in and outside the medical profession challenged cardinal premises that had underpinned the earliest plague tracts derived largely from Aristotelian, Galenic, and Arabic thought. In the late fifteenth century, Marsilio Ficino's tract reinvigorated antique authority on ideas of pestilence from the 'universal causes' of epidemics to recipes of the theriac. The 'superior causes' began with God and moved on to planetary configurations, eclipses of the sun and the moon, then earthquakes and other disturbances from below that caused mutation of air and poisonous vapours. In turn, these caused plague in their interaction with bodily humours and constitutions.[147] Some, such as the notaries Benedetti and Canobbio, explicitly rejected these remote causes. For others among the new community of lay writers on plague, their rejection was more implicit: the Jesuit Bisciola, the aristocrat Centorio Degli Ortensi, the gate-guard Besta, the merchant Panizzone Sacco, and the proofreader poet Borgarucci avoided the planetary and atmospheric notions of air altogether, beginning their descriptions

---

[143] Podiani, *Preservatio a peste*, 4r.

[144] Ibid., 5r–v. Also plague ordinances at Milan in 1576–7 saw fountains and other sources of drinking water as conduits of plague and demanded they be kept clean; *Gride diverse*, no. 138, 1577.vi.17.

[145] Benedetti, *Raguaglio*, 485v.   [146] Canobbio, *Il successo*, n.p.

[147] On Ficino's notions of pestilence as 'poisonous vapours' created by malignant constellations of planets, see Pennuto, *Simpatie, fantasia e contagio*, 394–6.

with the origins and spread of the plague in human terms and its contagion through other humans or goods, from one city or village to another.

Aided with health-board reports and hearsay, they dated the process as closely as they could and charted plague's progress with death counts. Contagion here was key, and probably Fracastoro's analysis and categorization of it was influential even to non-physicians, who now wrote on plague but did not cite him. Notions of contagion or its new emphasis on it, however, did not need to rely on Fracastoro; as a concept it had been present before the Black Death but developed rapidly in medical tracts and writings of non-physicians immediately afterwards.[148] Although the direct confrontation between 'contagionists' and 'miasmatists' may not have spread across Europe until the nineteenth century,[149] the two notions did not always coexist so peacefully as some have held for the early modern period.[150] The plague of 1575–8 provoked one of these moments in the history of medical thought when the two notions of disease transmission—one by people and goods, the other by mutation of air—were clearly in opposition, even if many physicians stuck to both.

These explicit and implicit challenges to the Renaissance model of plague did not, however, come exclusively or even principally from outside the medical profession. They began in fact to appear with the previous plague of 1555–6, but in muted form, at least in comparison to the explicit assaults on Galen and Ficino seen in 1575–8. One doctor writing of the 1555–6 plague raised questions about the 'future signs' of plagues. Referring to the ancient histories of the Romans, Bassiano Landi said it was 'easy to predict' future plagues from events such as earthquakes; however, in his town, Padua, immediately before the present plague no earthquakes had been reported, and indeed it was not reasonable to say that the city's air was putrid.[151] But he did not go on to criticize Galenic notions of corruption of the air and pestilence. Instead, he took the opposite tack, explaining why putrefaction of the air led first to large animals contracting the disease and then humans, and why war and unburied corpses caused corruption of air, then plague. Later his tract discussed in good Galenic logic influences of wind direction, humidity, and heat as causes of plague.[152]

In a tract of the same plague, another Paduan professor, Bernardino Tomitano, took his evidence from the Venetian health board to argue that the present plague had not depended on mutation of air alone; otherwise the Venetian islands

[148] See Cohn, *The Black Death Transformed*, 114–19; Winslow, *The Conquest of Epidemic Disease*, 94–96; and Singer, *The Development of the Contagium Vivum*, 3–5, who cites several early sixteenth-century physicians who anticipated Fracastoro's three categories of contagion and distinctions between infection and contagion.

[149] See for instance, Evans, *Death in Hamburg*, 237ff.

[150] See for instance, Pullan, 'Plague and Perceptions of the Poor', 112–13; and more recently, Kinzelbach, 'Infection, Contagion, and Public Health'.

[151] Landi, *De Origine et causa pestis Patavinae.*   [152] Ibid., 469v, 472v–3v. (BAV)

Murano and Giudecca would have been afflicted, and they were not.[153] Referring to the current plague in Venice (to which he devoted the second half of his tract), he refuted another Galenic principle: the plague had not been caused by the poor eating bad food. He pointed out that the peasantry around Venice were worse off than the urban poor but had not been seriously affected;[154] nor had this plague 'depended on celestial influences'. Instead, it had been caused 'purely and simply by contagion' from goods and people 'possibly coming from Soria'.[155] His view, however, was not intended to contradict Hippocratic or Galenic theories, which remained intact along with notions of configurations of stars, planetary movements, and eclipses as the causes of plagues. In fact, the first half of Tomitano's tract was devoted to these themes and followed the standard Galenic principles of corrupted air, vapours, humours, putrefaction, bad food, and so forth. Venice in 1555–6 was simply an exception.[156]

During the same plague, yet another Paduan physician, Lodovico Pasini, scoffed at the general set of clichés that had grown through the Middle Ages regarding future signs of plague, at least for this one specific plague: 'no comets, nor any sort of reptiles had emerged from putrefaction and multiplied; nor had underground animals suddenly surfaced; nor had birds flown their nests, leaving their eggs behind; nor had there been a conjuncture between Saturn and Mars . . . '. He concluded with an implicit critique of Galen, against 'the hot and humid signs' and with the conviction that the air in Padua was not corrupt. But Pasini did not draw any generalizations from this one plague in his city in 1555 or lodge an attack against the doctors and philosophers of antiquity or the Renaissance.[157]

Later, in 1570, a publication by another professor from Padua questioned notions of plague taken from antiquity, especially as concerned his own city. Beginning with Avicenna, Oddo degli Oddi first related the causes and prognostic signs of the most recent plague in Padua—constellations, climate, corrupt and putrid air, multiplication of frogs, reptiles, mice, flies, and other such animals and birds flying from their nests to the ground. But he admitted, like Pasini before him, that the climate and air of Padua had been clear and clean before the plague; no mice, rats, or other reptiles had been seen coming from their holes and multiplying; nor had smells emanating from the air, an eclipse of the sun, bad food, or notable constellations occurred in the plague year or immediately before.[158] These inconsistencies between ancient theory and the observed realities of his native city, however, did not move Oddo to question ancient authority. His

[153] Tomitano, *Il consiglio sopra la peste*, 11r ; also, see 'Catalogo: le teorie mediche sulla peste', 60.
[154] Ibid., 19r.   [155] Ibid., 31v.   [156] Ibid., 4v–16v.
[157] Pasini, *De Pestilentia, Patavina anno 1555*, 5r.
[158] Oddo degli Oddi, *De pestis*, 33v–5v. He does not clarify whether the plague in Padua was that of 1555. Corradi, *Annali*, I, 535–67, and IV, 456–86, records no traces of plague in Padua between 1555 and 1570 (the date of Oddo's tract, published posthumously by his son). The plague of 1564 does not appear to have expanded east of Piedmont.

next section, 'De Prognostico Patavinae pestis', went about-face, upholding the search within planetary constellations for the long-term signs of future plagues.[159]

Attacks against astrological explanations of plague or other 'superior' causes of plague became more frequent and fundamental in 1575–8. The *Dialoghi sopra le cause della peste universale* by a little-known physician from Lucca, Alessandro Puccinelli,[160] was not fixed on inconsistencies with the Galenic model from a specific plague at a single place and time. Instead, his tract was a resounding criticism aimed specifically against the canonical notions of plague causation supposedly found in Galen but most famously formulated by the Florentine humanist and doctor Marsilio Ficino in *Il consiglio contra la pestilentia* (written in 1481 and reprinted at least six times during the sixteenth century alone, more than any single work on plague in sixteenth-century Italy). As Puccinelli proclaims at the outset, 'Ficino was followed by most of those writing about plague'.[161]

During the 1575–8 plague, Puccinelli was practising medicine in Lucca, where it is uncertain if this plague arrived;[162] its threat, however, was certain: he talked of the difficulty of treatment 'in these times of little security and great fear, when the suspicion of plague was ever present'. The central theme of his dialogue concerned the astrological determinism of Ficino and those who followed him, seeing malignant configurations of stars and, in particular, the conjunction of Mars and Saturn, and lunar eclipses as the firmament of plagues.[163] Possibly Puccinelli did not know that these notions did not originate with Ficino but reached back at least to the *Compendium of the Medical Faculty of Paris* of 1348 and was steeped in the Arabic medicine of the early Middle Ages. Nonetheless, on the eve of the 1575 plague, Puccinelli argued that these ideas were the orthodoxy among physicians and were 'in error'. How, he asked, could anything 'so beautiful, saintly, and blessed as the stars influence something so lowly and pernicious as the *peste*'? For the same reasons, he also rejected eclipses of the sun and conjunctures of planets, as was 'the common opinion of doctors and so prevalent in Ficino'. His argument, however, did not derive solely from these aesthetic considerations but also from observation and 'recent memory' ('n'ho a memoria di fresco'). He charged that conjunctures of Mars and Saturn had occurred in 1568 and 1570 but no plague resulted. In 1570, moreover, there

---

[159] Ibid., 35v.

[160] Little is known about him, not even his dates of birth and death, and the above is his only known publication.

[161] Puccinelli, *Dialoghi sopre le cause della peste*, 1r. His claims seem justified: sixteenth-century authors of plague tracts cited Ficino more often than any other 'modern' (post-1348) authority.

[162] For instance, numerous Milanese *gride* issued by the city's health board banding travellers and goods from plague-stricken cities and regions such as Venice, Mantua, Trent, Padua, Messina, and other places in Sicily and Calabria, mentioned neither Lucca nor Tuscany; see *Gride diverse*, 1576.viii.7; 128, 1576.vii.7; 130, 1576.vi.22; and 143, 1577.iv.20. Nor have I spotted any from Bologna or Verona to do so.

[163] Puccinelli, *Dialoghi sopre le cause della peste*, 13r–v.

had been two long eclipses of the sun lasting three hours each but still no plague. 'Before and after Ficino many other conjunctures of the planets had occurred without causing any plague; whereas 1576 saw no eclipses or conjuncture of Saturn and Mars and yet plague struck throughout Italy and other places.'[164] The one doctor, according to Puccinelli, not to fall into 'these errors' was his near contemporary Girolamo Fracastoro (although here Puccinelli was in error).[165] From Fracastoro Puccinelli repeated the three modes of contagion—human contact, goods and clothing, and over distance—and his third dialogue explored the mechanisms by which plague spread: it was set not in the skies but in human interaction and commerce.[166]

In the same year, the Paduan-trained doctor Massucci, then practising in Jesi, another region perhaps only lightly touched by plague, sparked similar scepticism against the astrologers and remote signs of impending plague: 'from our daily experience how can we say that conjunctures or oppositions of the Sun, Moon, and the Stars cause plague?' He cited Plato and other antique sources to proclaim that the stars are of the most perfect and beautiful nature without any perniciousness. Like Puccinelli, he asked: 'How then could they be contagious and pernicious with things beneath them?' And he called doctrines that blamed the stars for any disorder arising from below ('murders, wars, fires, floods and many other evils') 'the madness of the astrologers ('la gran pazzia de gli Astrologi'). Instead, he asserted (perhaps without clarity), contagion and the pestilential quality of the air caused plague, and contagion could not pass from stars, planets, and other heavenly bodies as though they were contagious and malignant beings. Massucci lashed out against the antique authorities—Ptolemy, Alchabitio, Avicenna, and many others—'who have pointed to the skies as the cause of our disorders below'. They 'have deceived the world with a thousand lies'.[167]

Still other physicians writing during the 1575–8 plague went further, challenging the old constructions head-on. For instance, David de Pomi, in a published letter presented to the doge on 27 February 1577, read the next day to the College of Physicians and sent to the health board, questioned the astrologers

---

[164] Puccinelli, *Dialoghi sopre le cause della peste*, 14r.

[165] The Veronese clearly believed in the influence of the stars in generating germs and spreading diseases, especially the conjunction of Saturn, Mars, and Jupiter; Fracastoro, *De contagione*, 60–1, 64–5, and 148–9. In fact, he accepted the possibility of diseases caused by mutation of the air; ibid., 56–7 and 238–9. Where discussing the treatment of 'true pestilence', he contended: 'This contagion often has its source in the air'. In another place, however, he maintained: 'But it very seldom happens that the plague infects us from the corruption of the air' (112–13). On the other hand, in her analysis of Fracastoro's *De sympathia e antipathia*, Pennuto, *Simpathia, fantasia e contagio*, xxxv, 3, 11, 48–69, 300, and 395, maintains that he opposed 'magico–astrologche' doctrines rooted in the medicine of Ficino, Pistorius, and other physicians of the late fifteenth and early sixteenth centuries.

[166] Also see Augenio, *Del modo di preservarsi*, 20–1, who was sceptical of astrologers who saw the stars as inimical to human life. He argued that plague could not be caused by a firmament of the sky and less so by the circulation of the sun and was equally sceptical of comets causing plague (55).

[167] Massucci, *La preseruatione dalla pestilenza*, 55–8.

who predicted from the stars that 1577 would be a period of plague in Venice. He argued instead that the plague was presently in decline and confined to the poor living in three neighbourhoods (*contrade*). His argument for the ebb and flow of plague depended on transmission and control of goods and the infected.[168]

Others such as Andrea Gratiolo di Salò used experience of contemporary plague history to overturn the Renaissance model. Beginning with the standard universal causes—God, influences of the heavens, air, abundance of corrupt humours—he analysed two plagues intensely: that of 1567 in Desenzano, near his home town of Salò, and the one then spreading at the time of his writing, that of 1576.[169] He departed radically from other doctors, not only before the plague of 1575, but many who came afterwards. He started with the first cause of plague—God—and quickly dismissed it as irrelevant. As far as medicine and the examination of natural causes went, the influence of God was not even a proper question for doctors to be asking:

Not being a theologian, I am not in a position to say whether or not the plague of Desenzano proceeded from the will of God. I will therefore proceed as a doctor and discuss natural causes and those that can be directly observed to speculate on what causes gave birth to this disease.[170]

His next chapter considered whether the present plague 'derived from the stars'. He dismissed the hypothesis quickly, saying that he observed no compelling reasons to confirm it. Then he attacked the Galenic framework more broadly—the 'universal corruption of the air'. In Salò, where he was treating plague patients, he maintained that the air was always 'pure and clean [*limpido*], never foggy or misty'; yet there was now plague.[171] He also showed that doctors (such as Marsilio Ficino, 'gran Filosofo') who had tried to force their observations into this schema of universal causes of plagues had contradicted one another. While Ficino 'held that pestilence arose when the air was thick [*grosso*], swampy, foggy, and stunk', other physicians maintained that the pestilential putrefaction sprang first from clear or 'thin' air but lasted longer when it was dense. Gratiolo attacked these speculations, seeing no reason for any such development or connection between this contradictory rise from thin air and duration in dense air.[172] He then questioned another cornerstone of sixteenth-century Galenic medicine, that plague derived from corrupt humours generated from bad food. Here again, history served him. He turned to the last great famine in his region, that of 1559 and 1560, one which had been long and grave but had not produced plague;

---

[168] *Breve Discorso contra l'opinione di alcuni che vanno predicendo futura peste alla Magnifica Città di Venetia; nel prossimo anno M.D.LXXVII*, within de Pomi, *Brevi discorsi*, 303v–306r (BAV).

[169] Gratiolo, *Discorso di peste*. In addition to these two plagues, he ended his tract with a long 'Catalogue of the most famous plagues', 95–132.

[170] Ibid., 19. Palmer, 'The Control of Plague' 254, argues that in the medical debates of 1576–7, God became much more dominant with the influence of the Counter-Reformation. He does not, however, show it. From my reading of the plague texts, I find the opposite.

[171] Gratiolo, *Discorso di peste*, 20.   [172] Ibid., 22.

nor could the plague's absence be attributed to 'continuous honest living' during these years.[173]

Beyond the standard models of plague, Gratiolo also questioned other correlations and universal causes drawn more recently by sixteenth-century doctors, such as that plague always followed closely outbreaks of smallpox or measles ('varuole, ferse').[174] 'After practising medicine for many years', Gratiolo recorded that in Salò almost every year, usually in autumn, cases of smallpox and *ferse* arose but had not provoked outbreaks of plague. From conversations with other doctors practising in Venice, Padua, and Mantua, he held that the same could be said for these regions.[175] He questioned other correlations and causes that had been repeated since antiquity such as plague springing from unburied corpses or dead fish stinking the air.[176]

Finally, Gratiolo questioned the ease of tracing the plague's contagion from one place to another through rumours that one individual or another was responsible for the transmission of plague into a large city. His questions arose not from doctrine but from detailed examples and stories he had collected from his and others' practices to plot possible avenues of plague transmission from Trent to other places that had set off the plague wave of 1575–8 through northern Italy.[177] Supposedly, a woman said to be from Civezzano in the district of Trent carried the plague from Trent to Desenzano. Because of her devotion, they said, she did not become ill but came in contact with many in the Trentino and infected them. Through commerce the contagion then spread. Gratiolo said this opinion was widespread but untenable. The woman had taken a small and tightly-packed boat with eighteen others from Riva di Trento to Desenzano, a distance of thirty-two miles, with one sleeping on top of the other as was customary in these 'boats of passage'. Another woman from this place had slept with her head in the alleged carrier's lap all night. Given these conditions, all or most of the passengers should have landed with the infection, but, Gratiolo maintained, this had not happened. Neither the carrier nor the woman she supposedly first infected showed pestilential signs and symptoms. Instead, the second woman was examined and found to have only a 'simple case of *petecchie*' that proved not to be contagious. Moreover, neither her husband nor their four children, all of whom slept in the same bed, were taken ill. Besides, no other

---

[173] Gratiolo, *Discorso di peste*, 28.

[174] Fracastoro, *De contagione*, 34, used the same term for *morbillo* or measles. It could have been any childhood disease with spots or rashes such as scarlet fever; see *Grande Dizionario*, V, 869.

[175] Gratiolo, *Discorso di peste*, 26.   [176] Ibid., 26.

[177] Ibid., 28–9. Gratiolo's and others' attempts to track the plague should sound a cautionary note for historians today who believe that the first carriers of plague can be so easily identified in sources such as burial records; see Scott and Duncan, *Biology of Plagues*; idem, *Return of the Black Death*; and the criticisms in Cohn and Alfani, 'Household and Plague'. Similarly, the accounts of Canobbio, Benedetti and others contradict Fenlon's conclusion (*The Ceremonial City*, 218) that the narrative structure of such works was a 'search for a single individual as the author of the crime' of introducing and spreading the plague to a particular city.

person she saw or served when she was sick caught the disease. Further, Gratiolo questioned: had she been so contagious, the authorities of Trent would not have allowed her to continue circulating with others in the territory. Finally, plague had not yet infected the district.[178]

Thus Gratiolo's *disorso* questioned almost all received medical theory as well as contemporary stories and rumours about plague, its causes, origins, and transmission from God to the local news. His tract was not, however, entirely negative, a sweeping aside of all theory and speculation. Chapter thirteen, 'the true reason for this plague has been the filth in houses' ('le sporcitie delle case'), continued to examine specific aspects of his contemporary plague of 1575–8 and entertained other theories that were not a part of the general sixteenth-century canon of Galenic-Hippocratic plague tracts before 1575. For instance, in this region worms on bodies were said to have been a characteristic of plague victims, and a Carmagnolese doctor, Pietro Giacomo Zovello, had associated an incidence of plague with an increase in silk worms. Gratiolo did not accept or reject the hypothesis but thought it worthy of mention and of empirical investigation.[179]

He then discussed the particular aspects of the plague in Salò based on the reports and statistics assembled by the officer in charge.[180] His descriptions were not unlike those of plague seen in other places and other periods of the sixteenth century—continuous fevers, small bumps (*petecchie*), sometimes with buboes and *carboni*, sometimes not,[181] but almost always accompanied with lassitude, bodily weakness, laziness, head and backaches, swings from somnolence to sleeplessness with delirium, loss of reason, red eyes, loss of appetite, continuous nausea, vomiting, 'corrupt excrement', a multitude of worms, especially among those afflicted with *petecchie*, and many more accidents, concluding with 'all died within four days, and many sooner'. He added that he had known only three plague cases involving bloody noses, and in no case was there spitting of blood, 'although it is seen with a multitude of others not afflicted with this disease, especially children'.

His list was one of the longest seen with these plague doctors, but what is significant here is Gratiolo's reluctance to generalize from the Salò experience. From his own observations, he discussed the effectiveness of various medications and cures, the existence of carriers who did not become ill, and babies who nursed from afflicted mothers but did not become infected. By contrast, infants nursing from mothers infected with *mal Francese* inevitably became infected.[182] Gratiolo continued to cite Hippocrates, Galen, Avicenna, and Al-Razi, and moderns such as Ficino and Fracastoro, as well as local doctors such as 'il nostro' Boccalino d'Asola. But by sweeping aside the canonical universals, he was able to make new observations and comparisons in a fresh and empirical struggle to understand

---

[178] Gratiolo, *Discorso di peste*, 28–9.   [179] Ibid., 31.
[180] Signore Michele Faliero, Proveditor di Salò and Capitano della Riviera.   [181] Ibid., 33.
[182] Ibid., 91–2

the sixteenth century's big killer. As with many other writers of the 1575–8 plague and as his chapter heading stated boldly, most fundamental of the causes of plague were filth, poor living conditions, and social deprivation.

A similar spirit can be detected with other physicians writing on plague in 1575–8. When it came to the ultimate origins and causes of plague, Donzellini's attitude was much the same as Gratiolo: 'let's leave that to the theologians and astrologists, but as a doctor, let's not jump to conclusions about these influencing elements below [*questi elementi inferiori*] or about corrupt air.' He proceeded to cast more doubt on generalizations from astrologists as well as from doctors of the Galenic tradition: 'as for this year—a plague year—for the entire year, it has been dry and crisp with little rain; nor has the summer been excessively hot and there has been plenty of wind.'[183] He criticized other aspects of Galenic thinking and causes of epidemics. According to Donzellini, no famine had occurred during that year forcing plebs to eat spoilt food. Instead, the Veronese put his finger on the cause he found most relevant: 'Thus it remains that the cause of this horrible death can be no other than contagion and that it has been carried from one place to another.'

As with Gratiolo, Donzellini turned to history as a new key for understanding plague and epidemic disease:

it can be confirmed from history and the real connections [*& vera relatione*], that the disease came from Trent to Venice, Mantua, and Verona via infected goods. And it can be shown that this pestilence had the same accidents and effects [in all these places] beginning weakly and then gaining force as it snaked through the people, in part through their frequent intermingling, in part by imprudence and greed in the handling of the goods of the plague-stricken.[184]

Through these interpersonal connections and micro-histories, Donzellini the academic physician makes explicit the criticisms that the notaries Canobbio, Benedetti, Besta, and others brought against the rhetoric and logic of Mercuriale and the Paduan Medical Academy. Contagion and the plague's progress itself replaced notions that the disease derived from 'superior causes' of changes in air. Finally, he turned to cures and preventives, parting company with plague manuals since the Black Death: the course of the plague was so quick, running between two and three days, that it did not leave enough time for purgatives or bleeding.[185] For Donzellini, and by implication many other doctors of the 1575–8 crisis, preventative medicine could triumph over plague. The remedies of this medicine, however, were lodged in governmental decrees and public health and not traditional recipes prescribed for the individual administered at the bedside. With this new scepticism of Galenic and Renaissance universals as well as the entrenched remedies for treating plague, no simple dichotomy divided laymen on health boards from academic physicians who wrote treatises.

---

[183] Donzellini, *Discorso nobilissimo*, 313v (BAV pagination).   [184] Ibid., 314r.
[185] Ibid., 316r. Here, he contradicts his earlier attacks in 1373 against Calzavelia.

This scepticism of and challenges to assumptions of antique and Renaissance medicine continued in plague tracts with the next big plague in Piedmont in 1586. In that year, Francesco Alessandri completed a second tract in Turin, supposedly an Italian translation of his earlier one in Latin written during Piedmont's previous plague of 1564, but new sections now appeared and old ones such as the lists of recipes disappeared. One of the new sections considered the signs and predictors of plague. Alessandri consoled his readers that not all those signs claimed by ancient and modern doctors as 'sad omens' were in fact justifiable. Rather, it was contagion, spread by commerce of foreign merchandise or by human infection that caused plagues. When the disease spread 'as with a fire lighting dry wood', alarms should sound awakening a population to recognize the presence of plague. Without citing Fracastoro, he then explained the three ways in which plague spread.

Moreover, he attacked other theories 'with dialogues, and bearing funny names' ('e cognome di burla') that presumed to explain the appearance of plague by the configurations of planets and infected air. He cited Galen chapter and verse, but in spite of these citations charged that it was absurd to think that plague derived from poisoned air. Otherwise, he reasoned, 'plants, fruit, and other things would be poisoned'. He ended in the nominalist spirit of his fellow citizen Agostino Bucci,[186] asking rhetorically: is it not better to try to observe with great diligence, even if not everything can as yet be discovered, than to find a hidden agenda in the skies, a cause that defies being seen ('qual antivede')?[187] At least from the plague of 1575–8 to the end of the century, the evidence from physicians' plague tracts conflicts with the present orthodoxy in the history of medicine: challenges to the ancients 'had few repercussions in the sixteenth century' in any field of medicine, except anatomy[188] and had to await a Protestant Paracelesian alliance north of the Alps during the seventeenth century.[189] The plague of 1575–8 instead jolted physicians writing on plague from the bedrock of antique and Renaissance medicine perhaps more significantly than with doctors and surgeons writing on any other medical subject, including anatomy, during the sixteenth century.[190] Clearly, this generation of plague doctors had yet to construct grand theories to replace Galen or Ficino. However, with confidence they felt compelled to cast aside old generalities and instead to trust their own clinical and epidemiological observations. Armed with empirical data collected by their health boards and with a wealth of historical cases, they began to search for new correlations. Some of these might now strike us as quaint or absurd, but overall their new empirical reasoning led them to seek the causes of plague as embedded in sanitary conditions and the nature of contagion. These

---

[186] See above, 179.   [187] Alessandri, *Trattato della peste*, 37r–v.
[188] Palmer, 'Nicolò Massa', 402.   [189] See Epilogue.
[190] On the theoretical conservatism of anatomy during the sixteenth and seventeenth centuries and its adherence to Galen's tripartite division of physiological function—liver, heart, brain—see among other places, Wear, 'Medicine in Early Modern Europe', p. 285.

ideas now began to replace stars, weather, bad air, humours, and even God for understanding plague and disease.[191]

GOVERNMENT REACTIONS

With the plague of 1575–8, governments followed suit with their own publications in Bologna, Milan, Verona, Venice, and probably many other cities. Broadsheets posted on street corners, called *gride* in Milan, *bandi*, *manifesti*, *editti*, *provvisioni*, *proclami*, and other names in other towns, decreed by princes, their lieutenants, directors of health boards, senates, bishops, and cardinal legates multiplied in far greater numbers than with any previous plague (see Fig. 1.2.) These legislated and advised on a wide variety of issues during the plague—regulating trade and provisioning the city, issuing *bollette* controlling the movement of people and goods, penalties for falsification of *bollette*, election of plague guards, notices of plague in other regions banning foreigners suspected of disease, regulations on burials, funerals, bell-ringing, penalties against the sale of contaminated goods, regulations and advice on cleaning houses, clearing rubbish, keeping streets tidy, sequestration of plague victims and those suspected of plague, the locking of houses and the means for guarding them, penalties for disobedience, quarantines of entire populations and of special groups such as women and children, allocation of funds and materials for the building of plague huts, new charities, and more.[192]

Plague legislation goes back to 1348, the famous Ordinances of Pistoia,[193] and can be found soon afterwards in Mantua, Venice, Milan, Pavia, and other cities in northern Italy as well as in Spain and France.[194] Such laws were promulgated and revised at regular intervals from those of Bernabò Visconti in the 1360s in Milan to the early modern period.[195] But nothing earlier compares with the explosion of decrees, government broadsheets, and printed *gride* to control plague as seen in Italian city-states in 1576 and 1577, especially in Bologna, Milan, and Verona.[196] To judge from Edit 16, inventories of ordinances at Bologna, and

---

[191] For others during the 1575–8 plague, who attacked or dispensed with the 'universals' of Galenic and Renaissance medicine, such as Udine's communal doctor, Gioseffo Daciano, see Chapter 8, 253–5.

[192] The most extensive of these that I have found are for Milan, *Gride diverse*.

[193] 'Gli Ordinamenti sanaitari del Comune di Pistoia', also partially translated in Horrox, *The Black Death*, 194–203.

[194] See for instance the plague ordinances for Rouen in 1512, references to similar laws passed in Paris in 1510; *Les ordonnances. . . Pour eviter la dangier de peste*; *Ordonnances contre la peste*, i; *Ordonnance de la police de la ville & faulxbourgs de Paris*; and in Lyon, *Conseil des medecins de Lyon*. Broadsheets of ordinances were not common in sixteenth-century France; instead laws were circulated in inexpensive octavo editions; Pettegree, 'Centre and Periphery', 113.

[195] See Carmichael, *Plague and the Poor*, 110–16; Bottero, 'La Peste in Milano nel 1399–1400', p. 18; and Testa, 'Alle origini dell'Ufficio di Sanità'. For Venice, see Palmer, 'The Control of Plague'.

[196] For Milan, see *Gride diverse*; for Bologna, *Bononia Manifesta*; for Verona and Venice, ASVr, Sanità, nos. 33 and 34.

the archives of Verona, examples of such legislation before the plague of 1575–8 were by comparison rare.[197]

These plague decrees of 1575–8 for the most part also dispensed with grand theories and universals and went straight to matters that could be seen with practical, direct, and public remedies. As the published inventories of these records for Bologna—the only such published inventory I know of—attest, the 1575–8 plague was a watershed. Before, the Bolognese authorities published only five plague broadsheets—one in 1550, another in 1565, and three in 1572. In the final quarter of the century, that number soared to 102 with most issued in the plague year 1576 (26).[198] For Milan, the number of these notices on plague for the years 1576 and 1577 was even more impressive; the city published and posted at least 138 of them in these two years alone, copies of which survive in the Biblioteca Braidense.[199] These were not only 'instructions' on what could or could not be done, such as the enforcement of quarantines;[200] they also gave simple and practical information on how to preserve the health of the community based on common-sense observation such as not to take water from communal wells that stank of mud;[201] 'instructions on how to disinfect every sort of object easily and securely'; ways of perfuming the house, letters, and books; how to cleanse the house, how to wash items with sand or salt water and, once cleansed, how to dry them. They even included instructions on how to boil water.[202]

In the archives of Verona, similar instructions are seen in plague *proclami* issued by its health board in 1576 that strove to teach 'the inhabitants' how to rid their houses of bad smells and waste, 'to keep them clear of every sort of rubbish', to keep scented herbs in their rooms and how to make perfumes and incense to clean the air and wash their walls with water and hot vinegar.[203] Other Veronese *proclami* gave common-sense advice ('Avertimenti d'esser osservati nel tempo del contagio') on fleeing crowds in city squares, public places, and especially schools during plague time, avoiding areas of stench and garbage, advice on what to eat, making fires, washing the face, hands, and mouth with vinegar or vinegar diluted with water and cleaning inside the nostrils, as well as supplying recipes for protecting against plague recommended 'by all ancient and modern authorities'.[204]

In addition, the inventories of Bologna highlight the 1575–8 plague as a turning point for other related concerns with hygiene, cleanliness, and safe water.

---

[197] One example regards the few plague statutes printed in Nevizzano, *Summarium decretorum Sabaudiae*.

[198] *Bononia Manifesta.*

[199] *Gride diverse*, contains 142 of these broadsheets, but four are misfiled from later plagues of the late sixteenth and early seventeenth centuries.

[200] See *Gride diverse*, and individual decrees collected in *Bandi & Constitut. diverse di Bologna*, nos. 99, 100, and 110–120.

[201] *Col nome del Spirito Santo* and *Ottimi remedi per mantenersi sani nel tempo della peste.*

[202] *Col nome d'Iddio . . . che s'hanno da tener in sborar ogni sorte di robbe infette.*

[203] ASVr, Sanità, no. 33, 127r.   [204] Ibid., 137r–8v, no date, arranged with the 1576 *proclami*.

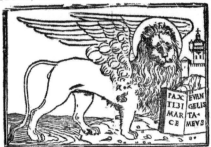

COL NOME D'IDDIO·

MODI, ET ORDINI CHE S'HANNO
DA TENER IN SBORAR OGNI SORTE DI
ROBBE INFETTE, ET SVSPETTE FACILMENTE, ET SICVRAMENTE.

M· D· LXXVI· IX· NOVEMBRE·

 O L E N D O i Clarissimi SS. Sopraproueditori,& Proueditori alla Sanità dar facile, et sicura strada à ciascuna persona di poter nettar ogni sorte di robbe che per occasion del presente Contagio fossero infette,ò sospette,manife stano con l'autorità del Senato, à commune utilità, gli infrascritti modi, ricordati senza alcun premio amoreuo mente da M.Marc'Antonio Lancia Qua

mescolandole con bastoni,& lasciandole tãto che l'acqua habbia le uato quattro bolliti almeno,poi da persone nette siano cauate,& g tate in acqua fredda,poi si spremono,& asciugano,& restano nette
    Modo di nettar le robbe d'importantia col sabbion .
S I mettono le robbe che si uogliono nettar in luogo scoperto,oueo al coperto sopra terreno che sia fresco, uicino a pozzo,oueo in na gazzeni freschi,facedo in detti luoghi un suolo di sabbion asciut o, t to sei dita,& sopra da persone infette si stende un lenzuolo mondo so

Illustration 7. Venetian broadsheet: *Methods for cleaning every sort of infected good*.

Certainly early modern Italy did not invent street cleaning or other governmental policies for personal and public hygiene. In Florence, such ordinances reach back at least to 1324,[205] Pisa to 1287,[206] and Bologna to 1245.[207] Emergency statutes in Venice, Florence, Lucca, and most famously, Pistoia, in 1348 illustrate well that government officials saw the new disease as highly contagious and propagated through unsanitary conditions. These decrees anticipated policies that would continue to be developed through the late Middle Ages and the early modern period—regulations about burials, limited participation at funerals, restrictions on and removal of dirty industries such as the tanning of hides during plague, bans on contacts and commerce with territories under suspicion, laws against the sale of second-hand clothing, and in anticipation of Fracastoro's notion of *fomites*, bans of various types of merchandise, especially cloth.[208]

---

[205] See Carabellese, *La peste del 1348*, 145–7.

[206] *Bibliografia cronologica di leggi sanitarie toscane*, 5–10.

[207] Maragi, 'La santé publique', 84, cited in Henderson, 'The Black Death in Florence', 143.

[208] The literature on public health in Italy following the Black Death is vast. The most detailed to date with the most acute comparisons unfortunately remains unpublished; Palmer, 'The Control of Plague', esp. ch. 1–3, 5 and 6. Various short works by Cipolla have vividly illustrated the financial, social, theological, and institutional problems confronting individual health boards during plagues of the seventeenth century. His work, however, does little to chart the development of public health over the late

In the 1930s Ernst L. Sabine discovered that the Black Death of 1348 was a fillip to the organization and enforcement of city cleanliness in London with new and more frequent ordinances on street cleaning and controls over food supplies, and especially meat.[209] The impact of the 1575–8 plague on such controls was more immediate and dramatic. In Bologna—the one Italian city where the published warnings posted on street corners allow us easily to quantify change—only two broadsheets appear before 1575 that ordered urban residents 'to clean the streets, squares, porticos, and other public places' of waste and excrement or keeping streets cleared of other impediments to commerce.[210] With 1575 until the end of the century such broadsheets appeared almost yearly and in some years such as the plague year of 1576 as many as five times. Moreover, after 1575 these became more specific with regulations that the streets, squares, and porticos had to be cleaned at least once a week.[211] Along with these ordinances, bans were issued on keeping canals and other sources of city water clean, prohibiting swimming in them and forbidding washing of vegetables and silk worms ('bugati') in city wells and fountains.[212] These broadsheets appeared yearly in Bologna through the last quarter of the century (when the inventory ends).

The effect of the plague of 1575 as a watershed was not simply a matter of print culture. Throughout the sixteenth century Verona (unlike Venice, Milan, and Bologna) printed few of its *proclami*, especially those issued by its health board.[213] But from 1555 to 1600 its health board issued at least 282 such ordinances, only nineteen (less than 7 per cent) of which were printed.[214] With these archival documents the importance of 1575 was even more pronounced than in Bologna. Only four decrees from the health board antedated 1575,

---

medieval and early modern periods or to compare developments within Italy or between Italy and other regions, except to say that Italy was more advanced and that health defences in 1630–3 were more robust than in 1348; see his *Cristofano and the Plague*, 118; and *Public Health*, 18. As Palmer, 'The Control of Plague', argues, health policy in northern Italy after the Black Death to the seventeenth century was not, however, a steady or linear development. For the general outline of developments such as the first permanent health offices, quarantine, and lazaretti, also see Carmichael, *Plague and the Poor*, ch. 5; idem, 'History of Public Health'; Cipolla, 'Origine e sviluppo degli Uffici di Sanità'; idem, *Public Health*; and Cosmacini, *Storia della medicina*. For Milan, see Albini, *Guerra, fame, peste*; for the mobilization of a health board during the plague of 1575–6 in a town in the Milanese territory; see Capasso, 'L'Officio della Sanità di Monza'; and *Atti dell'officio della sanità di Monza*. For its late development in England, see Slack, *The Impact of Plague*. For the absence of permanent health boards in Spain, see Bowers, 'Plague, Politics'.

[209] Sabine, 'Butchering in Medieval London'; 'Latrines and Cesspools of Medieval London'. Also see Gottfried, 'Plague, Public Health and Medicine'. Earlier, Thorndike, 'Sanitation, Baths, and Street-Cleaning', was less attentive to the importance of plague but his examples of medieval sanitation, street cleaning, and cleanliness mostly postdate 1348.

[210] *Bononia Manifesta*, nos. 720 (1570) and 813 (1573).   [211] Ibid., no. 1921 (1588).

[212] The earliest ban against washing plants and silk worms in city fountains was in 1567; ibid. no. 520; with 1575, they appear almost yearly. The first broadsheet on cleaning canals and locks was also in 1567; ibid., no. 532. The first prohibiting swimming in the canals was not until 1584, ibid., no. 1530.

[213] See ASVr, Sanità, nos. 33–4; and Archivio di Comune, no. 211.

[214] There were more but many of these were duplicate *proclami* or ones repeated on the same day (ASVr, Sanità, no. 33). This *fondo* also includes thirty-seven printed decrees from Venice.

and one of these originated from Venice and another initiating a visitation of Verona's hospitals appears not to have concerned plague. By contrast, the health office issued forty in 1575, all concerned with plague and on average over ten a year for the remainder of the century, even though Verona was not directly threatened by another plague until 1629.

Although the 1575–8 plague did not initiate networks of correspondence on suspected plague areas and printed bans against persons and goods coming from these cities, the Bolognese decrees show that 1575 was again a crucial turning point: not only did such bans multiply vertiginously; the networks of information became increasingly more international with notices of plague and bans placed on goods and persons from villages and towns in Spain, Portugal, France, Provence, Germany, Sardinia, Austria, Switzerland, and England.[215] The decrees of Verona's *Sanità* concentrated even more intensely on these prohibitions and by the 1580s became increasingly international, targeting cities and regions throughout Flanders, Austria, Switzerland, Germany, Spain, France, Holland, Zealand, and England.[216] Of its 282 decrees, 99 pertained to the exclusion of trade and entry of persons from places where plague was known or suspected and to the quarantining of goods that had already been transported to Verona by specific international merchants.[217] All derived from the plague of 1575–8 or afterwards. In a quantitative sense the 1575–8 plague scored here another first.[218] Furthermore, they set the stage for international cooperation, warnings, and surveillance of plague that would endure to the nineteenth century.[219] As with

---

[215] See for instance, *Bononia Manifesta*, nos. 1383, 1388, 1415, 1416, 1792, 2024, 2033, 2542, 2568, 2579, and 2634. Also, Palmer, 'The Control of Plague', 154, suggests that the years 1576–7 moved Florence's health board to send regular reports on the plague in Venice to Lucca, Genoa, Ancona, Bologna, Ferrara, and Naples.

[216] Moreover, these do not include thirty-seven late sixteenth-century printed *proclami* issued by Venice's health board on suspected places, which Verona's health board kept in their archives. The Veronese were particularly sensitive about those from suspected places who attended the annual fair at Bolzano. The earliest of these decrees, however, does not appear until 20 August 1575; ASVe, Sanità, 21r.

[217] Not every place, however, shows such a clear transformation with the 1575–8 plague. For Florence, where this plague did not strike (and perhaps for this reason) very few *bandi* regarding plague or sanitary measures are seen in its surviving sixteenth-century laws, notices, or proclamations, whether published or not (even though a permanent health board was established in 1576 and earlier *bandi* survive). Instead, the watershed for Florence came with its first plague since the 1520s, that of 1629–31. See Archivio di Stato, Firenze, Ufficiali di Sanità, Decreti, nos. 1–2; *Legislazione Toscana*; *Bibliografia cronologica di leggi sanitari. . . dalla Biblioteca nazionale centrale di Firenze*; *La Legislazione medicea sull'ambiente.*.

[218] With initial work in the Bibliothèque nationale de France and the Bibliothèque Sainte-Geneviève, I have not found any comparable survival of plague broadsheets for France. Moreover, the publication of plague ordinances for Paris and Lyon shows a much more limited structure for plague control with no plague passports, systems of plague intelligence, intricate instructions for guards, or the surveillance of the plague suspected within cities. The plague laws of Paris, promulgated periodically through the sixteenth century, show little development; rather, they were repeated almost verbatim; see *Les ordonnances. . . Pour eviter la dangier de peste*; *Ordonnances contre la peste*, i; *Ordonnance de la police de la ville & faulxbourgs de Paris.*

[219] The broadsheets reproduced in their entirety from the Neinken Collection for the cities Bologna and Brescia, 1610–1800 and 1613–1796, respectively, show no new innovations or changes in character from the broadsheets of Milan, Verona, Venice, and Bologna seen during the last quarter of the sixteenth

the academic plague tracts, governmental concerns with practical and observable measures of public health and hygiene multiplied and at times modified or indeed ignored altogether theories of the mutation of air and the universal causes of Galenic and Renaissance medicine. The massive increase in plague writing by academic physicians and the laity that began to challenge Renaissance medicine with the plague of 1575–8 influenced and accompanied a new surge in Italian states' intervention into concerns over health. These then widened the gap, setting Italy apart from the rest of Europe, not only on governmental and health-board practices, but also on the consequential patterns of pestilence itself through seventeenth and into the eighteenth century.[220]

century, except for reports on cattle plague in the 1730s (although the Veronese ones report one from 1599) and bans that penetrated further east and into Africa. For these later broadsheets, see Jarcho, *Italian Broadsides Concerning Public Health*; on international controls of diseases during the eighteenth and early nineteenth centuries, see Restifio, *Le ultime piaghe*.

[220] See n. 99 above.

7

Plague and Poverty

Despite bitter controversies and recriminations sown by the plague of 1575–8, one issue drew considerable consent: plague writers increasingly stressed the social and economic causes of the plague and its transmission. As we have seen, despite the questionable character of Raimondo's water theory to explain the Venetian plague in 1575, his critics did not dispute his premise that plague arose within the poorer working-class districts of Venice because of their reliance on contaminated water. His critic Andrea Glisenti concurred and added that plague originated and spread among the poor because of social conditions, principally wretched and overcrowded housing.

Plague had not always been seen as a disease of the poor,[1] and indeed the few records of a statistical nature for the Black Death and the first recurrences of plague in the second half of the fourteenth century suggest that the disease was not one predominantly of the poor until as late as 1400.[2] One chronicler after another across Europe described the plague as killing indiscriminately without regard to age, sex, or social class. The Florentine Matteo Villani, writing of the Black Death of 1348, along with an anonymous German chronicler describing a plague in the 1370s, claimed that the poor may have been among the first victims but the pestilence eventually levelled populations equally, killing 'men of every condition, age, and sex'.[3] Few saw the rich surviving any better than the poor in 1348–9, and the exceptional few who did, such as Geoffrey of Meaux, seem to have been persuaded by the logic of the stars rather than by what they actually observed on the ground: 'the lesser stars signify . . . the common people, and therefore the effect of the illness which they brought touched those people more'.[4] Others in 1348, however, thought that 'the planets looked down on rich and poor alike', and saw them dying equally, even if the poor may have died first. According to these doctors, one reason the rich were momentarily protected was

---

[1] De Witte and Wood, 'Selectivity of Black Death Mortality', comparing skeletal remains from the East Smithfield cemetery with samples from two medieval Danish sites, have concluded that Black Death skeletons had more lesions and were more fragile. They do not, however, take into account that London had been suffering dearth and famine since 1346 and that principally London's poor were the ones buried in the new mass plague pits.

[2] See for instance Carpentier, 'Famines et épidémies'.

[3] For these and the following citations see Cohn, *The Black Death Transformed*, 126–8.

[4] Horrox, *The Black Death*, 170.

because of their gluttony and eating rich foods, which generated 'heat or fumes' blocking the fumes of the plague.[5]

For subsequent plagues of the fourteenth century, chroniclers even saw the disease striking the rich more than the poor. For the next plague in 1358, it was the 'good and notable citizens of Orvieto who received the greatest damage'.[6] For the same plague in Germany, the pope's doctor, Guy de Chauliac, said it began with commoners ('populares') but ended with killing more of the rich and nobility.[7] The chronicler of the Grey Friars at Lynn called the plague of 1361 'a great pestilence . . . of children, adolescents, and the wealthy'.[8] The Sienese Donato di Neri pointed to fathers, heads of households, grand citizens, and merchants as the ones who died in the plague of 1363 at Pisa.[9] Neri reported that the next plague of 1374 singled out grandees: ten cardinals at Avignon, and at Siena, the podestà, his son, six judges, all his knights, notaries, and police, so that hardly anyone in his service was left.[10] The *Anonimalle Chronicle* maintained that the plague of 1374 'killed a great number of the citizens of London, the best sort and the richest of the city, including many valiant officers of the Chancery, Common Pleas, and the Exchequer'.[11] Thomas Walsingham said the plague of 1379 rapidly stripped England of its best men, and 'of the middling groups '(mediocribus') nearly every house had been evacuated so that hardly any remained.'[12] As late as 1400 others such as the anonymous chronicler of Tournai continued to see the plague as lacking any distinct class bias.[13] At least one doctor during the sixteenth century, Giovanni Filippo Ingrassia, reflected on these historical differences in the social evolution of the disease. In 1576 he remarked that Italian plagues of the 1360s were different in their social patterns from the disease today: now the disease is confined to the poorest plebs ('poveretti plebei').[14]

When did this change occur? The plague of 1400 was the last I know in Italy for which a contemporary claimed that the disease lacked a social bias in its mortality or that the rich may have been more susceptible. At Florence, this was also the first plague for which records of a quantitative sort exist to show that the plague had taken a decisive class bias across an entire city. In addition to the vast majority of that year's plague victims not possessing family names or upper-guild professions, the topography of death prefigured what would become common with plagues in sixteenth century as reported in many plague tracts.[15] The plague

5 'An astrological German tract written soon after the Black Death', in ibid., 179.
6 *Ephemerides Urbevetanae*, 84.   7 Guy de Chauliac, *Chiurgia*, Tract. II, cap. 5.
8 Horrox, *The Black Death*, 86.   9 *Cronaca senese di Donato di Neri*, 604.
10 Ibid., 654–5.   11 *The Anonimalle Chronicle*, 77.   12 *Thomae Walsingham*, 319.
13 *Chronique des Pays-Bas*, 332.   14 Ingrassia, *Informatione*, 15.
15 For this analysis, see Cohn, *The Black Death Transformed*, 173, and 209–10. A concentration of plague deaths among the poor may have also been the case with the plague of 1390 in Arezzo: the named occupations of victims in the burial records of the city's Misericordia were predominantly street vendors, servants, barbers, and prostitutes; ibid., 171. According to Carmichael, 'History of Public Health': 'Only during the fourteenth century do descriptions of plague note the loss of many principal citizens. After that period, elites seem to have worked out effective patterns of flight . . .' (198). Yet, despite their recourse

not only struck Florence's poorest parishes on the periphery, such as Santa Maria in Verzaia and San Frediano, the worst; it infected these communities first and continued there throughout the plague cycle.

Even though the plague in Florence of 1400 killed as many as 12,000 or more than a fifth of the city during the late spring and summer, it hardly touched the inner city within the original Roman walls, where the houses and palaces of the elite were concentrated and where few textile workers or artisans resided. With plague raging through working-class districts of the city, mortality rates within the centre, instead of rising, dipped even below their averages during recent non-plague years, suggesting that those who could, followed one dictum of the plague literature—to flee as quickly as possible. But given the overwhelming proportion of the poor who died, even from the outset when the cause of death was not yet certain, and given the numbers of servants who perished within elite households without the subsequent deaths of their patrons, flight cannot have been the only reason for the steep class gradient of plague mortality. In fact, as Giovanni Boccaccio's *Decameron* attests, the rich and nobles had begun to flee cities with Black Death itself in 1348, and yet the disease was not then, or later during the fourteenth century, one almost exclusively of the poor. Rather, by the beginning of the fifteenth century the plague had assumed the trend of many other infectious diseases that eventually strike primarily those with poorer nutrition and worse living conditions. This disease as one of the poor is given further support by the close correlation between bad harvests and famine and the eruption of plague—a pattern that Henri Dubois and others have shown became well entrenched by the fifteenth century but not before.[16]

Despite these trends, it is remarkable just how little notice doctors and others in their plague writings gave to it or speculated on its causes before 1575. In Karl Sudhoff's abridged editions of 288 plague tracts from 1348 to 1500, only three saw the poor as the prime victims—a tract of a Florentine doctor written in 1382, one by a Parisian doctor and medical professor writing in the first half of the fifteenth century, and another written for the duke of Milan in 1477. All of

to flight, elites continued to die during the last stages of the plagues in early modern Italy. In 1575–7, 1629–30, and 1655–6. See, for instance, Canobbio, *Il successo*, 17r, who commented in September 1576, even the elites, who had escaped to their villas in the Veneto, began to die. Moreover, in earlier plagues of the sixteenth century, members of the middle classes and elites died of plague as seen with members of Niccolò da Massa's family, although typhus (*petecchie*) was a greater threat to the upper classes; see Palmer, 'Nicolò Massa', 388–9. North of the Alps this chronology may have been different. According to Grell, 'Plague in Elizabethan and Stuart London', 425, the topography of London's plague mortality did not show a class bias until the seventeenth century. Slack, *The Impact of Plague*, ch. 5, however, shows that a distinct social pattern in plague mortalities had emerged in towns such as Exeter, Bristol, and Norwich by at least the second half of the sixteenth century as well as in London; idem, 'Responses to Plague', 458; in London the poor were blamed for it: the 'sins of the suburbs'.

[16] According to Dubois, 'La depression', I, 327, from 1437 to the end of the century, plague was consistently accompanied by bad harvests. Blockmans, 'The Social and Economic Effects of Plague', 863, has found the same for the entire fifteenth century. For the sixteenth and seventeenth centuries in Italy, see Cipolla and Zanetti, 'Peste et mortalité différentielle'; and for England, Slack, *The Impact of Plague*.

these relied on Galen pointing to bad food, food poisoning, or famine to explain the poor dying in greater numbers.[17]

By the second half of the fifteenth century Milan's necrologies show indisputably that the plague had become consistently a disease of poverty. By the early sixteenth, according to John Henderson, Italian city-states began to discover 'a closer association between poverty and disease, with the poor seen increasingly as the cause of disease as well as being its victims'.[18] Yet, surprisingly, even in the sixteenth century before 1575, plague tracts rarely connected famine, poverty, or living conditions with plague or tried to explain the correlation. In fact, before this plague, observations on poverty or famine and plague or the absence of noblemen and the rich among plague victims appear as rarely as during the first 150 years after the Black Death. Only four tracts suggested such a relationship, and only one a causal link between poverty or famine and plague, and three of these were written during the plague of 1555–6. As we saw in the previous chapter, the Venetian Niccolò Massa connected the 1555 plague with poor living conditions and the habits of the poor in that city. In addition, for the same plague, the doctor Vittore Bonagente simply stated that 'in a real plague [*peste vera*] such as the one now afflicting Padua, the poor and destitute [*pauperes miserosque*] were the first to be infected'.[19] Slightly more profoundly, Bassiano Landi saw the origins of the 1555 plague springing from the war Francis I, king of France, was waging along the Ticino river. From this destruction plague soon followed and spread through the regions of Piacenza, Cremona, and Ticino. Citing Galen, Landi saw plague and famine as interconnected, that it arose from bad or spoilt food ('vesci cibi').[20] The fourth tract came later, provoked by a plague of 1564 that spread through Switzerland (especially in the canton of Graubünden), parts of Piedmont, and northern Lombardy (especially Chiavenna).[21] Agostino Bucci advised that 'at times of heightened danger of plague, it is best to force the lowest classes ('la plebe minuta') and the useless poor and beggars from the city, consigning them to a place where they can recover.[22]

By contrast, with the plague of 1575–8 numerous plague writers discussed the relationship between plague and poverty and offered a wide variety of explanations for it, grounding their arguments in social, economic, and material conditions. First, like Landi, the 1575–8 plague writers saw a clear connection between famine or bad harvests and plague. The Veronese doctor Donzellini cited a Greek proverb: 'first famine, then plague'.[23] From Cremona, Somenzi held that famine had been a precondition of plague in Trent in 1575 that set off the contagion across northern Italy.[24] The Milanese gate-guard Besta saw famine

---

[17] 'Leve Consilium . . . a Francischino de Collignano', 365–84; 'Brevis tractatus contra pestem', 77–92; and 'Ein Pesttraktat eines Magister Berchtoldus', 77–95.

[18] Henderson, 'Charity and Welfare', 78.   [19] Bonagente, *Decem problemata*, 8v.

[20] Landi, *De Origine et causa pestis Patavinae*, 470r–v (BAV pagination).

[21] Corradi, *Annali*, I, 516–18.   [22] Bucci, *Reggimento*.

[23] Donzellini, *Discorso nobilissimo*, 310r.   [24] Somenzi, *De morbis*, 1v.

and plague working together to produce mounting mortalities in Milan,[25] as did the Veronese druggist Bellicocchi in his tract addressed to the rulers of his city in 1576. He advised the provisioning of good food to the poor as an effective 'antidote' to those dying of plague, if done in time. Based 'on ancient authority, experience, and observation', food, he asserted, was one of the basic 'remedies' to cure plague.[26] In his poem on Venice's affliction, Borgarucci claimed that the ensuing hunger in 1576 killed as many as the disease itself.[27] With the abandonment of crafts and industry and unemployment caused by the plague, the notary Benedetti saw hunger as one of the major disasters of the Venetian plague. Similarly, several poems in praise of Verona's plague-time podestà, pinned famine and its fear as two of the *pestifer Dragon's'* seven heads to be slain.[28]

Others went further, seeing famine as the longer-term cause of plague and of prognostic potential. For the artisan autodidact Giovanni Ambrogio the origins of Milan's 1576 plague were food shortages ('la calastria de viver') dating to 1570 followed by famine that weakened the population, making it and especially the poor more susceptible.[29] Even for the theological writer Cardinal Borromeo in his advice to the clergy of Milan in 1576, famine, and not the stars, eclipses, or configuration of planets, was a prognostic sign of plague: 'when a large famine and poverty strike a region, especially where a great multitude of people lack basic foodstuff and are forced to eat many corrupt things . . . contrary to nature'.[30] Finally, the historian Tranquilli, in an attempt to correlate plague with prodigies over 2309 years of history, found famine to be the most usual cause of plague across time and especially during the sixteenth century.[31]

Beyond famine, plague writers of 1575–8 understood poverty more generally as a root cause and charity as a principal plank in the struggle against plague. For the Milanese poet Goselini, such charity involved more than just 'feeding and nourishing the poor in general'. Governments needed to ensure that artisans were kept employed during plagues so that they could live by their crafts; otherwise, 'the pains of famine and then plague were invited'.[32] As far back as the plague of Ethiopia and Athens to his present plague in 1576, the Bresciano doctor Glisenti saw pestilence's first cause as poverty: the loss of work and the inability to gain one's living led to 'ugly and fearsome famine' and the necessity to eat bad food.[33]

Equally important, numerous plague writers in 1575–8 began to describe what plague officials and doctors on health boards across various Italian cities had known for a century or more: plague afflicted principally the plebs. The pharmacist Bellicocchi reported that plague 'spread [*serpendo*] first and foremost among the poorest [*minuta plebe*] and people in need'.[34] In his tract of 1575 the

---

[25] Besta, *Vera narratione*, 14v.   [26] Bellicocchi, *Avvertimenti*, 427r–v (BAV pagination).
[27] Borgarucci, *L'afflition di Vinetia*, 8.   [28] *Raccolta delli componimenti*, 14r, 19v, and 36r.
[29] 'Le "Memorie" di Giovan Ambrogio', 9.   [30] Borromeo, *Avisi comuni a tutto il Clero*, 150.
[31] Tranquilli, *Pestilenze che sono state in Italia*, 10–11, 19–20, and 22.
[32] Goselini, *Componimenti Christiani in materia de la peste*1.
[33] Glisenti, *Il summario delle cause*, n.p.   [34] Bellicocchi, *Avvertimenti*, 411v.

bishop of Verona observed that noblemen and ladies were not being infected; rather it was then spreading exclusively among plebs.[35] The Venetian David de Pomi maintained that during the summer of 1576 anyone who ventured to investigate the plague dead or those presently infected would find that the victims were either plebs or those who had had recent contact with them.[36] Donzellini observed that the plague struck more the poor and needy plebs than the rich and nobles and those who could live comfortably.[37] In his poem on the 1576–7 plague in Milan, Bernardo Bertholio saw plebs alone as the ones 'invaded' by this 'most calamitous plague'.[38] A poem by Antonio Pasini also pointed only to the plebs as afflicted 'so furiously' ('Plebe grassatur furibunda tabes') in the plague at Verona.[39] The Milanese historian Bugati made the same assessment: 'only the plebs and populace caught and spread it among their friends and kin and occasionally to those they served'.[40] By August 1577 he estimated that around 10,000 had died of plague, all of whom, he asserted, were commoners, and many of them, women and children.[41] Finally, throughout various parts of his long plague treatise, Ingrassia observed: 'for the most part the contagion struck the plebs; it was extraordinarily rare that even a poor nobleman would catch the disease'. One explanation he advanced was that 'without any effort, the nobleman would receive help and assistance'.[42] In 1576, Gratiolo da Salò explained the correlation between class and plague as the consequence of the lack of cleanliness: 'Finally, as continued experience clearly shows us, the more dirty and foul the individual, the more likely he is to be afflicted, certainly more so than the clean and the noble.'[43]

Plague doctors and writers of later plagues in the sixteenth century continued seeing plebs as the repositories of pestilential infection and to give reasons for it. In 1587 Francesco Tommasi, a doctor from Colle Val d'Elsa, but practising at Rome's largest hospital, Santo Spirito, certainly was not without moral prejudice in his observations of the plague striking most frequently 'the filthy plebs and those who were dirty, such as Jews, butchers, cooks, tailors, and then the greedy and unclean and disorderly types, gluttons and libidinous men, whose activities gave rise to putrefied blood'.[44] With fewer moral overtones, however, the Sicilian Pietro Parisi, who had become an honorary citizen of Palermo because of his medical service during the 1575–7 plague, claimed in 1592 that plague struck the lowest classes ('la bassa plebe'), because they were the ones who in times of famine and plague were 'forced to eat bad and corrupt food, stinky bread, grass, and unknown roots'.[45] In a chapter 'On the universal prognosis of plague'

[35] Valier, *Commentariolus*, 76r.   [36] De Pomi, *Brevi discorsi*, 302r (BAV pagination).

[37] Donzellini, *Discorso nobilissimo*, 310v.   [38] Betholio, *in urbe Mediolani*.

[39] *Raccolta delli componimenti*, 118v.   [40] Bugati, *L'aggiunta*, 149.   [41] Ibid., 164.

[42] Ingrassia, *Parte quinta*, 19. Similar assessments are also in his *Informatione*, parts I and II: 61, 64, 76, 225, 264; part III: 4; and part IV, 141.

[43] Gratiolo, *Discorso di peste*, 18.   [44] Tommasi, *Tractatus de peste*, 14.

[45] Parisi, *Avvertimenti*, 5.

of his *Trattato della Peste* (published in the same year), he maintained that 'the appearance of poor malnourished girls and old starving and unclothed women' were the signs of coming plague and this was especially true of the present plague in Sicily (1592): 'their miserable bodies were particularly disposed to receiving the disease and changes in the air'. From them, the disease then passed to the plebs, 'swallowing them up like ravenous wolves'. Parisi then gave his observation authority by citing classical texts of Oribasius,[46] Paolus,[47] and Aëtius.[48] Gerardo Columba of Messina placed the plague of his city in 1596 within the context of famine, which had reigned throughout Sicily during the previous two years; even if its victims were not exclusively the plebs, it 'spread poorly among men of the upper classes [*viros primarios*]'.[49]

For Piedmont's plague of 1599–1600[50] Roffredi identified Turin's victims as concentrated in 'the city's vilest neighbourhoods', where leather-workers, grooms, stable boys, working girls ('muliercularum'), the lowest of the whores ('meretricum sintina'), and the meanest of the plebs resided, where the house of prostitution called 'il Bori' was found. This area was hit first and most savagely, leaving few survivors. It was the area of the most pestilential air and the most squalid housing, called 'habitacula', where inhabitants wore the vilest clothing 'accustomed to drawing in plague'. Their food was 'fatty, corrupt, and spoilt', and as a consequence 'their bodies were often smeared in excrement'. Their streets were filled with waste; their latrines overflowing 'without means for washing away the fetid odours that brought the disease seeping through their nostrils'.[51]

---

[46] Along with Alexander of Tralles (525–605), these three were the principal Byzantine compilers of Galen from the third to the seventh century; see Durling, 'A Chronological Census of Renaissance Editions', 231. Oribasio di Pergamo (325–403) was the personal physician of the Roman emperor Julian and the author of a seventy-volume medical encyclopaedia, *Collectiones medicae*, which was an extended summary and commentary on the medicine of Galen. According to Temkin, *Galenism*, 64 and 95, he marked the *terminus a quo* of Galenism in medicine.

[47] The Byzantine compiler Paul of Aegina (625–90) wrote an *Epitome* of medicine in seven books largely based on Galen and Oribasio; see Durling, 'A Chronological Census of Renaissance Editions', 231.

[48] Aëtius of Amida (*c.* 550) was a physician to Justinian I, who compiled a medical encyclopaedia in sixteen books. Parisi, *Trattato della peste*, 105. On these compilers and Byzantine medicine, see Castiglioni, *A History of Medicine*, 250–7.

[49] Columba, *Disputationum de Febris pestilentis*, 1r.   [50] Corradi, *Annali*, I, 702–3.

[51] Roffredi, *Pestis, et calamitatum Taurini*, 21. Except for those who spoke of reptiles, scorpions, other animals, and occasionally mice coming out of their holes presaging future plague, he was one of the very few sixteenth-century plague writers to point to mice or rats (*mures*) during plague: as a consequence of the killing of all the cats in Turin as a preventative measure, 'rats multiplied more than ever, crawling out from under desks, without any fear, swarming in new colonies, infesting everything and gnawing away, ruining all our property' (31). Similarly, Ingrassia, *Informatione*, 69 and 279, noticed that after all the cats had been killed that mice [or rats (*topi*)] increased in number. The point remains: late medieval and early modern plague, if anything, gave rise to increased rat populations, unlike *Yersinia Pestis*, which decimated rats before people, leaving sickly rats and their corpses, not emboldened frisky ones to swarm everywhere. Historians wishing to argue that medieval and early modern European plague was *Yersinia pestis*, have yet to find any references to a sudden increase in dead rats; instead their efforts have produced the opposite: the occasional appearance or increase of living rats during plague time. See for instance Slack, *The Impact of Plague*, 238–9.

Contemporaries' awareness of the tight relationship between poverty and plague certainly continued with plagues in the seventeenth century.[52]

As some of these passages suggest, the doctors of 1575–8 and thereafter not only saw plague arising from commoners and their neighbourhoods but also began to speculate on what these social patterns indicated about the character of the disease—its causes, the reasons for its spread and intensity, and its prevention. One line of interpretation found support in Galen and Hippocrates: epidemics and plagues were associated with bad food and food poisoning and could be fuelled by malnourishment. For instance, a tract from Asti written during a plague at the end of the sixteenth century saw victims dying of hunger and thirst because of the economic constraints in provisioning basic necessities; plague arose from malnutrition and the corruption of food.[53] In his *Avvertimenti*, to argue that famine and bad food led to plague in his time, Parisi noted that 'ancient histories narrated that pestilence has its origins in the eating of spoilt food'. He cited Galen on Roman plagues, when people had been constrained to eat spoilt vegetables and other food including frogs, the extremities of trees, and leaves ('frittici?'). After Galen, he added other authorities and historical cases from the ancient Hebrews, a famine in Marseille in 363 AD, the Italian plague of 1523, one of 1570, to that of his own experience during the current plague of 1592. Only as an aside did he admit, 'of course God was the first cause' and cited Marsilio Ficino for this and the configuration of planets as causes.[54] Similarly, Somenzi and Glisenti cited Galen and the plague of Athens to argue that poverty and bad food brought on plague.[55] Others such as the historian Tranquilli, who certainly knew the works of Galen, may have had him in mind when he reported the causes of plague in 1575. Although Tranquilli held that the disease had been carried to the extremities of Italy by ships originating in the Levant, 'even more so' its rise at Mantua and Verona in April 1575, he claimed, was fuelled by 'a great disease [*gran male*] brought on by the poor eating an extraordinary quantity of fish caught in a dried up [*risecata*] part of their lake'.[56]

WATER

Doctors and other plague writers of 1575 and afterwards, however, went beyond Galen and medieval physicians to understand the social facts of their present plagues and to explain why pestilence began in the worst neighbourhoods and afflicted principally the poor. Although Galen mentioned 'bad drink' along with

---

[52] See for instance Rondinelli's remarks regarding Florence's plague in 1629–31: 'La strage maggiore del male è stata nel popolo minuto, ne' poveri, e nelle donne; della nobiltà n'è morta pochissima . . .' cited by Lombardi, '1629–1631: crisi e peste a Firenze', 37.

[53] Arellano, *Trattato di peste*, 28.   [54] Parisi, *Avvertimenti*, 1 and 5–6.

[55] Somenzi, *De morbis*, 20v; and Glisenti, *Il summario delle cause*, n.p.

[56] Tranquilli, *Pestilenze che sono state in Italia*, 21–2.

'bad food' as consequences of pestilence, the writers of the 1575–8 plague investigated more fully questions of water supplies and contamination across cities. As we have seen, Raimondo devoted an entire tract to explain plague as infecting the poor because of their reliance on bad drinking water, but he was not alone in suspecting a correlation between polluted wells and other sources of water and the concentration of plague victims as the poor.

Without tying his argument to specific events exclusive to Venice such as sea-water flooding wells, Somenzi pointed to polluted supplies of water in the working-class districts of Milan and Mantua to explain why plague first infected the plebs in these and other cities. More than contaminated food, water supplies did 'maximum damage' to the poor. He further argued that water was the principal source of the disease—its malignant juices imperceptible to the poor 'procreated' the disease. In addition, those who ate fruit and vegetables washed with polluted water succumbed to it.[57] As a charitable act in plague time, Somenzi recommended distribution of abundant supplies of wine to the poor.[58]

Ingrassia also saw the many fountains and streams ('fiumicelli') that ran into the city of Palermo as a source of the 1575 disease. As early as 1560 he was one of the few before 1575 to point to contaminated water as a cause of plague and contagion. He pinned the flooding of the previous winter as a cause of an epidemic of 1558 in Palermo, 'because the ground became kneaded [*impastata*] with a viscous mixture of putrefied stuff', the atoms of which evaporated in rivers, fountains, and wells during the summer, adding to the putrefaction of the air.[59] He maintained that Naples did not suffer from these problems, not because its water was any better, but because its aqueducts were covered along public streets so the water did not evaporate filling the atmosphere with putrefied fumes. Thus corrupted water was a concomitant cause of plague, not because of drinking it but because of its contribution to bad air, and because of this analysis, he did not in 1560 link water supplies to any particular social group or neighbourhood afflicted by plague.

In 1575, his thinking about pollution, water, and contagion evolved, even if his classical sources and references remained much the same. Like Raimondo, he also connected flooding with pollution, but not in Raimondo's peculiar view. More precisely and emphatically than Raimondo or any other author of the sixteenth century or before, Ingrassia connected water supplies with the social geography of the city and its patterns of morbidity and mortality that resulted from the *mal contagioso*. Polluted drinking water was now seen as the source of disease. Water washed down the rubbish ('le bruttezze') from butcher and leather shops along with all the dirt and grime ('tutte le sporchezze') from cloth production in the city, and the bilge ('le dette billacchie') polluted the ground where there were

---

[57] For Galen, however, the eating of spoilt food was a consequence, not a cause of plague. I thank Vivian Nutton for this observation.

[58] Somenzi, *De morbis*, 32v and 39v–40r.   [59] Ingrassia, *Trattato assai bello*, 23v.

Cc. 27. (C.)

NICOLAI MASSA VENETI

ARTIVM ET MEDICINAE DOCTORIS

LIBER DE FEBRE PESTILENTIALI,
ac de Peftichiis, Morbillis, Variolis, & Apoftematibus
peftilentialibus, ac eorundem omnium curatione,
necnon de modo quo corpora à pefte
præferuari debeant.

OPVS SANE VTILISSIMVM,

cui nuperrime Auctor tum pleracq alia, tum præcipue doctri-
nam addidit de rebus, quæ peftilentem contagionem
fufcipere, uel non fufcipere posfint.

Cum indice rerum notabilium in fine operis appofito.

AQVA NON SI-

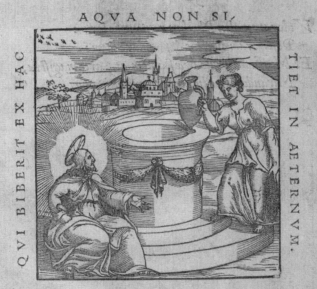

QVI BIBERIT EX HÁC   TIET IN AETERNVM.

VENETIIS, APVD ANDREAM ARRIVABENVM,
Ad fignum Putei.   M D L VI.

Illustration 8.   Nicolò Massa, *Liber de febre pestilentiali* (1556).

many wells. 'Little by little' this trash polluted city wells, 'especially those used by the plebs'. Ingrassia revised his earlier view on water pollution as a 'universal' cause of bad air affecting all classes equally. Now he saw the rush off of industrial waste, excrement, and rubbish as affecting the water table and thereby polluting wells and other sources of drinking water that mainly served the plebs.[60] In an elementary fashion (but unfortunately without maps, tables, or quantification), Ingrassia next anticipated John Snow's findings on the wells of London during the cholera epidemics of the 1850s. The neighbourhoods of Palermo with high rates of infection from the present disease, he argued, correlated closely with polluted wells. He noted that the contagion of 1575 did not spread to those who drank from the well of 'Garraffo' for instance and 'other similar sources of purer water' but instead was found in those neighbourhoods where the poor were forced to drink polluted water.[61]

HOUSING

Unlike previous authors of plague tracts, those of the 1575–8 plague investigated and speculated on the housing and living conditions of the poor to explain the rise of plague and its intensification within certain neighbourhoods. Previously, writers such as the Venetian doctor Niccolò Massa might have advised their readers to keep air circulating through their houses and to keep them clean and pretty ('& alia quædam pulcherrima')[62] or to close windows at night and open them in the mornings to circulate the air. He also went beyond other plague writers of his generation in arguing that plague arose principally among the poor because of their habits and cramped housing,[63] but he stressed mostly the habits of the poor and saw no topographical correlations between poverty and plague or that plague clustered in certain neighbourhoods because of bad housing or social conditions such as poor plumbing. In 1576 plague writers went further. Canobbio saw a positive correlation between neighbourhoods of overcrowding and bad housing with high plague mortality. This was especially pronounced in the city's Jewish quarters. He reported a case of one *torazzo* (tenement) in the Jewish *contrada* that housed fourteen families, all of whom died of plague in 1576. He reported that 300 such homes in the city were similarly overcrowded with fifteen to twenty of the same family: here, all family members died of

---

[60] Ingrassia, *Informatione*, 64.

[61] Ibid., 61. The Veronese *sanità* also were suspicious of the spread of plague through wells and drinking water. In a decree of 25 September 1576 the supply of water to those in the *contrada* of Tomba, the neighbourhood of its lazaretto, were limited to one well; ASVr, Sanità, no. 33, 56r.

[62] Massa, *Liber de febre pestilentiali*, 70–6. Many plague tracts of the late fourteenth and fifteenth centuries gave advice on when to open and close windows and doors to keep air circulating and to keep the house closed from the pestilential vapours; see for instance, Tommaso del Garbo, *Consiglio contro a pistolenza*, 19–20; and Benzi, 'Trattato', 88.

[63] See Chapter 6, n. 60.

plague.[64] His third book pertained to the causes of plague deaths and concentrated on the poor, their abandonment and lack of food and medication. But above all else, 'death was a social disease',[65] in this case linked to their miserable housing ('casucccie') and neighbourhoods.[66]

Udine's public health doctor during the 1576–7 plague, Daciano, pointed to the need for cleanliness, especially in periods of plague. But he realized that these matters were more difficult for the poor than the rich, 'who enjoyed every comfort and happiness, who possessed beautiful rooms and well-built abodes, could light odoriferous fires and keep their homes continuously perfumed with sweet scents, who ate abundantly with the best and most delicate foods and most precious wines, who could enjoy vast spaces almost without end'. He contrasted their conditions with those of 'the miserable poor' and stressed their shoddy housing: 'at best they led their lives within cramped, narrow, dirty hovels'. He claimed that the health board had done its best given its resources to alleviate the pain and suffering of the poor and that without its charity many thousands more would have perished in the plague; not only those sequestered under suspicion but others from famine and the cold.[67] Towards the end of the century, the Sabaudian doctor Roffredi, saw the 'pestilential air' in Turin hovering within neighbourhoods that were 'filthy and possessed indecent housing' ('ubi immundiores domus, spurce areae'). No doubt his observations and those of others who correlated plague and poverty were tinged with social prejudice. Roffredi also contended that the plague infected 'the filthy poor, the ill-dressed, and those who were sexually licentious'.[68]

Others such as Donzellini may not have broken completely from social stereotypes, but they could nonetheless question ancient formula as with Galen's that plague originated from famine. As for the plague in Venice in 1576, Donzellini was unequivocal: 'there had been no extraordinary food shortage that molested the plebs and poor any more than the nobility or the well off'. Rather, it was the plebs' bad housing on ground floors, along with their normal life style, their bad living that made them more susceptible. Like others in 1575–8 he pointed to the sources of food, water, and contamination. Their food was 'of bad sustenance'—greens ('herbe'), fruits, roots, sour foods ('fortumi'), cheese, clams, leftover fish and meat, and 'what is worse', bread poorly risen and baked. They drank cheap wine, blended and adulterated, or salty water from the drain-off of floods or polluted wells. 'Negligence, untidiness, and imprudence of these manual workers (*di tai [sic] persone mechanice*), who failed to protect themselves from dirty things (*che non fanno schifar il male*)' worsened their conditions. Such habits characterized especially children, greedy women, the lazy ('ociose') and less cautious men.[69] Gratiolo, however, focused more clearly on housing

[64] Canobbio, *Il successo*, 12r.   [65] The phrase is Coleman's, *Death Is A Social Disease*.
[66] Canobbio, *Il successo*, 23r.   [67] Daciano, *Trattato della peste*, 45–6.
[68] Roffredi, *Pestis, et calamitatum Taurini*.   [69] Donzellini, *Discorso nobilissimo*, 314r.

as the principal menace: the 'filthiness of housing produces the plague', and it came from 'a multitude of people living together', in other words overcrowding, resulting in great stench (then understood as the source of contagion). Those living in such conditions lacked the means to change their clothing or to keep themselves clean.[70]

The Cremonese physician Somenzi showed less prejudice and placed less importance on supposed differences in the behaviour of rich and poor. Instead, he concentrated on housing as the principal cause of the plague's concentration within neighbourhoods of the poor. First, because of their indigence, many were forced to share accommodation in small houses ('domunculis'). Secondly, the disease spread easier in these houses because they were already unhealthy ('insalubritas'), and thirdly because plague could spread so much easier in such cramped spaces, it spread here more quickly through and to other neighbourhoods. According to Somenzi, the rich avoided plague, not because they were wealthier per se, but because their homes were larger and cleaner, allowing wind to pass through them. They were therefore able to keep the contagion away for much longer and were better positioned to prevent the pestilential air from seeping in or being carried there by others. In short, overcrowding caused plague to spread in working-class quarters, and because it spread there with such deadly effect, Somenzi argued, it satisfied Galen's definition of a 'popular' epidemic and therefore was 'true' plague.[71]

Others connected the plague's spread with failure to remove filth, rubbish, and excrement. Local plague ordinances such as those enacted at Bologna in May 1576 saw the removal of waste and cleaning of sewers as central to the struggle against the spread of plague. The ban gave Bolognese residents three days to clear every bit of excrement ('ogni quantitata di letame') from their stalls and adjacent alleyways, public streets, and other places, along with any trash, waste, chunks of earth, or mud—dry or fresh—lying either in the house and areas of habitation or outside as under porticos, attached to columns, and in streets. Violators were to be fined 10 *scudi* per infraction, to be paid by both landlords and tenants.[72] On 10 November and 'reiterated' the following day, another Bolognese ban made clear that mud and other waste increased 'the danger of infection'. The ordinance required residents to clean the streets in front of their houses and carry the mud, earth, excrement, and other filth outside the city. Every fifteen days they were to sweep the streets and clean the pilasters, columns, and porticos in front of their houses. Anyone caught throwing washing water, piss, water with ashes (used in washing) or other filth from windows or any other place was fined 5 *lire* a throw.[73]

[70] Gratiolo, *Discorso di peste*, 16–18.   [71] Somenzi, *De morbis*, 31v–32r.

[72] *Bandi & Constitut. diverse di Bologna*, 341v–42r, bando no. 100.

[73] Ibid., no. 119. Milan passed similar ordinances during this plague; see *Gride diverse*, no. 138. Earlier plague ordinances such as those promulgated in Rouen on 26 November 1512 were not nearly as detailed.

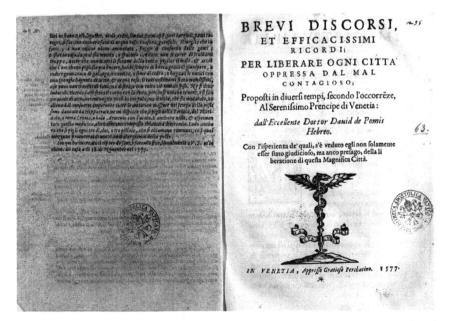

Illustration 9. *Brevi discorsi et efficacissimi ricordi per liberare ogni città oppressa dal Mal Contagioso* by Dottor David de Pomis Hebreo, 1577.

By 1575, the doctors raised similar alarms about public filth and housing. After pointing to the corruption of wells that served the plebs in the months leading to the outbreak of plague in 1575, Raimondo turned to housing: the poor were forced to live in hot rooms that were small and smelly. These conditions, combined with bad food and water, 'weakened their constitutions and humours', making them more susceptible to plague and, if they caught it, more likely to die from it than the better-off. He also attempted to explain the greater mortality of women in many Italian cities by the sixteenth century.[74] Again, housing was critical. Because of their 'weaker constitutions', women were more likely to become ill from the bad water and to die from plague, 'especially those deprived of doctors, medicine, and good housing ('di buone stanze')'.[75]

They only fined those for throwing excrement or garbage into the streets and for failing to keep streets clean, *Ordonnances contre la peste*, n.p. [1r]. Also, see Rouen's laws on street cleaning not passed as plague legislation on 7 December 1507 and 24 July 1513, ibid., 9v and 10v.

[74] In the Milanese necrologies during the plagues of 1452, 1468, 1483, 1485, 1503, 1523, and 1524, women consistently died in greater numbers than men; however, in predominantly rural areas of Nonantola (Modena), men and women died in equal numbers; see Alfani and Cohn, 'Nonantola 1630', 108–10.

[75] *Discorso*, 391v (BAV pagination).

David de Pomi writing a year earlier was more precise in connecting plague to the poor and their housing.[76] With the summer heat in 1576 he witnessed the explosion of the plague, 'a massive putrefaction of the humours', which was especially severe among the plebs, who were poorly controlled 'in their way of life', and crowded ('stando strettamente') into small houses without air ('che non hanno sboro'). He then drew a direct correlation between these conditions, neighbourhoods, and plague. To end the plague, he argued for the evacuation of those living in these courtyards and houses that lacked proper air; otherwise the inhabitants who remained would become infected and would perish. Moreover, the disease would then spread to houses on higher storeys. In need of manual labour those higher and better-off would have to descend to these houses for help, thus risking infection.[77] De Pomi wrote to the president of the *sestiere* of Santa Croce proposing that the city forcefully remove all the poor, even those who were at present in good health, from their dark dwellings and temporarily rehouse them in other parts of the city while their homes were thoroughly cleaned. He estimated the cleaning would require between fifteen and twenty days and that around 3,000 in each sixth of the city would have to be evacuated. This, he argued, was preferable to sequestrating the population, because by his plan, the artisans could continue working, benefiting themselves and the public. No doubt over-optimistically, he argued that the 'Magnificent City' could begin celebrating their liberation from plague only fifteen to twenty days after the operation had been completed. His ideas were taken seriously. Later that year, between 9 and 13 July 1576, Mercuriale and the Paduan professors made similar suggestions based on housing and Venice's poor,[78] and in August 1576 the Senate accepted that the spread of the disease hinged on poor housing ('casette molto ristrette et anguste') and made provisions to move 10,000 of the poor from the worst areas to a site at Lizzafusina. The plan, however, was never realized.[79]

The Milanese doctor and professor of medicine at Pavia Archileo Carcano, at the age of 21, published two plague tracts in 1577,[80] and went further: he saw the home as essential to whether plague would spread to or within a neighbourhood; householders should regulate and 'correct' the air within their homes and prevent smells evaporating from latrines and sewers from seeping through the home. It was not just important to ensure that such fetid discharges were removed from the house but especially from particular places and cubicles within it (the lavatories?).[81] The last section of his second tract divided preventative measures against future plagues under three rubrics—'men, the city, and the house'.[82] For both the city and the house, he emphasized the importance of regularly cleaning

---

[76] De Pomi, *Brevi discorsi e Ricordi*, 302r–3r. This section of de Pomi's report was submitted on 3 August 1576. According to Edit 16 only one copy of this publication survives, BAV.

[77] Perhaps class divisions were aligned more vertically in Venice than in Palermo.

[78] Pullan, *Rich and Poor in Renaissance Venice*, 318.   [79] Palmer, 'The Control of Plague', 144.

[80] He died in Milan in 1588 at 32. In his short life he published four books.

[81] Carcano, *De peste opusculum*, 20.   [82] Carcano, *Trattato di peste*, 13r–19v.

sewers, latrines and commodes ('gli odiosi vapori de i cacatoi, & de condutti, o cloache'), the removal of excrement especially from bedrooms and not only during the summer months.[83]

Issues of proper plumbing—public and private—now entered other plague tracts for the first time. In addition to the old advice about leaving windows open, especially those on the north and east to allow sun and wind to circulate through the house, Ingrassia stressed that the house had to be cleaned regularly and thoroughly with every sort of waste removed and stressed cleaning of one's own latrines and toilets ('lebellache').[84] He also poured scorn on Palermo's public latrines and other modes of removing waste from the city. Throughout the harbour area ('città di marina') a public latrine emptied into the sea above the water line, where everyone went to empty their excrement. The sea served further as a waste bin for every other sort of trash including dead animals. This hazard had been ordered to be cleaned two months previously, but it worsened daily.[85] Ingrassia also pointed to the total lack of plumbing and the consequent habits of the poor as a reason for plague emanating from their wretched houses ('nelle loro casuzze'): they kept vases full of their excrement in their rooms, under their beds for almost the entire day. 'They must learn to empty and clean their rooms often.'[86]

PLAGUE ADVICE AND LAWS TARGETING THE POOR

From the start, medieval doctors knew their new scourge was highly contagious, and by the fifteenth century, they advised patients to avoid places where crowds gathered such as city squares and especially enclosed areas such as churches. However, in pointing to such places, plague writers before 1575 did not discriminate socially, that is, seeing some places worse than others according to the social geography of the city. In 1575 and afterwards they did: areas where the poor gathered and resided were now viewed as dangerous sources of the disease. Ingrassia advised fleeing all interaction with the plebs during the Sicilian plague of 1575; 'their bodies and clothes were foul and unkempt, ugly and filled with filth', and by these means they infected many. It was especially dangerous to be amongst them 'in their multitude and confusion' during the heat of summer. In his role as *Protomedico*, he pressured the archbishop of Palermo to prohibit funeral services during the late summer of 1575 along with Palermo's summer festival in mid-August called 'de i Cirij'. Despite his religious zeal—Ingrassia had been a member of the Sicilian Inquisition and expressions of religious piety fill his medical writings—he advised abandoning squares and crowds, 'even' churches

---

[83] Ibid, 18r.   [84] Ingrassia, *Informatione: Parte terza*, 4.   [85] Ibid., *Parte una*, 44.
[86] Ibid., *Parte terza*, 6. Also, Alessandri, *Trattato della peste*, 23r, stressed the need to clean privies (*cessi*) during plague time.

and attending mass were to be avoided: 'as far as was possible, it was best to stay away from others'. This was especially the case with 'crowds of the plebs'.[87]

As we have seen, published legislation, bans, or *gride*, proliferated during the plague of 1575–8 for various cities in the north of Italy.[88] Despite changes in attitudes to the poor, begging and new forms of urban welfare that reach back a century or more, plague laws and statutes had not targeted the poor, at least not to the extent now seen with the outpouring of such ordinances published in broadsheets in 1576–7.[89] The first Bolognese *manifesti* outlawing various forms of low-life—*forfanti, vagabondi, comedianti, cingari et giocatori*—from entering the city do not appear until 1566, and are repeated on three occasions before 1575.[90] By contrast, during this plague and afterwards to 1600, at least thirty-eight such ordinances were printed and posted.[91] Moreover, they became more extensive, prohibiting begging within the city, placing distribution points of charity beyond city walls, prohibiting 'poor peasants' from entering the city,[92] and preventing soldiers returning from wars to enter.[93] The same appears in Verona, where its proclamations remained mostly unpublished. The earliest statute issued by the city's health board against the poor, beggars, low-life, those without employment and disbanded soldiers appears only with the first days of the city's discovery of plague in August 1575. They were given three days to leave the city. In one respect Verona's charge against the poor may have gone beyond the harshness of the decrees in Milan and Bologna: early on during the plague the poor from the city or territory of Verona who wished to enter or re-enter the city were barred whether or not they carried a *fede* (certificate), attesting to their good health and that they had not been to a place under suspicion.[94] In the remaining years of the sixteenth century, such injunctions at Verona were repeated with increasing details on persons to be excluded and of the threats and punishments to be inflicted on the poor, including torture. In addition, boatmen, carters, and others responsible for transporting such people to cities were equally threatened with severe punishments.[95]

In sixteenth-century plague treatises, the only recommendations for special laws or treatment regarding the poor before 1575 that I have found come from the advice of the Torinese doctor Bucci in his first tract of 1564. It is one of

[87] Ingrassia, *Informatione, Parte terza*, 4.   [88] See Chapter 6, 202–7.

[89] See for instance, Michielse, 'Policing the Poor'; Henderson, *Piety and Charity*, 359–64; and Pullan, *Rich and Poor in Renaissance Venice*, ch. 3.

[90] *Bononia Manifesta*, no. 457, 8 and 17.i. 1566. An earlier broadsheet of 1564 (no. 397) prohibited vagabonds and others forming crowds but did not expel them from the city or prevent them from entering.

[91] Ibid., nos 1006, 1102, 1162, 1200, 1255, 1299, 1366, 1450, 1724, 1786, 1880, 1927, 1972, 2020, 2039, 2069, 2134, 2146, 2158, 2248, 2280, 2411, 2485, 2491, 2508, 2613, 2730, 2789, 2821, 2821, 2867, 2997, 3014, 3033, 3057, 3085, 3155, and 3197.

[92] Ibid., nos 2248, 2280, 2508, and 2789.   [93] Ibid., no. 2753.

[94] ASVr, Sanità, no. 33, 28r–29v.

[95] Ibid., 34r, 1575.ix; 132r, 1577; 258r, 10.ii.1590; 259r, 17.vi.1590; 260r, 24.v.1591; 262r, 1591.viii; 1591.viii; 338r, 1596.ix.5; 382r, 1598.ix.19; 396r, 1598.ix.19; 399r; 19.ix.1598; and Archivio Comune, no. 211, 24.vii.1578.

the few before 1575 to regard the prevention of plague beyond the personal and to enlist what de Pomi would later call 'the Arm [*Braccio*] of the state'. Under threat of plague 'not only persons but also materials, merchandise, and letters should be banished'. 'In times of maximum danger', the lowest classes and unemployed ('la plebe minuta et inutile') along with poor beggars are to be driven from town and consigned to a place where they could recover. He then tempered this harsh measure by enjoining the state first to spend sums from the public purse for their benefit. Clearly, he saw intermeshed the well-being of the state and the community as a whole, including his elite clientele and readers with that of the poor.[96] In his later tract written in the midst of Piedmont's worst sixteenth-century plague, that of 1585, Bucci elaborated further on the state's role in prevention, control, and cure of plague, what he called (following the divisions of Ingrassia's tract of 1577) the three principal and necessary means: gold, fire, and the hangman's noose ('Oro, Fuoco & Forca'). Again, the fate of rich and poor were intertwined.[97] During the plague of 1585, another Piedmont doctor elaborated on the state's role during plague, emphasizing more *forca* than *oro*. In Francesco Alessandri's tract a human cleaning was to accompany the physical purging of excrement from streets: beggars who sing on street corners, quacks ('cerretani'),[98] whores, and houses of prostitution were to be 'swept from the city'. In addition, he called for banishing certain honest and skilled artisans because of their pollution. Dyers and leather-workers were to be moved 'far away'; and butchers whose shops were close to the river were to be moved immediately downstream.[99]

In decrees and commentaries of 1575–8, emphasis on the poor was also more draconian than the measured response of Bucci in 1564. As early as March 1576, when plague struck Monza but months before its entry into the city of Milan, officials of the Milanese health board acted against the poor and other suspicious elements within the city: 'Because there are many scroungers [*scrocchi*], beggars and vagabonds in this city, who cannot be cared for in hospitals, they are ordered to leave the city.' From fear of plague igniting the tinderbox of overcrowding, bad habits and odours of the poor and the disorder caused by scroungers and beggars, the Milanese health board sought to control also other sectors of the poor. 'Porters, mountain people, women rag dealers [*cimere*], and similar persons who lodged in bed-sits [*una sola camera*], kept their clothes unwashed and greasy, and gave off the worst stench', were at particular risk 'of causing a big epidemic [*un gran male*]'. Therefore, with plague on the city's outskirts,

---

96 Bucci, *Reggimento*, n.p.

97 Bucci, *Modo di conoscere*, 18r. These three political 'remedies' were repeated (citing Ingrassia) by the doctor Geronimo Gatta in his plague tract during the Neapolitan plague of 1656; see Calvi, 'L'oro, il fuoco, le forche', 458.

98 On the origins of this word from the religious sect of the castle at Cereto in the duchy of Spoleto, see Pullan, 'Plebi urbane', 1012.

99 Alessandri, *Trattato della peste*, 30r–v. Also, see Chapter 8, 256–8 on Alessandri's public health ideas.

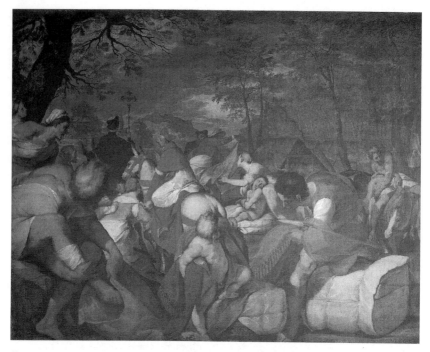

Illustration 10. Giovanni Battista Crespi, called Il Cerano, *Carlo Borromeo Distributes His Clothing and Furnishings to the Plague-Stricken*, 1602.

the government passed new injunctions outlawing any occupancy of more than four people to a room or more than two in a bed. Such persons, moreover, were required to keep their rooms cleansed ('purgate') and clean. The ordinance did not specify how such a law would be enforced; nor did it allocate resources for those suddenly to live cleaner and in less crowded conditions.[100] In March, still before the plague had struck the city, the health board prohibited the entry of tricksters, gypsies, negroes, knaves, herbalists, street-singers, comedians, whores, and similar odd sorts ('furbi, cingari, ghitti, furfanti, herbolari, cantainbanco, commedianti, meretrici e simil sorti de genti stravaganti con fede'). The guards and health officials were to visit often the city's Jews and the poor of St Peter's to ensure that their houses were being kept clean.[101] These prohibitions against 'oddballs', beggars, and certain categories of the poor may not have been carried out sufficiently for once plague entered the city in August similar *gride* were posted again. On the 17th a 'bando' against beggars and scroungers required 'the city to be purged not only of mud and excrement but also of people who

[100] Centorio Degli Ortensi, *I cinque libri degl'avvertimentii*, 13–15.   [101] Ibid., 21.

were unclean in their bodies or clothing'.[102] Those who went begging in front of churches, along streets, or from house to house were to be punished by whipping or imprisonment and their names submitted to the parish elders.[103] According to Bugati, in September 'all the vagabonds, beggars, and scoundrels' were rounded up and driven from the city to a place called Vittoria beyond the Porte Romana, near Melegnano.[104] On 18 February 1577, the health board reissued bans against poor beggars coming to the city. Another *grida* issued the same day stressed the importance of cleanliness for 'liberating the city from the evil contagion', arguing that beggars and poverty were the generators of the disease among themselves and to others. Thus the health board governors ordered the poor along with the blind accustomed to begging to remain at home.[105] Later, on 18 October 1577, the health board outlined instructions to the deputies who guarded the city gates not to admit 'scroungers, beggars, vagabonds, women of ill-repute, or similar persons, who were a threat to the public'. Similarly, those providing useful services but who were on the lower rungs of the occupational ladder, 'porters, women rag-dealers, repairers of old shoes [*Ciavatini*], street sweepers, coalmen, or similar sorts from the mountains as well as any dirty or unkempt people, even if they carried plague passports', were barred at the city's gates.[106]

CHARITY TO THE POOR

Health authorities, city councils, princes, and the Church in Milan and in other Italian cities did not, however, confront the social-epidemiological realities of sixteenth-century plague only with social control, repression, and exclusion. Michel Foucault's 'great confinement' of the mad, poor, and other marginals, justified and accelerated by epidemic disease during the early modern period, as John Henderson has rightly emphasized, had another side often ignored by historians.[107] While clearing cities of its waste and pestilential odours also meant driving vagabonds, beggars, comedians, the poor, and other undesirables from town, governments also passed plague decrees to shore up and protect the indigent. In three cities whose plague *gride*, *provisioni*, and *proclami* I have surveyed—Milan, Bologna, and Verona—again, these provisions became visible

---

[102] Ibid., 77.   [103] Ibid., 78.

[104] Bugati, *L'aggiunta*, 149. Perhaps this was the ordinance of the health board issued on 17 September 1576 that survives in *Gride diverse*, no. 102, giving the 'Frontatori and Scrocchi' six days to leave the city. For a rosier picture of this same event, see Bisciola, *Relatione verissima del progresso della peste*, 6r, who viewed it as charitable kindness initiated by Carlo Borromeo.

[105] Centorio Degli Ortensi, *I cinque libri degl'avvertimenti*, 331; and *Gride diverse*, no. 37.

[106] *Gride diverse*, no. 12.

[107] Foucault, *Madness and Civilization*, 63–4. Henderson, *The Renaissance Hospital*, xxx–xxxi, 261, and 331, also argues that confinement in Counter-Reformation Florence must be seen in the broader context of medicine and charity delivered to the poor and not simply as repression; also see 108.

only with the 1575–8 plague.[108] As ruthless as were the decrees of Verona's Sanità against the poor, expelling them with threats of torture and death, the government at the same time issued other decrees deploring the plight of its 'poor workers and artisans because of the suspension of trade and industry and especially that of the silk business'. As a result, early on during the plague, at the end of September 1575, its health board demanded that Verona's citizens come forward within four days to give charity to the poor,[109] and in October, the city's legislative Council of Twelve passed an ordinance beseeching citizens to raise and distribute charity to feed and support the poor.[110] In August, with threats of fines and corporeal punishment, it demanded that surgeons, doctors, and other carers treat any with fevers or suspected pestilential symptoms.[111] The afflicted were overwhelmingly the poor.

The Milanese government took similar actions: 'deploring the damages brought on by plague not only in the city but in several places throughout the duchy', it allocated funds as early as 27 September 1576—less than two months after the first plague cases appeared in the city—to mitigate the economic hardship and losses engendered by plague.[112] On 25 October, the governors instructed on provisions to be distributed to the poor through *signori* designated for each parish of the city, specifying the daily rations of bread, rice, salt, grain, meat, and other food to be distributed to men, women, and children, along with subsidies to wet nurses to attend orphans of plague victims and to those who cared for the sick.[113] The health board zealously and meticulously recorded these allocations and other charities, listing all the inhabitants of each parish, house by house, each person by age and sex, and the number of families in each house. They noted which families shared the same wells, stairways, and other communal properties as well as the amounts they received in charity.[114] Daily visits to households were to be made to ascertain the numbers in each parish, to inspect whether any had fallen ill, and to report such cases to the doctor in charge of that gate. Those diagnosed with plague were sent either to the plague huts or the lazaretto of San Gregorio, where they were washed and given new clothes. On 17 July 1577 the Milanese health board tried further to mitigate the economic stress and loss of work: 'Beyond the difficulties born of the plague and its inconvenience', the city's governors recognized the strain on artisans and workers to pay rent for their shops during quarantine and allowed them to

---

[108] Clearly such measures had been taken with other disasters such as famine in the past and probably plague. For instance, in calling for charity and piety from the church and its citizens in 1575, the Veronese Council of Twelve recalled previous 'calamitous times' when its citizens had come to assist its poor in 1539, 1559, and 1570; none of these, however, were plague years; ASVr, Archivio di Comune, no. 89, 108v–9r, 1575.x.10.

[109] ASVr, Sanità, no. 33, 61r, 1575.ix.27.

[110] ASVr, Archivio di Comune, no. 89, 109v, 1575.x.10.

[111] ASVr, Sanità, no. 33, 17r, 1575.viii.18.   [112] *Gride diverse*, no. 4.

[113] Ibid., no. 65.   [114] Ibid., no. 26, 1577. iii. 10

withhold a third of it.[115] The decree was extended on 11 September to those renting houses, shops, and taverns if prevented from occupying them because of suspicion of infection.[116]

Other decrees that on first glance may have seemed harsh and repressive against the poor had a silver lining. For instance, the law removing 'all the vagabonds, beggars, and scoundrels' from the city to Vittoria near Melegnano, eight miles from Milan, according to the Jesuit plague chronicler Bisciola, was an act of charity. These were poor ones 'without housing or certain habitation', who stayed in hostels or taverns, or servants whose lords had sent them away because of suspicion of plague and now were forced to live from handouts, or they were unskilled labourers ('di qualche arte leggier') currently out of work. At Vittoria they were given decent lodging in a palace earlier constructed by the King of France. Here, 400 of 'these destitute people' were well fed from the charity of certain gentlemen and dressed in suits of red and purple from funds raised by Cardinal Borromeo: 'all their needs were met'. In addition, the young were taught to sing the Litany and play musical instruments so that after the plague, when they returned to the city, they would be better equipped to collect charity by singing 'with the greatest consolation for all'. Furthermore, at Vittoria, 'the good pastor' (Borromeo) cared for the spiritual needs of the sick and dying.[117] Unfortunately, historical records have not preserved the voices of the inmates to gain their impressions.

On the division of labour in ministering to the needs of the city during plague, the Church played a vital role, and in Milan, as in other places, its energies were not confined to spiritual health alone. Because of the remarkable ecclesiastic leadership of Cardinal Borromeo—for which he became a saint—the Church's intervention in the daily affairs of the state during the plague may have been, however, greater here than elsewhere. His leadership and innovations such as his march of the Holy Nail, his organization of Milan's jubilee, and invention of practices such as the Forty Hours of Devotion, stamped his name on the 1575–8 plague beyond Milan's borders as the plague of San Carlo. In addition, Borromeo wrote plague tracts and regulations that enjoined clergy and citizens to offer charitable services to the poor and plague-stricken.

His handbook for the parish clergy and others to care for the infected, published in the early stages of the plague in 1576, listed numerous charitable acts to be rewarded by plenary and other categories of indulgences.[118] These may have

[115] Ibid., no. 3. The decree paid particular attention to the problems of bakers.

[116] Ibid., nos 4 and 16. On 25 October that year the board reported 'innumerable controversies' between landlords and tenants that had arisen from this statute. A group of senators was elected to adjudicate the cases; ibid., no. 17.

[117] Bisciola, *Relatione verissima del progresso della peste*, 6r. According to Besta, *Vera narratione*, 16r, the Cardinal raised 'a general charity' of 600 *scudi* for the hospital of Vittoria.

[118] Borromeo, *Pratica per i curati*; and idem, *De cura pestilentiae* [1577] in *Constitutiones, et decreta sex prouincialium Synodorum Mediolanensium*, 20.

begun with the clergy but, despite the title of this work, concentrated on the laity. Again, the recipients were overwhelmingly the poor:

We grant plenary indulgence to those below for every day that they perform any of the offices or duties below . . .

> To those who administer any sacrament to the plague-stricken
> or to the suspected in any place, whether at San Gregorio,
> the plague huts, or in their houses.
> To physicians who take the pulse [of the plague-stricken].
> To nurses [*comare*] who help [the physicians], touching the
> plague-stricken or the suspected.
> To the wet nurses who nourish infected babies. . .
> To barbers who bleed or treat the infected medically.
> To servants who assist the infected, touching
> them when the need arises.
> To those who carry or lead the sick to the hospital or the huts.
> To those who bury, carry, or lead the plague dead to their graves.

Borromeo conceded lesser indulgences to many other ordinary citizens and residents for smaller acts of charity and service: 'To those who would visit, console, or encourage [*essortarà*] the plague-stricken or the suspected, to those who bring them messages, food, or medicine. . .and similar acts of charity', and the list goes on.[119]

Borromeo's tract was intended to rouse ('de' eccitare') everyone to practise simple acts of charity, 'so important to the poor and the plague-stricken'.[120] He began with moral and religious duties, that 'his people' should go to the altar and confess their sins. But even this advice had a practical medical angle: it was to alert them to the dangers of hiding the disease. If the disease were exposed earlier, he preached, they had a better chance of survival and would cause less danger to others, and perhaps most importantly they stood less chance of dying without last rites.[121] In this vein, his tract addressed local authorities—the elders, syndics, and consoles of the parish—along with the fathers of families to stay vigilant in their watch over the spread of the plague, to report any cases immediately to the secular and health authorities. He exhorted the populace to obey all the ordinances decreed almost daily by the health board magistrates and admonished secular authorities from city commissioners and elders of the parish to lowly *monatti* or plague cleaners and carters to perform their duties without robbing or extorting money from the afflicted, to clean infected houses and huts thoroughly, and to burn all the straw within the huts once the infected had departed dead or alive.[122] He also expressed moral concerns over plague visitations, especially as regards the inspection of women's bodies: it should be done only if necessary and

---

[119] Borromeo, *Pratica per i curati*, 7.   [120] Ibid., 7–8.   [121] Ibid., 8r.
[122] Ibid., 18r.

only by the appropriate professions—barbers, doctors, and, if possible, other women.[123]

Borromeo only then turned to his own dependants, calling on parish priests to visit all the poor daily, attending not only to spiritual but also to all their bodily needs, rapidly procuring for them any remedy through all available avenues, to see if their parishioners were in need of clothing and bedding, or of any assistance, or if they were being mistreated in any way. They were to ensure that their parishioners received the services of doctors, barbers, nurses ('comadre per le paiole'), and wet nurses, and that the plague cleaners buried the dead and purged infected houses. This patrol of priests also 'kept an eye on' the morals ('all'honesta') of women and the young, locked in their homes, the huts, or the lazaretto. During periods of quarantine his priests were to be especially vigilant in condemning sin and attacking violations of quarantine. In their sermons, they were to preach to their parishioners and especially to soldiers and guards of the city gates 'against blasphemy, dancing, singing, games, theft, laziness, drunkenness, idle pastime [*i trattenimenti vani*], dishonesty but also against neglecting their duties towards the sick and others'.[124]

Borromeo appointed his priests to dangerous posts as residents of the plague huts, ordering them to withdraw from any contact with the community at large while in this service. In addition to caring for the spiritual needs of this sequestered community, they were to ensure the maintenance of the huts—that they remain adequately covered with straw and their inmates kept comfortable, supplied with enough beds, mattresses, sheets, matting, stretchers ('lettiere'), medication, and protected against the cold during the winter.[125] Furthermore, he took to heart the safety of his priests, both those who worked in the huts and those who stayed in their communities. Not only were they to flee from any sign of contagion, but they were to avoid contact with the plague-stricken in their rooms or in the huts. He gave specific instructions on how best to protect their health while ministering to the needs of the plague-stricken, whether performing spiritual or corporeal duties. Confessions were to be heard at the doors of the infected or at a similar safe distance; priests were 'to be on guard' ('et star in tanto un poco discolto'). While at the altar, the priest should place a gate around it to protect him from the congregation.[126] When giving communion, he should avoid touching the clothing, beds, and sheets of the infected and should make sure that they did not touch his clothing. He should take every caution to avoid the breath of the afflicted and employ methods and preservative medicines approved by doctors such as washing one's face and the hand that gave Holy Communion with vinegar. He should wear under his gown a sponge bathed in vinegar tied to a little cord around his neck and should keep certain aromatic herbs and similar preventative medicines in his mouth.[127] He was given

---

[123] Ibid., 29r.   [124] Ibid., 22r.   [125] Ibid. 16r, 30v, 32r, and 43r

[126] Borromeo, *De cura pestilentiae*, 39.   [127] Borromeo, *Pratica per i curati*, 23r–v, 30r, and 45r.

permission not to enter rooms where he suspected any dying of plague. Further the suspected were to carry a white stick four *cubiti* long (about 1.60 metres) to warn priests and others of their presence.[128] He gave priests permission to perform baptism by infusion (which avoided touching the baby) rather than by immersion.[129]

In order to report cases of plague quickly and expertly and to give the last rites in time, Borromeo instructed his clergy on the common signs and symptoms of the plague: 'fever, notable pain or heaviness in the head, vomiting, and tumours in various parts of the body'.[130] He also realized that the clergy would be scarce in these trying times and gave authority for those outside the Church to hear confessions and without confession booths. Even women could be granted the right in such conditions.[131] His regulations played a major role in the distribution of charity throughout the city, and in particular for the building and provisioning of the plague huts along with the cleaning, purging, and burning of infected clothes and goods.[132] Priests were also ordered to keep parish records to be passed on to the elected parish plague doctors, reporting who had died and those suspected or infected.[133]

I have summarized these tracts and regulations at length, because I know nothing like them before 1575, either by the clergy or the laity. No earlier plague tracts gave advice or dealt so directly with the day-to-day practicalities in the administration of care for the plague-afflicted or those suspected, from the supply of medication and sheets to the thatching of plague huts or to the problems and methods of exhorting thousands of volunteers and professionals not to desert the afflicted, but to engage zealously in the risky work of curing, nursing, and patrolling plague patients. Not until 1575 had any other published work addressed the poor with such minute detail.

Borromeo's tract, however, was not unique among the writings of clerics addressing similar problems in other Italian cities in 1575–8. A cleric at Forlì (where there is no evidence of this plague arriving) published a selection of the ordinances promulgated by the bishop of his city, Antonio Giannotto. To celebrate the jubilee year, Giannotto organized processions of religious companies and of 'many barefooted men and women' singing of litanies and psalms, and called together all the poor of the city to examine their 'matters of faith'. When news of the plague's worsening in Venice and Padua arrived at Forlì, however, he crossed the line of the spiritual to engage in debates on the temporal, arguing against continuing ties with Venice, despite the importance of these links to the

---

[128] Borromeo, *De cura pestilentiae*, 40 and 44.   [129] Ibid., 44.

[130] Borromeo, *Pratica per i curati*, 36r. Borromeo's personal library suggests a strong interest in medicine and the new anatomy that had developed since the 1540s; see Belloni, 'Carlo Borromeo e la storia della medicina', 174.

[131] Borromeo, *De cura pestilentiae*: 'Permittendi sacram confessionem audire extra Ecclesie fines atque adeo etiam foeminis extra confessionalem sedem' (22).

[132] Ibid., 60.   [133] Ibid., 38.

economic well-being of his city.[134] To avoid imminent ruin, however, his actions were neither as bold nor as secular as those of Borromeo: instead, he ordered his citizens to face the danger 'with tears, prayers, fasting, charity, and other works of penitence . . . to atone for all acts of plunder and illicit gains'.[135]

Another tract, that of the Florentine Camoldolese monk Silvano Razzi, was certainly more traditional than those of Borromeo. The causes and remedies of the plague touched on Galenic points such as the bad quality of the humours, the corruption of the air, contagion, and other 'dispositions that bring on this infection'. But this was only a medical preface to an extensive survey of the principles and underlying causes and cures of plague. Many of these ran counter to the general advice doctors gave on attitudes and the psyche during plague time, that encouraged leisure, light thoughts, even frivolity. According to Razzi, the principal causes of plague were pride and arrogance, followed by blasphemy, heresy 'and its contagion'. Possessing prohibited books, robbery, abduction, usury, sacrilege, vanity, flirtation, and 'every sort of carnality' was for Razzi signs of plague and simultaneously the Antichrist. Also, activities such as indecent madrigals, disgraceful songs, lascivious dancing, indecent familiarity with others, luxurious dressing ('la delicatezza de' vestimenti'), and reading sexy books, 'especially when they contain biblical stories' brought on plague. The use of nude pictures under pretence of fine art was a covert means for inciting 'every sort of filthy concupiscence; such barbaric impiety revived ancient idolatry'. What perturbed Razzi even more was placing these nudes on altars, 'where the eyes and mouth should be most chaste in the presence of the Lord'.[136]

As for remedies to protect against the plague, Razzi's advice hinged largely on religious and ideological matters. He advocated prayers to the Mother of God, the celestial court, and especially to a town's patron saints, along with the plague saints Sebastian, Gregory, and Roch. Disgraceful books, ones of earthly love and other forms of vanity, magic, astrology, and especially 'the books of the rabbis and Jews, which contain blasphemy and falsehoods', were to be torn apart and burnt immediately, along with cards and dice.[137] He then turned to the duties of priests, confessors, and others who preach. They should ensure that doctors, surgeons, barbers, pharmacists, and prefects and assistants in hospitals were prepared to receive God's grace and organize processions with flags of saints; console and comfort the afflicted about to die; organize confraternities and other companies of the laity to process with their standards and read their holy books on various days of the week.[138]

But Razzi's plague compilations did not end with bigotry and moralistic admonitions. In addition, he translated the ordinances enacted by the bishop of Mantua, Marco Gonzaga, during the current plague. The first of these pertained

---

[134] *Ordine et modo tenuto da monsig. Antonio Giannotto*, 41.   [135] Ibid., 42.
[136] Razzi, *Cause et rimedi della peste*, 23–31.   [137] Ibid., 50–2.   [138] Ibid., 59–66.

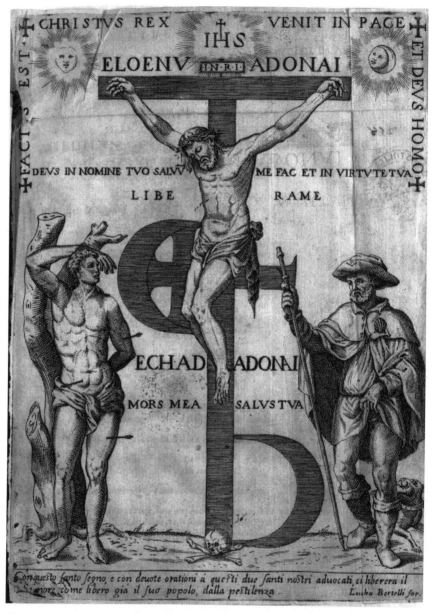

Illustration 11. Iconography of Plague Saints Sebastian and Roch.

to the well-being and property of the Church and its ministers. For instance, if a sacristan should become infected with plague, there would be no need to burn his vestments (at least not those of great value), and plague officials should take extra care when dealing with the holy relics as with cleaning parchments and other important registers recording litigation, peacemaking, legacies, and the memoirs of the founders and beneficiaries of monasteries and other religious orders. Like Borromeo, however, Gonzaga did not direct his attention solely to spiritual or clerical matters. Other provisions pertained to physical health, antidotes, *palle* or balls to be worn around the neck filled with incense and perfumes, and ways of purifying the air. On these matters as well as other medical remedies regarding diet, clothing, and habitation, clerics were advised to seek out 'good medical counsel'. More significantly, these provisions then turned to an area of activity where the ecclesiastical arm should play a charitable role in the health and well-being of the community. They advised secular magistrates to organize a public treasury ('un publico errario') with a specific plan to help the poor: in every parish a public oven should be constructed in an open place with a granary to provide flour and bread for the needy; a charity for clothing should be established; a doctor and surgeon with assistants should be assigned to each parish, and a register (*catalogo*) made of all the poor families within each parish 'as has been done and has currently been reinstated in Milan'.

The Mantuan bishop's provisions then directed the various groups within the Church on their specific duties for assisting the poor and infected. First, novices and those too old to help physically should be removed to places that were secure from the plague's contagion. Religious personnel providing assistance to those in infected houses should have a separate place to live during the plague so as not to infect others; clergy caring for the plague-stricken in hospitals and elsewhere should take precautions against becoming infected, 'guarding themselves from becoming too familiar with the laity'.[139] In addition to publishing his own ideas and those of Gonzaga, Razzi also translated or summarized compilations of other plague doctors from the Black Death period, such as Tommaso del Gardo, to contemporary doctors.[140]

Still other clerics such as the Milanese Franciscan Bernardino Busti published tracts during the 1575–8 plague that also went beyond the usual moral and spiritual causes and remedies for plague and crossed to the medical. His 'Sermon' of forty-eight pages summarized texts such as Avicenna on the twelve signs of plague and supplied cures and preventive measures from ancient and modern medical canons. Some of these contravened usual religious doctrine on plague, such as his advice to the healthy not to touch or come near the infected, and he repeated the old adage so contrary to Christian morality—flee from plague 'fast, far, and for a long time'.[141]

---

[139] Ibid., 69–73.   [140] Razzi, *Modo di conservarsi sano*.
[141] *Cause et rimedi della peste et d'altre infermità* (within the Razzi volume, 138–85).

Moreover, a plague tract by Bologna's archbishop Cardinal Paleotti began with prayers, litanies, and orations to Saints Sebastian and Roch, and to the present pope, Gregory XIII, and with other spiritual exercises such as saying five Ave Marias and five Paternosters before the cross. The tract, however, quickly turned to the social dimensions of the plague, instituting new plague-time organizations and encouraging the confraternities of Saints Sebastian and Roch to help 'the poor and the oppressed' with tasks such as accumulating 'stocks of money, grain, flour, wine, vinegar, wood and other materials' to be made available for the needy during the plague. The tract called for a new organization of the 'Misericordia' that would bring together rich bakers to be called 'the bakers of the Misericordia', doctors, barbers, druggists, and ministers of the Monte della Pietà, to organize food, services, and money for the poor, a one-stop shopping of charitable and medical service that was initiated on 2 October 1576.[142] Like Borromeo, Bishop Marco Gonzaga, and the Franciscan Busti, Paleotti saw charity not only in its spiritual role but for its practical medical significance. He even presented charity as a form of self-interest in the secular realm: the better-off should want to enter 'this Congregation to help the miserable plague-stricken, not only for the saintly purpose of paying their charitable debt to the poor, but to defend themselves and their city from infection'. 'If the afflicted are not helped', Paoletti warned, 'the disease will soon spread easily to the houses [of the well-off]'.[143] Governments such as Bologna's followed suit with their own measures to exhort their communities to assist the poor in plague time as with the posting of broadsheets in 1576 listing the 'Ways for assisting the poor of Bologna when the plague begins to make its demands'.[144]

Finally, writing slightly after the plague of 1575–8 but drawing on his experiences in Milan during this plague and with Carlo Borromeo as his guide, the Capuchin friar and director of Milan's lazaretto, Paolo Bellintani, emphasized throughout his unpublished plague tract the central importance of provisioning the populace during plague, first by stockpiling resources as soon as news of plague reaches a region, then, by creating a Monte di Pietà and by distributing daily rations of bread, wine, meat, and *minestra*, served to men, women, and children in varying quantities, which he specified.[145] Furthermore, as head of the lazaretto he was particularly concerned with the safety and well-being of its impoverished inmates as well as those in the huts and the city at large: he imposed draconian punishments against any attempting to rob or defraud the poor in their weakness and established a special core of police and spies for their protection.[146]

As seen in various *Successi della peste* by notaries, administrators, and others, the clergy were not the only ones to emphasize the importance of charity to

---

[142] *Bandi & Constitut. diverse di Bologna*: no. 114; Paleotti, *Sommario delle cose*, 375r–6v.

[143] *Lettera pastorale di . . . Paleotti*. Borromeo organized similar groups utilizing lay confraternities in Milan; *De cura pestilentiae*, 22–4.

[144] *Bononia Manifesta*, no. 1037 (1576).   [145] Bellintani, *Dialogo della peste*, 101–2 and 139.

[146] Ibid., 141–3.

combat plague. In addition, doctors of the 1575–8 plague also turned their attention from the exclusive concerns of the infected patient to the social welfare of the community as a whole and especially the poor. Despite clear evidence for over a century, not until the plague of 1575–8 did doctors consider and try to analyse in their plague tracts why the poor were the plague's principal victims. In so doing, they extended their cures and preventative medicines to the social, economic, administrative, and political realms of feeding, clothing, and caring for the poor. Ingrassia's *Quinta parte* of his *Informatione*—published a year after the first four parts in 1576 and when plague in Palermo had begun to subside—went beyond measures to be taken while plague flared. It endeavoured to find ways to prevent plague for the foreseeable future, even for ever. By 1577 plague for Ingrassia had become a question of social class: long-term resistance against it rested entirely on attacking the causes of poverty. The acts of city governments' health boards show similar changes in consciousness. In 1583 with no plague on the immediate horizon or even further afield—the next plague to threaten any region of Italy would not appear for another year—Verona's Sanità remembered Bishop Valier's fight against plague in 1575 with his services to the poor. With the bishop's example in mind, the health board then issued regulations to all the city's hospitals and hostels lodging the poor. Within fifteen days, all the priors and governors of these institutions were put under threat of heavy fines to clean their buildings, renew all their beds and coverings, washing blankets, sheets, pillows, stretchers, and so on, replace the straw and whitewash the walls of all the dormitories where the poor resided to avoid the risk of infection in the future.[147] Before arriving at this stage, however, the plague writing of physicians had transformed. We now turn to this genre shift, the origins of a new public health literature.

[147] ASVr, Sanità, no. 33, 201r, 17.iv.1583.

8

Towards a New Public Health Consciousness in Medicine

Charity to the poor as a weapon against the arrival and spread of plague was not entirely new in 1575–8. In fact, plague tracts written in 1575–8 referred to previous examples of charitable responses to plague in various Italian city-states. The Milanese gate-guard Besta, for instance, recalled the city's assistance to the poor during and immediately after the plague of 1523–4.[1] As we saw in Chapter 1, Vincenzo Tranquilli did much the same for Perugia, referring to the same plague, maintaining that Perugia was one of the worst places struck by it, where a third of the city died, most of whom were the poor. His brief account of this plague shows that in administrative structures and measures to control plague (although not as extensive as in Venice or Milan), perhaps little had changed by 1575–8. In 1523 Perugia elected three gentlemen over sixty years old to head a health board with five assistants, one for each *contrada*. (It is not clear that any of them were physicians.) They immediately passed ordinances to keep the city clean and to cast out thugs, vagabonds, and other undesirables suspected of harbouring and transmitting plague. The board prohibited commerce with foreigners and appointed twenty men to guard the town square and maintain the security of the shops. Funeral processions were outlawed along with visits by friends and family to the plague-stricken. Only those designated by the officials could visit the afflicted. The city created an area to sequester the infected and those suspected of plague; the latter were to wear a cap as a sign. As soon as anyone became ill or died with plague symptoms, officials were to be informed and the house of the ill or dead placed under quarantine and locked for forty days. Charity was given to the poor during this period but not to the rich or able-bodied suspected of plague. Officials kept records of those quarantined and the amounts spent on them as well as of those dying of the disease. From these records Tranquilli calculated that the plague peaked at 150 deaths per day and that during the five years of plague, from 1523 to 1528, 8,000 died in Perugia.[2]

Despite these developments in various other cities such as Florence, Venice, and especially Milan, whose health care and controls against plague have been

---

[1] Besta, *Vera narratione*, 30r.   [2] Tranquilli, *Pestilenze che sono state in Italia*, 19–20.

better studied for the late medieval and early modern periods,[3] physicians appear to have paid little attention to them at least in their written work or to make recommendations about plague and its public defences. Nor was there a corpus of other manuals penned by lawyers or government officials that addressed issues of public health in any systematic manner or made concrete recommendations. Less than a handful of the plague treatises published before 1575 had devoted more than a sentence or two to public health during plague; few addressed the administrative structures and decisions on the mechanisms of charity or the controls to be implemented in plague time.[4] Even those who had sat on city health boards and dedicated their tracts to them, such as Andrea Turini (1473?–1543?) from Pescia, personal physician to popes Clement VII and Paul III, wrote traditional tracts aimed solely at cures, treatments, preventatives, drugs, and other remedies for the individual patient.[5] Similarly, Pietro Mainardi wrote his plague tract in the midst of the 1523 plague for the benefit of his city, Padua, and dedicated it to the city's health board. In so doing, he began his tract with a citation not from Galen or Hippocrates but from Aristotle's *Politics*. Nonetheless, when Mainardi reached the sections on preservation against plague, his analysis and advice failed to break the traditional frame centred on the individual patient: instead, it pertained to the usual—what to eat and drink, on exercise and personal protection (as far as possible) against putrid vapours. As for public measures to be taken by the prince or health boards, not even Hippocrates' supposed advice of communal fires was mentioned.[6] A Florentine physician, Girolamo Buonagrazia, writing during the same plague at Florence (1522), describes a Florentine *provvisione* that mandated the election of six senior physicians or surgeons to form a body to advise the government on health policy during the plague. The author was in fact elected to head ('capitaneus') this makeshift health board, but Buonagrazia did not spare a word on his new role or shed any ideas whatsoever

---

[3] See Chapter 6, n. 205.

[4] Perhaps unpublished plague tracts to be found in archives might modify this impression, but thus far those that have come to light and which reflect on public policy—those of the Milanese artisan Giovanni Ambrogio, the Capuchin Bellintani, the Venetian notary Morello—were all drafted either during the plague of 1575–8 or shortly afterwards. Tranquilli refers to 'a certain *memoriale*' or diary kept by his father describing these years, but presumably this was a typical family diary with historical reflections and not a plague tract. Outside Italy, the Spanish-Dutch humanist Juan Luis Vives anticipated these changes but only in one respect by addressing the danger of contagion from a variety of diseases arising 'from crowds of paupers gathering in churches and at festivals'; he did not propose positive measures for protecting communities against plague or other contagious diseases. *De subventione pauperum*, 42v–4v; also see Michielse, 'Policing the Poor', 3.

[5] Turini, *Utile consiglio preservativo & curativo delle peste*. This work does not appear in Edit 16, but is found in BAV, R.I.IV.2114, 290r–304r. Written between 1505 and 1510, it was dedicated to the health board of Rome but made no recommendations to it. He wrote another tract on fountains and wells from a physician's perspective, dedicated to his patron Pope Paul III: *De bonitate aquarum Fontanae*. Filled with citations to Galen and Hippocrates, it also declined to make recommendations for public works or health. On Turini's later defence of Galen and correspondence with and criticisms of Fracastoro, see Pennuto, 'Introduzione', xxxii–xxxiii in Fracastoro, *De sympathia*.

[6] Mainardi, *De preservatione hominum*, n.p.

pertaining to health policy and plague control; his was again a traditional treatise directed to definitions, causes, cures, and recipes for the individual. [7]

By contrast, from 1575 to 1578, such concerns entered and restructured various forms of writing about plague even plague poetry. Earlier tracts addressed problems of cleanliness, stench, and filth that were in effect communal problems in attracting disease and fanning its spread. But earlier, as with Marcello Squarcialupi, who practised in Piombino during the 1560s, such questions concerned recipes directed toward personal hygiene: advice 'on washing the face, mouth, hands, and inside the nostrils first thing in the morning' and on airing and perfuming the house and washing its walls. [8]

Of the medieval plague tracts from the Black Death to 1500 abbreviated in Karl Sudhoff or in full by others, I know of none to address governments with recommendations for public health or that entertained possibilities for plague prevention that redounded community-wide. From my reading of over 300 sixteenth-century plague treatises, only four or five anticipated the post-1575 directives to control plague with specific communal and political measures, and these were brief, confined to a page or less. By contrast, the plague of 1575–8 suddenly widened the physician's remit and at the same time expanded the authorship of plague writing. Poets, gate-guards, theologians, bishops, parish priests, gentlemen, humanists, translators and editors, notaries, druggists, and surgeons supplemented, competed with, and challenged the traditional writers of plague tracts—university-trained physicians—and they did so by addressing the state with new concerns about public health. [9]

The first pre-1575 exception was written during or immediately after the plague of 1523, which swept through Rome, Perugia, Bologna, Milan and other places in central and northern Italy. It came not from a doctor but a lawyer, Girolamo Previdelli, born at Reggio, professor of juridical institutions at the University of Bologna, and a defence lawyer for Henry VIII in one of his divorces. Anticipating tracts of the 1575–8 plague and thereafter, Previdelli's metaphor for plague was war: 'we presently are vexed with a public and internal war . . . a vast pestilence has swept through many parts of Italy, a massacre no less disastrous than that produced by the sword'. [10] He then advised on the rights of the city to maintain its health in plague time: two or three guards should be posted at each city gate to prevent migrants and foreigners from entering and infecting the city. Foreigners staying as guests in the city or *contado* should be expelled;

---

[7] Buonagrazia, *De provisione et cura morborum pesilentium*. On Buonagrazia, see Henderson, 'Epidemics in Renaissance Florence'. Also, see the traditional tract of Emanuele, *Opus utilissimum contra pestilentiam*, written just after this plague in Rome and commissioned by its plague health board.

[8] Squacialupi, *Difesa contra la peste*, 30–48.

[9] Before 1575, over 90% of the authors of plague tracts in Italy had been university-trained physicians; only occasionally were they penned by clerics, and these (before 1576) focused on spiritual cures.

[10] Previdelli, *Tractatus legalis de peste*. Perhaps similar remarks and concerns with plague and the public realm can be found in other legal manuals before 1575 without 'peste' or a variation in their titles, but they do not appear in Zacchia's comprehensive *Quaestionum medico-legalium*.

as soon as signs of pestilence appear on anyone, the city has the right to expel the person as with lepers, Jews, and prostitutes; anyone suspected of carrying the disease or to have been infected by others can for the public good be expelled; anyone engaged in any occupation that might spread plague can be forbidden to practise it.[11] Most of this tract, however, dealt with one legal matter that was more personal than public: justification for reducing the number of witnesses required to testify last wills and testaments of plague victims, their rights to do so from doorways and windows, the legality of a testament redacted in the presence of a parish priest and two witnesses without a notary, and the possibility of a woman being a witness without the consent of two blood relations as required by municipal law under normal circumstances.[12] Although Previdelli's legal tract by definition involved government, only two folios concerned public health and these focused on the rights of the state to exclude foreigners and those suspected of carrying the plague. The positive role of the state and for disease control and prevention that would became the focus of plague tracts in the 1575–8—caring for the poor and the ill, building new hospitals, keeping streets, latrines, and water supplies clear of waste and excrement—were untouched.[13]

The second exception comes from a tract of 1527, republished in 1556 and again in 1576 by the Augustinian friar Napolitano, head of the city's health board ('governatore sopra li amorbati in Napoli de Reame').[14] Again, concerns about public health form only a small part of it, in this case just over a folio and parts of that small section also involved the duties of the individual. Like Previdelli, the friar defended the state's right to expel foreigners suspected of plague, but, unlike Previdelli's legal tract, the friar commented on the state's role ensuring public cleanliness: 'The government or the officials of the city have the duty to keep the land clear of every sort of garbage [*bruttura*] and of corpses of unburied dead animals, because such stench and garbage corrupts the air . . .'[15] Further, he recommended that council meetings, schools, and other gatherings be prohibited, that the state investigate the disease, that the infected be separated from the healthy and their clothing and other goods be quarantined.[16] Other doctors during the next big plague, that of 1555–6, such as Niccolò Massa, suggested that little could be achieved by human effort beyond prayer for a cold winter, although when employed to give advice to the Venetian Health Office, he may have made specific proposals.[17]

The next anticipation comes from an earlier work of the politically active Palermitan plague fighter of 1575–6, Giovanni Filippo Ingrassia. His tract of 1560, inspired by an epidemic of 1558, probably influenza rather than plague,

---

11 Previdelli, *Tractatus legalis de peste*, 3v–4v.   12 Ibid., 4v–10v.

13 Previdelli's opinions on these matters set guidelines through the seventeenth century on legal medical questions regarding plague; see Zacchia, *Quaestionum medico-legalium*, 261, 264, and 274.

14 Napolitano, *Opera et trattato che insegna* (1556).

15 Ibid., 6r–v.   16 Ibid., 6v–7r.

17 See Palmer, 'The Control of Plague', 113 and 118–9.

concentrated on two deformed babies ('monsters') born in Palermo with an added report given before the city magistrates about the city's epidemic of 1558.[18] His addition deals first and primarily with the history of plague and epidemics in Sicily during the sixteenth century, the definitions of pandemic and epidemic, the signs of plague, notions of contagion, and 'atoms' in the air, all supported with copious references to Hippocrates, Galen, Aristotle, and other classical authorities. The final two folios, however, concern remedies directed to the ruler of Sicily: prayers for forgiveness of sins; purification of the air by burning fires; removal of stagnant water in general; removal of stagnant water that was green and smelly at the drapery ('Panneria') under the church of Santo Spirito; covering the stream of the tanners; cleaning water troughs of waste usually filled with dead dogs, cleaning public roads, purging stench with perfumes and big fires, covering wells, canals and aqueducts to stop fetid vapours polluting the air, and provisioning the population with good bread and meat ('carne di gienco'), 'which will be of the greatest protection for the afflicted poor as well as the healthy during an epidemic'.[19]

The last exception is the most remarkable. It comes from Piedmont, a region that remained untouched by the plague of 1575–8 but was struck by two others, in 1564 and 1585, which raged through France, Spain, southern Germany, and the cantons of Switzerland but not beyond the borders of Piedmont to the rest of Italy. *The Regiment for protecting men, places, and cities from the spread of Plague*, published by Agostino Bucci in 1564, was divided into three chapters. Two of these regarded the standard fare of plague tracts—diet and behaviour for warding off or treating plague. The first chapter, however, was new: it addressed 'the ordinances and laws that should be published and observed in these times [of plague]'. First, health officers were to be elected; persons from places suspected of plague were to be banned from the region; houses of plague victims were to be locked, and those who had associated with them were to be sent outside the city for forty days along with their goods, merchandise, and letters; guards were to be posted at city gates, mountain passes, ports, and rivers; the city and other places needed to be cleaned, and public money was to be set aside to assist the poor. 'Every effort should be made to keep the city clean, purged of every sort of garbage and waste.' In times of major danger, the lowest classes, including poor beggars, were to be chased from town and given lodging at some distance where they could recover. The city should have barbers posted before plague enters, ready to follow physicians' orders in the treatment of the plague-stricken. Priests and other clerics should be assigned to attend to matters of the soul. Ditches, wells, and aqueducts were to be inspected and repaired.[20] Bucci's chapter also touched on problems of sequestrating, quarantine, and assisting the poor. His remarks, however, remained brief and without the details later seen with 1575 plague tracts or with his own tract composed in 1584 during the next big plague to strike Piedmont.

---

[18] Ingrassia, *Trattato assai bello*, 1r–19v.   [19] Ibid., 22v–4r.   [20] Bucci, *Reggimento*.

Finally, Bernardino Tomitano's *Il Consiglio sopra la peste di Vinetia l'anno 1556* almost emerges as another exception but instead illustrates more explicitly than any pre-1575 text the limits practising doctors imposed on themselves as to which subjects they might address. Tomitano's introduction makes clear the division of labour between doctors and secular authorities on health boards or other branches of government. At the outset he states that his 'discorso' was in no way intended to replace the diligent work of Venice's *Sapientissimi Proveditori*.[21] Later, his chapter 'Other provisions for maintaining Venice's air pure and good' touches government policy and in particular the work of the Venetian health board, but instead of making recommendations to it, Tomitano describes only its 'diligence in keeping the city clean during the present plague with the possible exception of the city's drainage systems [*Gattoli*]', which 'were at times full of garbage and stinking odours from the vegetables, melon rinds, and other putrid things'. Given these conditions, he added, it is amazing that the air does not generate pestilential fevers every year.[22] He pointed further at an area of town that was particularly polluted, 'where the plebs dump their trash and odours escalate from certain canals'. But here he abruptly ended any further hints of criticism or possible recommendations to the Venetian authorities: 'it was not a matter appropriate to my duties' ('Ma perche l'officio mio non è di affaticarmi in ciò)'. Rather it redounded on 'those worthy wise ones ('a quelli diginissimi intelletti') to pass statutes on such matters.[23] The chapter ends with the physician turning to his proper sphere of competence—cures and remedies for the individual patient.

PLAGUE WRITING IN 1575–8

With the plague of 1575–8, not just with one exception in a page or two, plague doctors and others suddenly addressed questions and gave advice to health boards, city councils, and the prince. On these concerns they not only went beyond doctors and commentators of the late Middle Ages; they surpassed those of the ancient world. As Nutton has observed: 'From a Hippocratic perspective it was not a city that suffered in an epidemic, but an individual, and one's energies should be channelled towards maintaining or restoring the health of that individual.'[24] As Hippocrates set out in his *Epidemics*, the art of medicine consisted of three factors: the disease, the patient, and the physician;[25] no mention

---

[21] Tomitano, *Il consiglio sopra la peste*, 3r: 'Ma io non intendo supplire con questo mio discorso a la diligentia de i vostri Signori Proveditori & ministri.'

[22] Ibid., 21r.   [23] Ibid., 20v–21v.

[24] Nutton, 'Medicine in the Greek World', 30–1. For the variety of medicine in the ancient world beyond Hippocrates and Galen, see Nutton, *Ancient Medicine*.

[25] Cited by Maclean, *Logic, Signs, and Nature*, 93, as *Epidemics*, I, 13. This reference, however, does not correspond with modern editions.

was made of the state. The only glimmer of a public health measure that these late sixteenth-century doctors could extract from the corpus of ancient medicine was Hippocrates' supposed advice to burn public fires to keep pestilential vapours at bay (which in fact was a part of his legend rather than writings).[26]

Even the most cited and revered of the moderns for the 1575–8 generation of doctors, Girolamo Fracastoro, hardly alluded to the public side of medicine in his *De contagione*. The closest he came to it was at the beginning of his chapter on 'the treatment of true pestilent fevers' in a vague statement stripped of details and concrete recommendations: 'Far greater care and attention, both public and private, ought to be paid to fevers that are strictly speaking pestilent.' The 'public' was not, however, spelled out. Instead, his remedies centred on the individual and began in fact in a spirit bereft of civic responsibility: he recommended flight and, if this were not possible, to avoid the ill at all costs and attend to matters of personal hygiene such as keeping the body clean and changing clothing often. A later comment on government action was descriptive and limited to a single historical example: when Verona had 'acted most wisely' by burning the furniture of the plague-infected in 1511.[27]

Several physicians' plague tracts in 1575–8 were dedicated almost in their entirety to questions of public health and political action. Of these Ingrassia's two works in 1576 and 1577 of over 800 pages were the most monumental. His recommendations were addressed directly to the prince, the duke of Terranova. As seen in previous chapters, these concerned a wide variety of state initiatives relating to charity, taxation, the building of hospitals, street cleaning, the conservation of safe drinking water, guarding the city from infection, and enforcing strict separation of the afflicted and healthy. The first section of his separate publication, *Parte quinta*, subtitled 'Regarding the general preservation of the cities and territory of a kingdom, while in good health', published in 1577 with plague on the wane, extended notions of public health further. Its fifty-seven chapters focused on the state and the mobilization of administrative structures to protect a kingdom from infection. As illustrated in its frontispiece, these were divided into what Ingrassia defined as the state's three functions—*Ora, Fuoco, e Forche*—gold, fire, and the hangman's noose. Under these rubrics, Ingrassia planned permanent measures the state should enact before any epidemic came on the horizon. His dominant metaphor was war. 'As in peace', so in health, 'his Excellency the Prince' should make surveys of the cities and villages in his kingdom to estimate the amount of money that could be raised. The first of 'three principal human remedies' against disease was gold: public expenditures were necessary for the prevention of epidemic disease and even more so once an epidemic had invaded. In addition, the prince was to establish networks to collect intelligence ('intelligenza') and obtain 'continuous advice from villages and cities' about infection.[28] The prince must delegate power to officials governing cities

---

[26] See Chapter 3, n. 9.   [27] Fracastoro, *De contagione*, 238–9.
[28] Ingrassia, *Parte quinta*, ch. 3.

Illustration 12.   Ingrassia, *Informatione*.

enabling them to direct the other two principal 'human remedies'—fire and hangman's nooses. Failure of princes to delegate power, according to Ingrassia, had caused 'cities and villages in the our kingdom to come to the greatest harm because their deputies lacked sufficient power to enforce justice; as a result thieves had spread the contagion with their trade in infected goods'.[29]

The remaining fifty-one chapters all centred on governmental health policies—recommendations of specific administrative structures to be funded and measures to be taken in periods of good health as well as infection. For instance, Ingrassia advised each city and village to maintain its own horse patrols ('cavalli di campagna') for surveillance of travellers within a twelve-mile radius, to control for infection and the spreading of plague 'by those wicked villains who intentionally disseminate the disease'.[30] Doctors should be hired not just during epidemics but on a permanent basis and assigned to each city gate in major towns such as Palermo, Messina, Catania, and Zaragoza. His recommendations, moreover, went beyond any measures presently seen anywhere in Italy, even Milan and Venice: plans should be made in advance for the mass migration of women from cities when plague strikes, the assumption being that they were the most susceptible and the plague's principal carriers. This notion backed by plague statistics in cities such as Milan, did not, however, move Ingrassia towards harsh measures against women as happened with the stricter quarantines imposed on them in Milan during the past plague. Instead, cities were to provide play parks for them ('giardini a spasso') and facilities for their devotion.[31] Ingrassia envisioned other new public initiatives to be taken in non-plague years such as public courses on pestilential signs and symptoms required of all doctors to enable them to identify plague immediately. He returned continually to metaphors of war and peace: 'just as castles and fortifications must be made and provisioned in peace time to maintain order in war', a programme of construction of new lazaretti must begin across Sicily. He followed with detailed instructions for their construction and organization,[32] and in later chapters discussed the election of the officials in charge of lazaretti, permanent staffs of doctors, surgeons, confessors, barbers, nurses, notaries, gravediggers, under-officers, 'captains of streets' who visited the poor, those who drove the carts of inflicted to the lazaretti. For these functionaries, high and low, he detailed their salaries and duties.[33]

Ingrassia then dipped deeper into questions of political authority and organization arguing that doctors and officials of health boards should be given greater authority to sequester the infected and suspected and to lock up houses; prisoners needed to be separated into places for the infected, suspected, and healthy.[34] Labourers who resided in cities and worked in the countryside were to be issued passports but without the restrictions placed on foreigners. Instead, these workers

[29] Ingrassia, ch. 4.   [30] Ibid., ch. 6.   [31] Ibid., ch. 10.   [32] Ibid., 18 and 19.
[33] Ibid., 32.   [34] Ibid., ch. 16.

would carry *un bollettino brevissimo* with their names, place of work, and dates of departure and re-entry.[35]

Reflecting on his experience over the past two years of 'pestilential contagion', Ingrassia made specific recommendations on cleaning, purging, and burning of infected houses and goods, how to improve Palermo's new lazaretto, la Cubba, to correct mistakes made there during the previous year, and how to restrict more effectively the mingling of population during plague. He recommended stricter closure of schools, prohibitions on famous preachers drawing crowds, and even restrictions on performing mass. He advised that sermons be restricted to small discrete audiences, that women and children be sequestered, and prostitutes and pimps prevented from plying their trades during plague time because of their intimate intermingling with the populace.[36] Finally, he turned to the long-term cause of plague transmission—poverty—and argued for government intervention, first with charity for the miserable; secondly for a system of self-help and a bank for the poor.[37]

In addition to Ingrassia's lengthy and elaborate examination of an entire public health system, the 1575–8 plague also produced specialized manuals of a public health character not seen earlier. A tract from a Neapolitan councillor ('Giureconsulto'), Pietro Follerio, addressed to city governments, princes, and officers of health boards, was dedicated entirely to instructions and mechanisms for public control against the spread of plague into a kingdom. It detailed procedures on issuing plague passports and instructions for guards and petty officers. Beginning with the premise that plague was worse than war, because it killed all indiscriminately, state control in plague time needed an organization akin to the military. Follerio called for the appointment of the best and most vigilant men to be stationed at city gates and at minor and major entrances to the territory. They were to be taught that 'within their hands lay the lives of their citizens'. At least two were to be stationed at a post at all times. Further, foot soldiers and cavalry should patrol the territory night and day as was then the case, the manual claimed, in the Province of Campania. Secondly, officers were to be appointed for the production of plague passports ('bullectinos') stamped with the public seal and issued to inhabitants with their names and place of residence. Those without one were banned from the city and other places in the territory. The manual then listed items that were suspected of transmitting contagion and those that were not, such as metals, precious stones, and gold money, and ended by explaining quarantine procedures to officers.[38]

---

[35] Ibid., 17. In Milan, the *bollette* or plague passports became more elaborate and detailed in 1576–7, because of parish officers issuing them too freely (see *Gride diverse*, no. 59, 1576.x.5). Plague laws supplied sample *bollette*, which were to include the recipient's parish and gate, name and family name, age, destination, reasons for departure, and a personal description; for instance 'Pietro Buzzo, of average height, with a short black beard, 25 years old, on horseback for Mazenta, where he owns his own house'.

[36] Ingrassia, *Parte quinta*, 25.   [37] Ibid., 47.

[38] Follerio, *Ad instructiones urbanas*. According to Edit 16, he authored forty publications, all on legal and governmental matters. His advice on plague remained strong as a source of legal precedents through

NEW SECTIONS OF PHYSICIAN'S PLAGUE TREATISE

This heightened attention to public health and public prevention of plague in 1575–8 was not restricted to the new forms of plague writing that proliferated during this plague as seen in works such as those by Ingrassia, the Jewish doctor de Pomi, the druggist Bellicocchi, the doctor and astrologist Raimondo, the notary Canobbio, the gate-guard Besta, the Milanese gentlemen Crotto and Centorio Degli Ortensi, and others whose texts have been examined above. The 1575–8 plague also transformed the divisions and structure of the traditional medical plague tract dedicated to definitions of plague, causes, remedies, and preventive measures stuffed with recipes for those of different complexions, age, sex, and social class,[39] some with complex prescriptions of various pills to be taken on different days.[40] The physician's plague tract suddenly took a new turn, to what can be considered the beginnings of a public health literature and a new consciousness of public health among physicians. These new sections were not a paragraph or two, as seen in the handful of earlier cited sixteenth-century anticipations above, but often comprised from a quarter to half of the plague tract.

Within the traditional structures of the medical plague tract, instructions for governments gained a prominent place, as with a tract by the Neapolitan doctor Ajello. After definitions of plague, indications of ways to recognize it, discussions on air, diet, exercise, rest, sleep, conditions of the soul and mind (Galen's six non-naturals),[41] Ajello inserted a new section—'What must be observed regarding the good governance of plague within the city, for prevention as well as cure'—addressed to cities, princes, and administrators. Its first chapter advised on waste removal: 'all sorts of excrement, especially that of pigs', the disposal of dead or ill animals, culling household pets such as dogs and cats, the dumping of waste far from the city, special cleaning of certain dirty parts of the city such as porticos, where 'almost everyone deposited their household excrement [*escrementi comuni*]'. Ajello criticized the hygienic practices of the city's monasteries, the fuels burnt in private houses that filled the air with noxious smoke, and the gutters of houses that poured rain water into streets to the annoyance of passers-by. He paid particular attention to the need for cleanliness of houses, hospitals, and taverns near the bay of Naples and other water sources, advising governments to promulgate strict decrees against throwing waste from windows into the sea.

---

the seventeenth century; see Zacchia, *Quaestionum medico-legalium*, 264, 275, and 747. Other tracts such as one by a doctor of Chieti in the Abruzzi, Briganti (*Avvisi . . . al governo di preservarsi di pestilenza*) addressed to the health board and government of the kingdom of Naples in 1577, devoted entire tracts to matters of public health.

[39] For such a tract, see Bairo, *Nouum ac perutile opuscolum de pestilentia*; or Napolitano, *Opera et trattato che insegna* (1527), 2v–3r.

[40] See for instance Calori, *Regimento como lhomo si debbe gubernare*.

[41] See Chapter 3 above, n. 1.

Special instructions were recommended for the cleanliness of fruit, vegetable, tripe, and fish stands, and for the producers of leather and other workers with skins.

As with doctors in the north of Italy, he discussed the importance of clean drinking water, the cleaning of wells, aqueducts, canals, and locks, and the need for agents to patrol them. He called for a system of street cleaning where the city's streets were all to be cleansed twice weekly to ensure that waste from one part of town was not simply swept into another. In times of suspicion, he insisted on tight controls of goods and commercial traffic with a system of licensing and gate-guards, and urged household heads to be responsible for cleaning and whitewashing the walls of their houses. He recommended that the inflicted and suspected be moved from the city to places with good air and ventilation, such as San Gennaro near Naples, as the best means of saving the inflicted and protecting the healthy. He proposed constructing 'da bene' 'a hospital of medicine' here with special cellars for vinegar, wines, and bakeries, to supply all the needs of the plague-stricken so that supplies would not have to be transported across the city in plague time. He called for the expulsion of beggars, filthy people, those dressed in rags, and those who were often drunk, but those who were dressed poorly because of their poverty could stay 'so long as they washed their clothes often and as best they could'.[42]

The second part of the plague tract of a Bolognese doctor, Baldassare Pisanelli, then practising at Rome's Santo Spirito at the time of the 1575–8 plague, was entitled, 'the teaching of remedies by which the individual can preserve himself from the plague and the methods of curing the plague-stricken'. The first part of this book, however, concentrated on the state and its initiatives in preserving its subjects from plague and consisted of instructions to gate guards, banishing vagabonds and 'the useless' ('tutti gli inutili'), cleaning the city, modes of garbage collection, including the disposal of putrid vegetables and corrupt water, and the banning of certain foods from entering the city such as spoilt fish and mushrooms. Without a clear transition, the book then abruptly crossed from Hippocratic communal fires to diet and remedies for individual patients—pills, electuaries, confections, syrups, theriacs, and other secret recipes he had learnt on his travels in Germany, Italy, and Africa—prescribed according to whether the patient was poor or rich.[43]

The physician of Jesi Massucci signalled the need to alert the governors ('i miei Signori Governatori') in cities, villages, castles, and other places to keep squares, public streets, and other places within city walls clean, removing stagnant water, muddy excrement, and unsightly animals, placing hemp and linen production outside the city, and burying plague victims as soon as possible.[44] A physician 'elected and sent by the duke of Savoy to Milan' in 1576, Giovanni Barelli,

---

[42] Ajello, *Breue discorso*, 41r–3v.   [43] Pisanelli, *Discorso*, 31–4.
[44] Massucci, *La preseruatione dalla pestilenza*, 73.

wrote a tract based on his experiences and successes there, claiming that 'his secrets' had cured most of the plague-afflicted.[45] The work began along the usual lines, ready to unveil recipes of 'marvellous secrets and cures'.[46] The first of two books, however, was not devoted to the individual patient at all but instead turned to governments with lessons no doubt learnt from serving Europe's most advanced health board of the sixteenth century. His proposals on 'the ways to govern a community to obviate the causes of plague' concentrated on sequestration and quarantine of persons and goods.[47]

The tract of Bassiano Complani from Lodi, then practising in Milan during the 1576–7 plague, contained a section on 'plague precautions'. It began with praise of Milan's health board and stressed the importance of the public obeying its decrees or *gride*. Complani then turned to health boards and advised them on the edicts they should pass in plague time, ones 'against the spread of slime, mud, dirt, and putrid smells in homes and streets within the city and suburbs'. He emphasized the importance of surveillance and record-keeping, instructing them to examine at least bi-weekly the conditions of households, to control vigilantly the goods and food entering the city, and judging when to impose quarantine—concerns, he argued, that were central to the state ('res publica').[48]

Andrea Gabrielli, practising in Genoa, included a section in his tract entitled 'Preservation from Plague deriving from causes from below' (natural causes as opposed to divine ones).[49] He began by praising the prudent safeguards implemented by the Genoese health board to confront the threat of that new plague then encircling Italy but yet to reach Genoa.[50] These included their vigilance 'day and night' in guarding the major thoroughfares into Genoa and its countryside; organizing hospices outside the city walls to separate the suspected from the healthy; moving beggars, pilgrims, jugglers ('praestigiatores'), and the like from the city to a place where they would be cared for with good Christian charity; establishing a house to sequester for forty days or more along with their goods those who have managed to enter the city from suspected places;

---

[45] Barrelli, *Thesoro inestimabile che insegna*, n.p., preface. According to Edit 16, this doctor appears in no repertories of sixteenth-century writers and is known only from this single publication found in two libraries.

[46] In fact, Bellintani was critical of these French doctors because they supposedly boasted of secret cures, which he found useless or harmful.

[47] Massucci, *La preseruatione dalla pestilenza.*   [48] Complani, *Pestilentis morbi*, 14–20.

[49] Gabrielli, *De peste*, 34v–8r.

[50] This tract does not mention the plague infecting Genoa; nor is there any mention of it in Corradi's exhaustive survey of plague tracts and chronicles; *Annali*, I, 591–625; and VI, 492–555. In addition, according to Contardi's, *Il modo di preservarsi*, 3r (written in 1576) the citizens of Genoa, 'hearing that plague was close by' asked the doctor to write a short manual on the plague, but Contardi never specifies just how close the plague may have been. The disease, however, entered the city at the end of 1579. In December, the health board of Rome prohibited the Genoese and their goods from entering the Papal States 'because of the *pestilenze* then raging' in the Genoese region; *Regesti di bandi, editti*, I, 69. Also, da Tolone, *Trattato politico da pratticarsi ne' tempi di peste*, 35 and 51, reports that the 'fierissima contagione' afflicted Genoa that year against which its citizens dedicated a votive church to the Immaculate Conception.

prohibiting all animals and goods from suspicious places; hiring men to clean streets and infected or suspicious goods, and others to observe the sun, moon, and conjunctures of the planets. The city and towns of the Genoese state were to be kept free from all forms of putrefaction and fetid smells, by enforced cleaning of stables, latrines, and sewers, and guarding the city from the importation of bad fruit and vegetables and other foul-smelling substances and chemicals ('chymicos') such as sulphur and arsenic. Cadavers of all sorts from sea or land were to be buried properly or burnt. The manure from geese, ducks, pigs, cows, and other animals were to be deposited far from city walls. Those in prison or in monasteries should be exposed to fresh air and their quarters cleaned regularly, their foul odours eradicated. The officers of the health board should investigate and keep records of all illnesses during plague, their symptoms and places of pain on the body, with animals as well as humans regardless of age, class, or sex. Finally, Gabrielli's was rare among the sixteenth-century plague tracts to express anti-Semitism outright. In plague time the stiff-necked Jews ('Hebrei dure cervicis homines') are particularly suspect and, because of their filth and sin, should be separated from Christians.[51]

As this work suggests, shifts in the concerns of the traditional plague tract occurred not only where plague seriously hit but also where plague threatened. During the plague of 1575–8, the archbishop of Lanciano in the Abruzzi, commissioned the town's public doctor, Sebastiano Tranzi, to publish a plague tract in Italian, 'accessible and beneficial' to the citizens of this mid-sized town. Although Tranzi did not finish his treatise until the end of 1586, it dealt with conditions in Italy in 1576 to 1577.[52] His dedication to the archbishop described the double-pronged spread of that plague from the Dalmatian coast through Lombardy and the Veneto in the north, and from Sicily to Naples and the province of Calabria in the south, where it was poised to invade the Abruzzi. Unlike doctors in other areas of Italy untouched by this wave, such as those in Lucca or Perugia, Tranzi tried to guard his readers from the fright of an inevitable spread of 'this most cruel plague' to their city. He appears unique among sixteenth-century plague writers in his confidence that plague had little likelihood of invading his town. (Perhaps, a decade earlier, his tone may have been different.)

His argument began by praising the city's location, climate, air, and clean and abundant water near its gates, and most of the city's houses had the luxury of possessing their own wells. According to Tranzi, the town benefited

[51] Ibid., 35r. It was one of the few medical tracts of sixteenth-century Italy that pinned the spread of plague on Jews because of their behaviour or beliefs. Another was that of the Florentine theologian Razzi; see Chapter 7 above, n. 136.

[52] Tranzi, *Trattato di peste*. According to Edit 16, only one copy survives in Italian libraries but it is in Genoa and not the Abruzzi. Although intended for the citizens of this mid-sized market town, it is not cheap print and crossed the Alps, where it now survives in the Bibliothèque nationale in Paris; see *Catalogue des sciences médicales*, I, 678.

from the fertility of its countryside and the well-balanced constitution ('di complessione molto temperata') and good health of its inhabitants. He claimed that in his twenty-four years of practice there, far fewer cases of illness had arisen here than in neighbouring towns. For further proof of the city's good health, he pointed to the multitude of its old people and their longevity. However, Tranzi's confidence in the present and future preservation of Lanciano from plague centred on its 'good rule and governance . . . that resembled an ancient republic', its magistrates and laws. Most importantly, he emphasized the formation of a public health board that had kept the city free from the plague's invasion in 1575–8: eight honoured citizens from the town's best families had been appointed to guard the gates, rigorously preventing goods and persons from entering from suspected places. A blockade on all trade from Ragusa and other towns on the Dalmatian coast and from Schiavonia had been declared and ordinances passed providing 'all the necessary things' for plague prevention.[53]

Further, Tranzi drew attention to mundane matters such as mattresses: that they be of good quality wool and cleaned of all dirt and be laid with clean and fine ('sottili') sheets to be changed daily, cleaned, and perfumed. The same went for clothing with instructions on washing with good quality soap and other ingredients. Advice was given even on wiping ('purging excrement from the body, which should be done in privacy' [*per secesso*]), along with washing, cleaning the mouth and nose, and combing the beard and hair with specific brushes, on types of combs to be used, materials with which they should be constructed, and the use of hot towels and perfumed soaps. [54] But, he made clear, concerns with individual hygiene were insufficient to guard against plague: 'it is not enough merely to furnish, conserve, and defend one's own household; care has to be extended to the neighbourhood, the walled village, countryside, city, and territory'. Tranzi emphasized that such care was the duty of government, 'whether of a powerful nobleman, a governor, or a baron'. 'Against contagion', the ruler 'was to use all his powers to guard and defend friends, vassals, and all others under his jurisdiction.' He was to provide the necessary resources for his subjects; prohibit commerce from suspected places, ensure its streets remained clean, guard against the importation of linen, hemp, and silk, and the movement of pigs, sheep, goats, and cattle into villages and towns within his realm.[55]

***

The 1575–8 plague tracts can supply many more examples of this new wave of public-health consciousness among doctors, with new sections devoted to new concerns and ideas about public medicine. Some appeared in otherwise traditional and conservative tracts. Thus a community doctor hired by the

---

[53] Contained in Tranzi's unnumbered six-page dedication to Archbishop Mario Bolognini.
[54] Ibid., 16.   [55] Ibid., 17.

commune of Massa Lombarda listed the conjuncture of Mars and Saturn as a sign of future plagues but, at the same time, devoted a large portion of his tract 'on the universal preservation of men in plague time' to public forms of plague controls and prevention.[56] Let us, however, sample three further tracts by university-trained physicians, two published in 1576 and one in 1586. Only one practised in a university town, and none came from any of the major metropolitan areas where this plague then raged and where the vast bulk of plague tracts were being produced in numbers never before seen.

The first is the *Trattato della peste et delle petecchie* published in Venice in 1576 by Gioseffo Daciano, a physician employed by the commune of Udine, capital of Friuli. During the plague of 1576 Daciano was elected as doctor of the health board charged with visiting the ill and diagnosing plague.[57] The text received recognition as an authoritative source from other plague doctors as early as a year after its publication, as seen in Ingrassia's *Parte quinta* (1577), and later was cited by the Piedmont physician Roffredi in 1600.[58] Daciano's letter of dedication to the officers of Udine's health board, signed 15 May 1576, reflected on the previous two plagues in his city, in 1566 and 1572, in which he valiantly served. (He gave proof by including a letter patent of 1573 from the health board that acknowledged his service treating plague and examining plague cadavers 'with no small risk to his own life'.) His experience as a doctor of epidemics on his city's health board, however, reached further back. As 'a very young man with little experience even with simple fevers', he had given his diagnosis to the board regarding *petecchie*.[59]

His tract begins in the traditional manner with definitions of plague but also of *petecchie*, distinguishing between the two. He continued with further discussion of 'true' plague and pestilential fevers, before turning to the 'superior' causes of plague with the stars and planets, followed by 'origins' or causes closer at hand, conditions of air, water, and ground, signs and seasons of plague. Later chapters advised individuals on how to live during a plague, prognostics of pestilential fevers and *petecchie*, and methods for hardening and breaking apostemes and other swellings, all amply supported with citations to ancient and modern authorities. To these, he added historical examples especially to recent plagues and suspected ones in Udine and Friuli, of which he had had first-hand experience.

[56] Sorboli, *Discorso del vero modo di preseruare*. For other examples, see Chapter 7, for instance, the works of Carcano, and Crotto whose *Memoriale delle provisioni generali*, 3v, 4v, and 6r–v, praised the work of Venice's health board in 1576–7 and outlined its provisions but also praised Ficino and his tract and stuck to Galenic notions of the mutation of air as the cause of plague.

[57] Daciano, *Trattato della peste*. In describing the organization of the health board during this plague, Daciano notes his position and tasks (44).

[58] Roffredi, *Pestis, et calamitatum Taurini*, 17, 34, and 43; and Ingrassia, *Parte quinta*, 10 and 13. Furthermore, the survival of Daciano's tract in twenty-four libraries across northern and central Italy suggests a wide diffusion.

[59] Daciano, *Trattato della peste*, 25.

Yet within this traditional format of the plague tract, Daciano, like many plague doctors in other parts of Italy at that moment, came to conclusions that broke with the prevailing Aristotelian and Galenic orthodoxies in explaining previous plagues. First, he denied that the plagues he had experienced in Udine in 1556, 1560, and 1572 had arisen from hot and humid conditions, since such conditions were 'universal' to all of Friuli and not only to the region of Udine where these plagues had flared.[60] Nor could war 'with bodies left in their blood and unburied with fetid vapours' explain these recent plagues, since there had been none. Nor could they be explained by corrupt air, because no 'universal illness' arose across the region; instead, the disease was confined to the city of Udine. For similar reasons, along with the absence of earthquakes, he dismissed corruption from water and land as causes. Instead, his explanation for plague in Udine in 1556 was 'pure and simple': it arose from contagion and the importation of the disease from another place. His explanation was tinged with anti-Semitism but did not depend on it. According to Daciano, this plague had originated from perfidious and damned Jews, who brought their infected goods from Capodistria to Udine on 26 March 1556, the day of their Passover.[61]

The truly innovative part of Daciano's tract, however, was chapter 13, 'The means for managing and governing the city and the lazaretto during plague'. Here, he moved from personal to community health and its remedies. Like Andrea Gabrielli and others, he took his cues from the practices of the health board of his home town.[62] His first recommendations were hardly new: 'first and immediately public prayers, devotions, and fasting' were required and then the continuous burning of odoriferous woods throughout the city. His second, however, set out further community-wide principles from his health-board experience. All public facilities ('tutti li redotti publici') and especially schools were to be shut immediately. Then all the streets and squares were to be cleaned of excrement, filth, and trash—above all, the meat and fish markets. Similarly, particular houses, courtyards ('nelli contini)', or other places where a death had occurred or with smelly sewers were to be cleaned and the stench removed. Washing linen used for butchering was to be prohibited in the city's public waterways ('fosse della città'). 'Third', the sale and import of all textiles—cotton, linen, wool, and silk—was to be suspended, along with the sale of spoilt goods ('cose guaste') such as bad wine. Beggars and others who readily fell ill should be sent from the city, not to the lazaretto, but instead to another healthy place segregated from the population but provided for by the state.

'Fourth' on pain of death, no one was allowed to walk about the city visiting friends and relatives, and anyone who fell ill had to report immediately to the health board. To collect information on plague cases, two officers per neighbourhood were to be elected to visit all their households at sunrise. They were to report back to the health board and its doctor (in fact, Daciano), who

---

[60] Daciano, 17.   [61] Ibid., 17–18.   [62] Ibid., 41–5.

would diagnose the illness. In addition, health officers would see to the charitable needs of the plague-stricken and visit the ill daily. No cadaver was to be buried that had not been examined in great detail by the health board's doctor. The clergy were not to carry off any corpse without approval of the health board's doctor. If diagnosed as a plague death, the body was to be buried in the lazaretto.[63]

'Fifth', those discovered to have had recent contacts with the plague-stricken were to be locked in their homes for at least twenty-two days, while those residing in houses of a plague victim were to be confined for forty days and their goods consigned to the lazaretto. 'Sixth' those with plague symptoms were to be sent immediately to the city's lazaretto. On entering they were to be washed with vinegar and rosewater, their clothes changed and burnt. The lazaretti were to be divided into three parts—rooms for the afflicted, the suspected, and the 'poverini sani', those who went begging in the city. Each section was to be adequately (even lavishly) furnished 'with every effort made for the inmates' comfort'.

Daciano's final recommendations widened the boundaries of public health to include charity, public order, and trust. It was to ensure that the poor ('quelli miserabili') received all necessities 'to live orderly and well' bodily and spiritually. The lazaretto's guards were to be good and diligent and prevented from robbing the ill or taking advantage of them by various fraudulent means 'which brings harm and ruin to cities, as can be seen in these times with those of little religion and no sense of charity'.[64] While further chapters addressed the individual patient, they also reflected on the well-being of the community at large. To combat the spread of plague, those who had had close contact with the infected were to strip off their clothing and wash thoroughly with rose water mixed with a little vinegar, especially the face, the pulse, the neck, the underarms, and groin.[65]

There is no evidence of the 1575–8 plague arriving at Lucca. Fear of its arrival, however, was present, as the Luchesse physician Antonio Minutoli makes clear in the dedication of his plague tract to a fellow physician: the disease 'had spread widely throughout Italy, causing many deaths with the most grave and fearsome consequences'. Minutoli offered his treatise for the benefit and protection of his city.[66] Unlike Daciano's and most other sixteenth-century plague tracts, this one did not begin with definitions and end with recipes and surgical practices. Instead, Minutoli's was divided into 'two principal chapters for protection in time of plague'. The first concerned the individual and ways to resist the forces of the disease; the second was on public health, as the best 'means for weakening the causal agent of plague'.

On the first, not much, if anything, was new. He advised keeping the body clean to prevent the humours from attracting the air's putrefaction, moderation

---

[63] Ibid., 43–4.   [64] Ibid., 46.   [65] Ibid., 57.

[66] Minutoli, *Avvertimenti*, dedication page. This was the doctor's only publication, which survives in five Italian libraries and at the Wellcome and British Libraries.

in diet and exercise; he prescribed pills, powders, and other medication with detailed recipes. He gave advice about air and winds from various directions depending on where swamps lay and stressed the connection between emotional states and susceptibility to plague. His second part was original, if not in the actual practices of health boards in the most advanced city-states—Milan and Venice—then in the advice doctors now suddenly dwelled on in plague treatises for their local communities (many of which had not yet formed permanent health boards). Minutoli began this second part by reviewing previous governmental provisions promulgated to preserve their cities and drew lessons from this recent history. First, as soon as a plague is seen spreading into a region, the government must immediately procure as much food as possible, along with great quantities of scented wood, and should discourage the intermingling of citizens. Secondly, preventing plague's spread depended on the prior good health and strength of inhabitants. Thirdly, 'in addition to the ordinary lazaretto for the infected', the city must provide another large public space to confine 'suspicious persons, not yet afflicted', and a third for sequestering suspected goods.

Minotuli then turned to the importance of clearing filth from the city (including beggars) and especially that which produced the most offensive smells. Water supplies must be kept flowing and clean, not only within the city but outside it, even over a considerable distance from the city. All unnecessary gatherings were to be prohibited, especially those in the sun. Foods that spoil easily such as ells and tench, as well as all fish that was not fresh, mushrooms, and any meat of poor quality were not allowed in the city and summer fruit admitted only in small quantities and if of the best quality. Finally, the people should obey the laws passed by the Senate and the magistrates for the well-being of the city.[67]

The third tract comes from Francesco Alessandri, personal physician of the duke of Savoy. At the time of its composition Alessandri was practising in Turin, where the 1575–8 plague never arrived. The most disastrous plague of the sixteenth century to reach Turin, instead, came a decade later in 1586, when the threat and turmoil of plague stimulated the physician to publish what he called a translation into Italian of his previous Latin tract of 1578. A comparison of the two quickly shows that the second was radically redrafted to include new sections. Most importantly, Alessandri relied directly on his position and experience during the current plague and reflected specifically on the new circumstances in Piedmont and Turin wrought by the 1585 plague. On 20 August 1585 he had been elected to a board of physicians and surgeons of Savoy to evaluate where the air was corrupt, if the disease was malignant, and whether cases were dubious or true plague.[68] From the experience, he added a new section comprised of thirty-six pages—a sixth of the tract—inserted in the middle: *Ordini et avvertimenti per gl'officiali et altri per tempo di Peste*. Addressed

---

[67] Minutoli, 15r–16v.   [68] Alessandri, *Trattato della peste*, 18v.

to the plague official and not the plague patient, it departed from the traditional academic plague tract by focusing on the political.[69]

Plague ordinances, it instructed, need to be announced with the sounding of trumpets and ample published copies posted around town. In plague time those wishing to repatriate from abroad should not be admitted without a period of quarantine; however, before banning a place or province, even if many are dying there, it must be established that the place has been infected by 'true plague'. To make certain, a gentleman along with a doctor with previous plague experience should be elected to travel to inspect the disease. Alessandri then summarized the symptomatic and epidemiological traits of true plague for the benefit of these new plague officers—the nature of the buboes, *carboni*, and spots; when all or most in the same household 'with these frightening signs and symptoms' die in a brief period; when the neighbours who have had contacts with the victims also begin to die from the disease. Not all those with swellings in the glands ('ghiandusse'), he instructed, were necessarily victims of plague. He pointed to other diseases with similar signs of *ghiandusse* such as *mal Indiano* or syphilis and continued: surgeons and doctors should be employed 'by public charity' in plague time to report immediately any cases, whether suspected or certain, of plague. Officers need to be elected to issue *bollette* and passports (*passaporti*). Gate-guards should have two deputies. Lists of all the infected and the suspected should be posted and printed. He gave instructions about the construction of lazaretti and plague huts: where they should be built, the divisions between the infected, suspected, and convalescents; the posting of armed guards to enforce the separation; instructions on the changing of clothes and on goods to be cleaned, purged, or burnt.

He then turned to the community at large with further political instructions: each parish should elect three officials, a gentleman, a merchant, and a common-er, to assemble every day at the ringing of the church bells to inventory suspected goods and record the details of the plague-stricken. During times of plague funer-als had to cease; even close relatives were to be prohibited from accompanying plague victims to the grave. He instructed on street cleaning, the removal of all rags, perfuming of everything, including graves of the dead, the suspected, and the infected. Yet officials in charge had to be mindful of not giving rise to conflict, insulting the lower classes ('il popolazzo'), or treating differently 'nobles and mechanics, citizens and peasants, the educated and the ignorant'. He added detailed advice to the servants responsible for perfuming rooms, grave-diggers, and cleaners ('monatti'), those who drove the plague carts, those who took care of the horses, those responsible for washing infected clothing, those who made the beds of the infected, and those who had to touch them. These servants were also to be separated from the healthy. They were instructed on what to wear and to change and wash their clothing often.

---

[69] His earlier Latin tract contained 40 pages of medical recipes (58–98)—a third of the tract—which was extracted almost entirely from the second one.

The suspected and convalescents should be able to come out of their lodgings occasionally for air but must paint their faces white or carry a white stick ('banderola'). He gave other advice on purging or perfuming various sorts of goods, metal objects, vases in brass, copper, and bronze, letters, money, and so forth, specifying the ingredients and quantities of lye and vinegar for various washings. He pointed to bread and *minestra* as means of passing on the contagion. As with Milanese and Bolognese legislation, certain groups and occupations—mendicants on city corners, charlatans, whores, and dyers—were to be banned from the city; others such as leatherworkers and butchers were to be moved from the town centre and from proximity to streams and brooks. Silkworms were suspected and removed from town. The movements of pigs, geese, ducks, rabbits, and cows in the city should be guarded, dogs and cats culled, then buried in deep graves covered with lye. Prisoners were to be moved often from one cell to another. Finally, he reiterated the legendary advice of Hippocrates on burning odoriferous woods throughout the city.

Alessandri's instructions to officers then extended beyond details of daily administration to address collective and political problems of a more psychological nature: how to maintain community morale during plague to stop the flight of doctors, clergy, and the rich, and abandonment by loved ones. He instructed officers at all levels not to frighten commoners but to be 'loving, tolerant and solicitous of their needs'. Further, he examined the economic conditions wrought by plague and urged rulers to provision the city with stocks of food, vinegar, oil, salt, and other necessities before a plague arrived. Yet he also advised that the *miserabile* be banished, especially foreigners.[70]

***

Afterwards, at least until the end of the sixteenth century, advice to princes and 'Republics' (Commonwealths) and discussions on government policy during plagues became a usual part of doctors' plague tracts as with book I of a handbook that people could carry with them (*Porta tecum*) by the Sicilian doctor Giacomo Argenterio, written during a plague of 1598.[71] It included a section on 'remedies for ending the plague'. Argenterio advised that 'the republic in times of plague' ought to stockpile various types of odoriferous woods to be placed in front of all the houses of the city to perfume all the *contrade*. With other dry and odoriferous woods, these householders would be responsible for keeping the fires going for seven or eight days.[72] He called for ordinances to prohibit the importation of codfish, fish oil, pilchard, and putrid herring along with corrupt grain, infected meats, and spoilt fish during plague time. Streams and fountains

---

[70] Alessandri, *Trattato della peste*, 16r–34v.

[71] It also incorporated the tract *Rimedi, preservativi, e curativi* of the doctor and astrologer, Auger Ferrier (1513–88). Perhaps this was an abridgement of *Remèdes préservatifs et curatifs de peste* (Lyon: J. de Tournes, 1548). Curiously, the Italian was translated into French in 1630 at Siena.

[72] Argenterio, *Porta tecum rimedii piu veri*, 37–8.

were to be cleaned of garbage and city streets cleared of mud, carrion, scraps of leather, and rags.[73] To keep infection at bay, ditches and other places had to be inspected for dead animals, accumulation of garbage, and corrupt water. The ill should be visited and, if signs of plague were found, were to be removed from their homes and separated from the healthy; their houses locked with the remaining inhabitants inside or, if available, transported to a place in the countryside. If plague broke out in a neighbourhood, its communication with the rest of the city was to be severed, fires lit, houses of the neighbourhood washed, and the stricken separated from the healthy.[74] Finally, against Galenic doctrine, Argenterio argued that the reason the poor were so often the victims of disease had nothing to do with their nature or morality but with the resources available to them: if they could afford the same medical treatment and drugs as the rich, they would not become overwhelmingly the victims of plague, and with *buon consiglio*, 'the administrators of the republic' could solve the problem.[75] Such public health concerns continued in Italian plague tracts through the eighteenth century culminating with Lodovico Muratori's *Il Governo della Peste* written during the plague at Marseille in 1720–1 and revised during Italy's last great plague at Messina in 1743.[76]

As early as 1583 the Italian experience and change in medical mentality towards plague formed during the crisis years of 1575–8 began to be exported beyond the Alps 'as much for the wisdom of its doctors as that of its magistrates'. Along with his own plague tract, Joachim Camerarius (1534–98), a prominent doctor and Nuremberg humanist, translated from Italian into Latin five Italian plague publications of the Italian 1575–8 plague: Donzellini's tract of 1577, sections from Ingrassia's first tract on plague in Palermo in these years, parts of Caesare Rincii's (Centorio Degli Ortensi's) description of plague legislation passed at Milan in 1576–7, the constitutions, laws, and edicts passed in Venice during this plague, and a short pamphlet on the drug Armenian bolus.[77] Camerarius ended his florilegium of Italian works with a Latin poem composed by the head of Milan's public health board in 1576, Hannibal Cruceius (Lodovico Annibale Della Croce). Except for the tract on drugs, all these Italian works stressed the importance of public health through government intervention, charity,

---

[73] Ibid., 38.

[74] This was an exceptional case in that the historical inspiration came from outside Italy. Argenterio called the above a policy ('una politica') similar to that recently practised in the small towns of Tolosa (in the Pays Basques, then under Spanish rule, as was Sicily).

[75] Ibid., 39. Panseri, 'La nascita della polizia medica', 155–96, despite its title, concentrates more on ideas about disease in the second half of the sixteenth century than on changes in attitudes or new ideas towards public health.

[76] See Epilogue.

[77] Camerarius, *Synopsis*. On Camerarius and the significance of this publication for the rest of Europe, see Nutton, 'Books, Printing and Medicine', 398. Armenian Bolo, from Persia and Armenia, is fine red clay; see Fracastoro, *De contagione*, notes, 319. Given the survival of the *Synopsis* across Europe with copies in at least seven libraries in Britain today, it appears to have been widely diffused. It was reissued in 1597.

new magistrates and controls for remedying pestilence. In addition, Camerarius provided his German readers with a long bibliography of other Italian plague tracts, the majority of which were written during and pertained to the plague of 1575–8 and contained new sections on public health. He used these Italian publications to draft his own plague tract, the first one I know outside of Italy to move significantly from the concerns of individual patients to address health policy, the state's role as a regulator and provider in plague time.

Unlike Georg Agricola, who a generation earlier had provided a short two-page description of the health board in Venice within a lengthy theoretical discussion of various forms of contagion for German-speaking physicians,[78] Camerarius addressed these Italian measures directly to the magistrates of his city for immediate implementation. He recommended the founding of public health boards in German cities based on the Italian city-state model with at least one doctor on the board and preferably two, and he outlined their duties: the quarantining of travellers to towns during plague for at least fifteen days before being allowed to mix with the population; the quarantine of incoming goods; isolation of the plague-stricken and those from the same household to be transported to a healthy place beyond the city walls; the building of plague huts for the suspected and convalescents to be examined by doctors and surgeons; state-funded medication for the afflicted and for the cleansing of contaminated goods, and procedures for burning other plague-infected property.[79] During the next two decades, doctors in France, German-speaking regions, and to some extent England would begin slowly to follow the example of the Italian doctors of 1575–8, extending their plague tracts beyond the dictates and recipes for individual patients' souls and bodies to advise on health policy and matters of state.[80]

---

[78] Agricola, *De peste libri tres*, 60–63. Also, see Nutton, 'The Reception of Fracastoro's Theory of Contagion', 213–4. According to Nutton, Guinther (Johann Winter), *De pestilentia commentarius*, 'also attests a different Italian influence. One should clean up streams and wells, and shut down bad smells, such as tanneries and geese farms (a local touch for Guinther's tract was published in Strasbourg)'. Guinther, however, ended his discussion on a pessimistic note: 'whatever practical steps might be taken, flight was still the best remedy' (ibid., 220–1). The section of the dialogue which touches this Italian experience (*Mos Venetorum*), barely fills two of the 294 pages of this tract (72–4) and appears within a theoretical discussion of the direction of winds and the circulation of air. The two dialogues of the second half of the work, which concern preventative measures, fail to mention public health concerns; rather, they address the patient with recipes for purgatives, theriacs, and the like.

[79] Camerarius, *De recta et necessaria ratione praeservandi*, n.p.

[80] According to Slack, *The Impact of Plague*, the first publication of this kind was John Stockwell's translation in 1583 of Ewich, *Of the Duetie of a Faithful and Wise Magistrate*, published in Latin the year before. Slack also notes that Thomas Lodge's treatise of 1603, based on a French original, included a chapter on public health. From the epidemic of 1593 onwards, 'English writers began to refer to the obligations of magistrates during epidemics . . . to keep cities clean and above all guard against the transmission of infection from person to person' (p. 45). Still, according to Wear, *Knowledge and Practice in English Medicine*, 284, medical writers in England of the sixteenth and seventeenth centuries accepted the status quo regarding the living conditions of the poor without any 'wholesale reform'. These matters would begin to change only in the nineteenth century. Ewich's *De officio fidelis et prudentis magistratus tempore pestilentiae. . .* differed from Camerarius' work. It was more of a religious and moral tract on the obligations of the magistrate placed in a Lutheran context.

The earliest example of a physician's plague tract that provided examples and instruction on public health that I have found for France was one by the Lyonnais physician Claude de Rubys published in 1577. He had been a student in Padua during the plague of 1555[81] and cited the experiences and practices of physicians and health boards in Venice, Milan and Lombardy during what was then the current plague of 1576–7 and their implementation in Lyon.[82] These included public provisioning for the poor even before the plague struck cities; knowledge that plague erupted first in the neighbourhoods of the poor such as Lyon's Saint-Nizier, where especial vigilance had to be maintained; the public hiring of doctors, surgeons, and barbers; provisioning of drugs and other medication to the poor during plague without charge; control of merchandise and persons coming into towns; use of passports and quarantine; separation of the healthy and the suspected with the construction of huts to quarantine the latter; cleaning of streets; operations of Lyon's plague hospital, Saint Laurens; and organization of religious processions and actions against the Calvinists. De Rubys's tract, however, remained more descriptive than prescriptive, and in contrast to Italy, neither the late 1570s nor any other decade of the sixteenth century stimulated an avalanche of new plague writing in France and especially ones that included new sections on public health and the politics of plague as was seen in Italy. Tracts such as those by the Parisian doctors Jean Cassal[83] and Françoys de Courselles,[84] and the Lyonnais Antoine Royet remained fixed within the structures of the traditional Renaissance plague tract.[85]

In Italy, on the other hand, physicians' concerns with public health and the need for political solutions spilled into other areas beyond plague. Like so much of the plague literature in 1575–8, *Sources of Water and Rivers of the World*, published by the Roman physician Andrea Bacci (1524–1600),[86] concerned water, trash, and excrement. His work centred on problems Romans then currently faced with limited supplies of 'tasty and safe drinking water', the threat of epidemic disease, and with flooding. All three problems, he contended were connected and had worsened in modern times in large part because of the habits of Romans abusing their natural sources of beauty and commerce as depositories for their excrement and waste. As with the 'remedies' for plague emphasized by this new generation of doctors, the political sphere was at the crux of Bacci's arguments and recommendations, and he addressed these directly to the state.

[81] De Rubys, *Discours sur la contagion de peste*, 9.

[82] Ibid., 34 and 38. Also, see the various contributions of physicians in *Curationes ad praevisionem pestis*; and Le Paulmier, *Bref discours*.

[83] Cassal, *Traicté de la peste*.   [84] De Courselles, *Traité de la peste clair et très utile*.

[85] Royet, *Traicté de la peste*.

[86] According to Singer, *The Development of the Contagium Vivum*, 7, in a work of 1596 Bacci made 'the first clear attempt to describe the organized basis of a ferment'; that is, vinegar fermented through the progeny of 'tiny worms . . . living atoms'.

He called for the revival of public magistracies such as the ancient *Curatores alvei Tiberis*, the need for large expenditures on public projects such as diverting the Tiber's tributaries, dredging its river beds, and improving its banks. But more crucial was his call for state intervention into the habits of Romans and the need for public control and political repression (in Ingrassia's terms, the call for the *Forca*).[87] Compare Bacci's political analysis and public demands with the earlier concerns of the Roman physician Andrea Turini, whose 1542 tract on Roman fountains and water supplies skirted entirely politics and the public sphere.[88]

By the end of the sixteenth and early seventeenth century, physicians such as Filippo Cavriana (*Discorsi* [1597]) and Andrea Canoniero (*Dell'Introduzione alla Politica* [1614]) widened the physician's intellectual remit still further. Employing medical methods and reasoning, they branched into pure politics, addressing the ills of the body politic. Canoniero projected Hippocrates *Aphorisms* from observations about ailments and cures for the ill to arguments about the best systems of government.[89] Lodovico Settala, one of Italy's most illustrative physicians of the early seventeenth century, who had been prominent in the fight against plague in Milan in 1576–7 as well as in 1630 and the author of a large scholarly plague tract, illustrates this movement from the patient's bedside to engagement in political theory.[90] In 1627 he published a work purely on politics, *Della Ragion di Stato*,[91] in which he justified himself as a physician engaged in this new arena: just as doctors have studied poisons to recognize diseases, to understand their causes, and to devise cures, these same methods should be employed to uncover the machinations of tyrants and devise remedies for the body politic.[92]

In expanding their professional ambit beyond the patient's bed to the political sphere, physicians of the 1575–8 plague and afterwards began to approach the radical views on medicine Rudolph Virchow envisaged almost 400 years later:

---

[87] Bacci, *Delle acque de' fonti et fiumi*, 106–11 and Libro terzo, 213–308.

[88] On Turini and his tract on fountains, see n. 5 above.

[89] For this shift at the end of the sixteenth century in the importance of medical models for political theory by physicians and non-physicians, see D'Alessio, 'Per una nuova scienza', and especially 23–6 on Canoniero's use of Hippocrates' *Aphorisms*. To be sure, metaphors of the body politic go back to Plato and Aristotle, are well founded in texts of the central Middle Ages such as John of Salisbury's *Policraticus*, and became more elaborate in some *Regimen sanitatis* during the late Middle Ages; on the last see Rawcliffe, 'The Concept of Health'.

[90] On Settala's role as medical deputy in charge of visiting the plague-stricken of Milan's Porta Orientale in 1576–7; see Belloni, 'Carlo Borromeo e la storia della medicina', 169–70.

[91] It is abridged in *Politici e moralisti del seicento*, 43–141.

[92] Ibid., 51. Metaphors about medicine and medical reasoning began to influence political essays north of the Alps as well; see for instance Francis Bacon's 'Of Seditious and Troubles'.

'Medicine is a social science . . . Politics is nothing but medicine on a large scale . . . the ultimate aim [of medicine] is eminently social.'[93]

[93] Cited by Félix Martí-Ibáñez, 'Forward' to Rosen, *A History of Public Health*, 13. Also see Henry Sigerist (1891–1957): 'If medicine is a science, then it is a social science', cited in Webster, 'The Historiography of Medicine', 39.

9

Plague Psychology

TUMULT AND DISCONTENT

As many tracts of 1575–8 suggest, regional states and city magistrates were forced to pass draconian measures in plague time: civil order deteriorated with the threat and disruption of contagion.[1] Against the praise of epic plague poets of the local podestà and 'the readiness of noble citizens and merchants to assist the poor', not all saw their rulers acting on their behalf, administering their duties during these trying times with utmost efficiency or benevolence, especially towards commoners. Nor did such criticism arise exclusively from the middling or lower classes. The bishop of Verona during the plague of 1576 gave a more mixed picture of the city's progress against plague than that of the poets. He pointed to magistrates' negligence in making payments to the lazaretto of San Giacomo, despite mounting plague cases and deaths; the problems of indecision, which arose from the government's refusal to use the 'formidable name' of plague; and subsequent social tribulations of uprisings, cases of fraud, theft, witchcraft, and sedition'.[2]

At the very outset of plague in Milan, the city's governor, Marchese d'Aimonte, had to send troops of 'harquebusiers, lances, and other soldiers' to seal off the boundaries of the Borgo degli Ortolani, where the first plague case had been discovered, and to threaten with the death penalty those who broke from their locked homes: 'all those in that neighbourhood put up a big defence [*feceno grande difesa*] not to be locked away'.[3] According to the Dominican chronicler Bugati, the conditions of quarantine in Milan in 1576, the absence of work, and the consequent levels of poverty 'unknown' to the government, 'necessitated' and hence justified 'sinister revolt'. Eventually, however, conditions improved through the intervention of Borromeo and new administrative structures organized by the Senate and Milan's health board. Magistrates of the parishes and the city gates began providing adequate food and services to the poor.[4] According to the parish

---

[1] For a discussion of class hatred during later epidemics, see Amelang, *A Journal of the Plague Year*, 15–17; Calvi, 'L'oro, il fuoco, le forche'; and Baehrel, 'La haine de classe'.
[2] Valier, *Commentariolus*, 76r and 82v.   [3] *Il diario di Giambattista Casale*, 290–1.
[4] Bugati, *L'aggiunta*, 157.

gate-guard Besta, the threat of sedition during the 1576–7 plague was the prime mover of merchant and noble generosity towards the poor in Milan and the reasons for state intervention on their behalf. Even before the general quarantine of October 1576, the depressed conditions for work and mounting misery had overwhelmed the benefits from individual acts of citizen charity: 'With such great expense necessary to feed such large numbers of people', many (citizens and merchants) judged the situation impossible. They feared that the plebs, 'lacking all means of livelihood, would have to revolt'. Therefore, the citizens exhorted magistrates and nobles to act, otherwise these middling sorts would have to leave town to save their skins.[5]

The plague of 1575–8 was hardly unique in fanning disorder, lawlessness, or revolt.[6] In Florence, as early as 1383 a mass exodus of better-off citizens during plague provided an opportunity for the recently defeated artisans and workers—the Ciompi—to regroup and revolt against the city to restore their three illegal guilds of workers.[7] Similarly, during the next big plague to invade central Italy after 1575–8, that of 1587, a doctor in Rome's principal hospital of Santo Spirito generalized: 'beyond all doubt, plague gives rise to fights among the populace, sedition, and revolt'.[8] With the plague of 1629–33 in Florence, plague-related crime increased to such levels that new plague tribunals had to be created.[9] Moreover, from 1348 through the early modern period, historians have noted the rise of factional violence, criminality, and rioting in plague time.[10] The difference in 1575–8 was that physicians and other plague writers began to address these questions as important and appropriate matters for publication, debate, and speculation on their causes and made new recommendations for their resolution.

Mismanagement and the arrogance and cruelty of individual deputies or commissioners (heard most loudly in Panizzone Sacco's 'lament') were not the only political issues to trouble plague doctors and other writers during the 1575–8 plague. Some challenged the wisdom of the systems and stratagems themselves that health boards had imposed on urban populations across the Italian peninsula, which, they alleged, caused discontent among the masses and disobedience to state regulations. Again, physicians' written arguments and advice on plague broke the frame of previous plague tracts, which before

---

5 Besta, *Vera narratione*, 25r. Henderson, 'Epidemics in Renaissance Florence', 182, argues that fear of the poor and disorder during the plagues of the 1520s in Florence had the opposite effect: 'charity now disappeared'.

6 For a general overview of threats from the poor and unrest during plagues, see Pullan, 'Plague and Perceptions of the Poor', 101–23, esp. 116–17; and for a particular case, Cipolla, *Faith, Reason, and the Plague*.

7 On this abortive revolt, see Cohn, *Lust for Liberty*, 62, 73, and 304.

8 Tommasi, *Tractatus de peste*, 19r.   9 See Calvi, *Histories of a Plague Year*.

10 For lawlessness and rioting provoked during plague at Barcelona in 1651 and other plagues in early modern Europe, see Amelang, *A Journal of the Plague Year*; for increases in criminality, see Chapter 5, n. 55.

1575 had focused on the individual patient.[11] For instance, the Veronese physician Raimondo argued that many who had fallen ill in the initial stages of the Venetian plague of 1575–6 had died because of the city's insufficient charity and the inadequate medical attention and medication provided to the plague-stricken, and the plague was fuelled by merchants closing their shops, depriving workers and artisans of their livelihood. For Raimondo, matters had deteriorated over the sixteenth century: 'Had the infected received proper medical treatment in 1575 and 1576 as they had in 1528, plague mortality in Venice would have been a tenth of what it was. The merchants would have given work to the poor so that they could have supported themselves and would not have died from hunger and fear.'[12] According to Raimondo, the disease in 1528 had been more deadly than in 1575, but those doctors who normally treated only the rich had then risked their lives attending the poor, while in 1575 and 1576, few did so. Also, matters had been better during the plague of 1556 than in 1575–6. The earlier plague was no less malignant than the later, but fewer died because doctors offered to treat the afflicted, and thus the plague-stricken were not as terrorized or abandoned. Further, for Raimondo, the Lazaretto vecchio had become a death trap, 'where to enter is to abandon all hope'. By his account, these conditions—failure to treat the poor 'lovingly according to their needs', along with the authorities' terrorization of the city—led to the city's great ruin and conditions 'worsened daily'.[13]

THE SOCIAL PSYCHOLOGY OF PLAGUE

As early as the second outbreak of plague in Florence in 1363 and the plague tract of Tommaso Del Garbo, the psychological dimensions of plague became important considerations to plague doctors trying to comprehend the enigmas of why some perished, others became ill but survived, and still others remained unaffected. Along with certain behaviour and activities such as immoderate exercise, gluttony, sex, and various dictates on diet, states of mind also influenced susceptibility to plague: anger, grief, hatred, anxiety, and fear made the individual more open to the disease, while happiness and serenity helped to keep it at bay. By the late sixteenth century, doctors even thought that fear of plague itself killed their patients.[14] Plague writers also continued to point to attitudes and activities such as prayer, song, and telling pleasant stories that could preserve the spirit and thereby the body from plague. For instance, a small tract of 1528 by the

---

[11] For an example of the traditional pre-1575 plague tract concentrating on remedies, diet, and procedures for the individual patient, see Baviera, *Trattato mirabile contra peste*.

[12] Raimondo, *Discorso*, 392v–3r.   [13] Ibid., 394r.

[14] Condio, *Medicina filosofica contra la peste*, 5r.

little-known doctor Bernardino Bocca[15] advised readers to flee from indignation, anger, sex, and other wayward things and, instead, urged them to stay happy and be courteous ('& usa le cose utende polite').[16] Marino Massucci advised shunning anger, melancholy, fear of plague, and troublesome business during plague to stay happy. The Capuchin Paolo Bellintani, who officiated over the lazaretto in Milan during the 1576–7 plague, Brescia's a year later, and Marseille's in the early 1580s, attributed his survival first to God, then to his state of mind and jovial nature.[17]

As for sex, it was one of the few if not the only place where Massucci disagreed with his major authority, Hippocrates. On this activity, moderation was not advisable: 'as experience during plague has shown', unquestionably 'sex was harmful and should be practised as little and as infrequently as possible'.[18] During the 1585 plague, which afflicted only Piedmont within Italy, the university doctor Bucci gave a more liberal view of what was good for the mind during plague, reminiscent of Del Garbo's advice in 1363[19] but with greater detail:

arm yourself with hope and confirmation in the faith of God; seek out jolly company; treat yourself to music, honest and pleasing games, ban all lugubrious and troublesome thinking. Make every effort to stay happy; dress in silk or in cloth with light and happy colours; wear a ring with precious stones; hang out sometimes with jesters; give an ear to comedies, games, and pleasing stories; read books, tell jokes and delightful stories.[20]

Others, such as the Sicilian Ingrassia, gave a more extended list of activities and attitudes that affect 'the accidents of the soul' during plague than any found for the Middle Ages: stay happy in an agreeable and bright place filled with ornate and beautiful paintings without any fears or melancholic worries; go about in varied, cheerful, and beautiful clothing, take on graces ('far del galante'), wearing jewels of gold and precious stones on the fingers, pushing aside every vision and thought of death . . . attend banquets and retire to parlours and terraces ('solazzi') with friends to play games, tell funny stories ('facetie') and fables, enact comedies, sing songs, play musical instruments, and engage in other similar frivolous pastimes ('sciocchezze').[21] Unlike the late fourteenth-century Florentine doctor Del Garbo, who recognized that not all could afford jewels and other beautiful things to lift spirits during plague, Ingrassia did not here reflect on such limitations. Yet he did not forget the poor. In these banquets of the rich, charity

---

[15] From Edit 16, this author is known only through this one publication in two editions.

[16] Bocca, *Diuini fioretti preseruatiui*, 44.   [17] *Dialogo della peste*, 175.

[18] Massucci, *La preseruatione dalla pestilenza*, 87–8.

[19] On Tommaso Del Garbo's advice, see Cohn, *The Black Death Transformed*, 241–2.

[20] Bucci, *Reggimento*, n.p. City authorities in Milan, Bologna, Venice, and elsewhere appear not to have agreed: they expelled jesters and comedians from their cities as dangerous in plague time; see Chapter 8.

[21] Ingrassia, *Informatione, Parte terza*, 23. For similar lists for happiness see Barrelli, *Thesoro inestimabile che insegna*, n.p.

should be raised for the poor. 'Our tones should be the organs of the church, and this music along with the songs of the religious orders should help dispel all sadness over our recently departed friends.'[22]

Plague tracts to the end of the century and beyond continued to address these 'accidents of the spirit'. In a tract published in 1600, Giulio Durante of Rome's College of Physicians advised 'fleeing affects of the soul' such as melancholy, anger, angst, heavy thoughts of fear, brooding over death ('grande imaginatione della morte'), and to abstain as much as possible from sex. But unlike many others he did not point to the thoughts and activities that fortified the soul against plague.[23] By the sixteenth century not all agreed on the particulars of this spirit or on its rationale. The Augustine friar who headed Naples's health board took a slightly different stance than most. In his chapter 'on exercise and the accidents of the spirit', he began with the usual list of attitudes to guard against—melancholy, anger, fear ('pagure'), and irritation—but he raised suspicion about happiness or at least grand happiness ('de grande allegrezza') with excessive laughter ('superchio ridere') as a dangerous state of mind in plague time: 'because such a state opened the mouth [*de cabba*] widely, allowing air which might be corrupt or stinky to enter the wind pipe [*canna*]'. In the same year, the Brescian doctor Glisenti raised similar objections, advising readers not to go to places where excessive mirth forced too much laughter, which opened the mouth and allowed much air to enter the body. Proof of this theorem, Glisenti maintained, 'could be seen this year when many excellent lawyers who loudly disputed their cases took in too much pestilential air'.[24] During the plague at the end of the century, a doctor from Revignano, near Asti in Piedmont, also warned against 'excessive happiness' and went so far as to claim that the 'over happy' died in greater numbers during plague than the sad: too much laughter overheated the humours. Still, the doctor upheld the basic tenets of the best spirits to have during plague. Anger was to be repressed: it inflamed the blood and in turn the heart. One should endeavour to stay 'honestly happy' by dressing in the noblest clothes one possessed, playing musical instruments, singing, playing games that were not tiring, and wearing gold rings with precious stones—sapphires, emeralds, and rubies.[25]

The Augustinian friar Giovanni Battista elaborated further on the state of happiness for preservation in plague time: all anxiety and business dealings should be pushed aside and in their place the plague-threatened should sing, play jocular songs, and read pleasant stories. On sex, the friar was more liberal

---

[22] Ingrassia, *Informatione, Parte terza*, 24. Viscanio, *Regimento del viver*, B 2v, also recognized that the poor could not feast their eyes on jewels and precious stones; for them he recommended 'walks in the country, with flowers, gardens and . . . in the hills with similar objects to delight the eyes'.

[23] Durante, *Trattato della peste*, 11r.   [24] Glisenti, *Trattato del regimento*, 292.

[25] Sale, *Trattato di epidemia*, 6r. Also, Puccinelli warned of the dangers of 'excessive happiness'; *Dialoghi sopra le cause della peste*, 47r.

than the physicians Bocca and Massucci: it was acceptable but must be done in moderation and by those accustomed to having it ('a chi ne uso'); for those who were not, it was expressly forbidden, and for this reason men should be cautious mixing with women or getting married in times of pestilence.[26]

With the 1575–8 plague, however, as in other respects, the psychological analysis of plague took on another dimension—a political and collective one. Plague doctors such as Raimondo pointed to mass fear and its social and medical consequences and not just for the individual. Such fear, moreover, was not simply brought on by an individual's thoughts or choice of activities, such as failing to tell sweet tales among a select group of friends or dwelling on death. Instead, they were the consequences of political and administrative structures and decisions enacted by civic health boards and magistrates. Descriptions of mass fear and terror and how they affected populations are almost totally absent from discussions in plague manuals prior to 1575. Again, an exception comes from the previous plague in Padua and Venice in 1555. But this tract by the Venetian physician Massa did little more than state the obvious: 'seeing so many men taken by the serious and deadly disease, not only those who were suffering from the disease and the people [*popolo*] but others, including those ruling the city [Venice], became terrorized . . . Not without reason' this plague terrorized the entire city and with great injury to the Venetian government ('di vostra Serenità').[27] Although Massa saw plague as a catastrophe that affected the community as a whole, he did not elaborate on the pros or cons of particular governmental policies to combat plague. These earlier plague tracts simply did not enter this terrain of politics.

The plague tract of the famous Bolognese gentleman-surgeon and alleged charlatan Leonardo Fioravanti also anticipated concerns that would become commonplace in plague writing after 1575.[28] His tract, published in 1565, 'corrected and enlarged' in 1571, and republished posthumously in 1594,[29] began with the intent of convincing governments of 'one of the most beautiful laws': depopulations of cities, destruction of the countryside, and the ruin of kingdoms result from the fear and cruelty that governments impose on their people. If they resolved not to frighten and treat their subjects cruelly, far fewer

---

[26] Napolitano, *Opera et trattato che insegna* (1556), 11r. [27] Massa, *Ragionamento*, 1r and 30v.

[28] The literature on Fioravanti is extensive: he wrote over thirty works, practised medicine in Palermo, Naples, Rome, Venice, and Bologna, became well known for crossing many boundaries in the history of medicine. Fellow physicians in Venice accused him as unqualified; he was imprisoned in Milan for supposedly dispensing drugs that killed his patients, but later was hailed as the leading Italian follower of Paracelsus. See Palmer, 'The Control of Plague', 263–6; Giordano, *Leonardo Fioravanti*; and Eamon, *Science and the Secrets of Nature*, 261 and 168–93. Some modern medical historians still consider him a heretic; see Cosmacini, *Storia della medicina*, 140; and Palmer, 'The Control of Plague', 263–5; or a charlatan (Gentilcore, *Medical Charlatanism*, 267), although not in the strict sense: 'he never mounted a bank—but he influenced generations of charlatans after him with his medical "secrets", his empirical knowledge and his continual peregrinations' (268).

[29] It is presumed that he died in 1588, but it is not certain.

would die and those who did would not die so desperately. Doctors would not be frightened and would attend to their plague patients; priests would not flee from their spiritual obligations, and relatives would not abandon their loved ones.[30]

Yet after these provocative remarks in the preface, his *Reggimento* proceeded in traditional fashion, first defining plague and its causes, then proceeding to long lists of syrups, purgatives, and other recipes—'miraculous perfumes for the house', remedies for purifying the air, and palliatives for defending oneself against plague. Despite his introductory promises, Fioravanti said little about government reforms and, unlike plague writers of 1575–8, proposed no specific ordinances. Instead, his chapter seven, 'Why the plague causes so much ruin and mortality', is not a proposal for new state intervention, reforms, laws, or social engineering but the opposite: it called for the dismantling of state initiatives in plague time and especially the cornerstone of health boards' regulations—enforced isolation of the infected and suspected. Moreover, plague huts and lazaretti developed in Italian cities such as Milan and Venice over the past century were to be abolished, and Fioravanti offered nothing to replace them. He contended that villages in the Bolognese countryside during the plague of 1527 had fared better than the city because peasants had not experienced such great fear. The usual town ordinances of locking up the infected and suspected in their homes or leading them off to the lazaretti, burning their property, and sending grave-diggers through the city, had 'spread terror and filled the hearts of men and women with Hell'. Fioravanti was a true believer of laissez-faire government, *avant la lettre*. He proposed that princes and cities 'remedy' matters by lifting all the above-mentioned policies, allowing their subjects to live and move about almost in any way they chose. Doctors should visit and treat the infected in the patients' own houses, and druggists should dispense their medicines there. Only then, he predicted, would 'doctors stop being frightened, priests fleeing, and relatives abandoning one another'. And as a result, cities would cease being depopulated and kingdoms would stop going to ruin.[31]

'With this new order', Fioravanti assured, 'the plague would lose all its force, because 'suddenly great joy would fill the hearts of the people'. Had his doctrine been employed at the beginning, Fioravanti claimed, plague mortality would not have been so great, its force dissipated by the 'great power of happiness ('grande la potenza di tale allegrezza')'.[32] In other words, Fioravanti's 'nuovo ordine' was hardly new; rather, it was a reversion to policies in existence before the development of health boards, special plague ordinances, the circulation of

---

[30] Fioravanti, *Il reggimento della peste*, 11r. The first edition was published in 1565 but substantially enlarged in 1571, then reprinted in 1594 and at least twice in the seventeenth century (1626 and 1680). These later editions have the same pagination. The tract was also translated into German (*Regiment und Ordnung der Pestilenz.* . . [Frankfurt-am-Main, 1632]). In addition, Fioravanti was one of the few in the sixteenth century to suggest that medicine had progressed since antiquity, at least in developing drugs; Fioravanti, *Il reggimento della peste*, 7v; in 1565 ed., 6r.

[31] Fioravanti, *Il reggimento della peste*, 10v–11r.   [32] Ibid., 21r.

broadsheets, and lazaretti; a return to what in fact still persisted in most places north of the Alps through the sixteenth century.[33] By contrast, when writers such as the druggist Bellicocchi criticized institutions such as quarantine during the 1575–8 plague, they proposed concrete reforms and new institutions with even more intricate administration and governmental intervention to replace them. Instead of suspending government, Bellicocchi called for the opposite: the majority of those dying during plague, he concluded, died of hardship, from the absence of treatment, medicines, and government assistance ('governo necessario'). The illness of plague becomes deadly, he argued, when such measures are not delivered, allowing famine to kill as many as the plague. When food is supplied to the famished and treatment to the infected in time, life is conserved.[34] By contrast, Fioravanti's doctrine of happiness saw no need for governments to intervene to assist the poor.[35]

FEAR

As Paolo Preto has argued, 'for the entire fifteenth century and most of the sixteenth, Italian and European medicine confronted the problem of plague without any obsessions with poisonings and diabolical intervention.'[36] But this began to change in 1576, 'the year of the first pandemic of the early modern period',[37] culminating in the plague of 1629–30 with hunts for plague spreaders ('untori'), Milan at its epicentre: medical and religious authorities alike pursued and prosecuted 'wicked' plague cleaners and grave-diggers as manufacturers of plague and the culprits in its dissemination.[38] In 1575–8, however, such frenzy had yet to infect states, and, as we have seen, for the most part they legislated against such rumours of plague spreading. Moreover, doctors and other authors of plague tracts did not often mention diabolic acts of plague spreading, wiping poison on keys, door knobs, and gates. And when they did, they were often sceptical of them (as was the notary Canobbio), branding them as rumours of the superstitious and ignorant.[39] The most notable exception came from Sicily's *Protomedico*, Ingrassia, who emphasized the need for gate-guards and controls through the countryside, not only to prevent the plague-stricken from entering

---

[33] On the spread of health boards, lazaretti, and policies of sequestration in France and England during the sixteenth century; see Palmer, 'The Control of Plague', 146ff.

[34] Bellicocchi, *Avvertimenti*, 427r–v.

[35] On Fioravanti's anti-modernism and desire to return to the pristine and simple practice he imagined in ancient times; see Eamon, *Science and the Secrets of Nature*, 192.

[36] Preto, *Epidemia, paura e politica*, 10. One could go further and say that the absence of such plague scapegoating in Italy endured from the last moments of the Black Death in 1350 to the end of the sixteenth century. Allegations such as Calvi's that these prejudices were a constant over the almost 500-year history of plague are simply wrong; see Introduction, n. 12.

[37] Ibid., 11.   [38] Ibid., 15.

[39] See for instance Bisciola, *Relatione verissima del progresso della peste*, 7r.

the city but also to stop 'the devil and his evil ministers from transporting the various seeds of contagion'.[40] By the end of the century, however, those in medical circles became less sceptical of evil ones spreading the plague. Writing during a plague in 1598, Asti's doctor Arellano alleged that the second cause of plague derived from 'wicked ones who diabolically spread their poisons through the world'.[41]

But even if mass fear did not lead to mass hysteria during the plague of 1575–8, descriptions of mass fear and terror in plague tracts and their social and medical implications were no longer the exception. Those chronicling the 'progress' of plague, such as the Venetian notary Benedetti, described 'the daily terror' of plague massacres, sights of sons, fathers, and mothers stripped naked in public for doctors' investigations of their corpses before being carted to unceremonious burials. Such plague scenes touched Rocco directly as he transported three of his relatives to their graves. As with Fioravanti's criticisms, Benedetti saw terror infused in state policy—the quarantine of the afflicted and suspected. Rocco lamented the miserable fate of those locked away to suffer alone without assistance in their illness. Yet, cognizant of the dangers of contagion, he did not then propose, as Fioravanti had, that state systems of sequestration be dismantled.[42]

The Brescian doctor Glisenti related his first encounter with plague in 1576, that he could not have imagined how dreadful and frightening the plague was: he was so wrapped up in it ('investigating, experimenting, and learning from one day to the next') that it was not until the disease had run half its course that he realized how frightened he was.[43] Mass fear was seen where the plague may not have even struck or at least devastated urban populations as it had in Sicily or in the northern cities. The Lucchese gentleman doctor Burlacchino Burlacchini dedicated his tract to the duke of Savoy. Neither region shows evidence of plague between 1575 and 1578, but Burlacchini explained that in his nineteen years of service to his country as a doctor, he had never witnessed 'such fear, ruin, and misery' as that caused by plague, which devoured not just a particular spot but entire peoples, cities and provinces, and for this reason he wrote his tract.[44] Similarly, 'the great terror' of this current plague, which now 'threatened all of Italy', prompted Giovanni Battista Giudici, practising in the small town of Camaiore, where this plague had not yet reached, to write his plague tract on cures and preservatives.[45] Some, such as the Paduan notary Canobbio, even saw a silver lining in mass fear: 'because of

[40] Ingrassia, *Parte quinta*, 6 and 23. Moreover, his longer tract of the previous year, *Informatione*, 170, accepted the report of the doctor Bonagente that 'un scelerato' had rubbed infected soap on clothing and on people. Preto, *Epidemia, paura e politica*, 11, claims that Ingrassia denied such reports but does not cite any passage to substantiate his claim.

[41] Arellano, *Trattato di peste*, 25, 105, and 109. For other examples, see Preto, *Epidemia, paura e politica*, 12–15.

[42] Benedetti, *Raguaglio*, 482v.   [43] Glisenti, *Trattato del Regimento*, 1r.

[44] Burlacchini, *Ragionamento sopra la peste*, n.p. in dedication.

[45] Giudici, *Il Trattato della peste*, 5.

this fear, people have changed their ways; many in concubinage have unloosened the knot with the Devil, leaving their illicit partners and taking back the legitimate ones; others have transformed their lives for the better in other ways; many enemies have voluntarily made peace; others now are engaged in devout prayer.'[46]

The Sienese biographer of Pope Gregory XIII, Marcantonio Ciappi, writing from Rome, where plague may have struck but did not wreak the devastation of either the north or south, began his tract on preserving community health where plague may be suspected, not by defining plague or describing its signs and symptoms, but by describing its fear and terror. Although war, discord among princes, famine, and popular rebellion caused 'a thousand tribulations and suffering', no other misfortune, he claimed, caused the same mass fear as plague. Beyond the infinite suffering of individuals with the sight of so many dying daily, plague brought every day the fear of death. Unlike the Paduan notary, Ciappi saw no silver lining beneath this mass fear; instead, hunted down by plague, men became cruel, and losing all humanity, wives came to abhor then abandon their husbands, and vice versa.[47]

The plague writers of 1575–8 saw this fear coming not only from the disease itself and mass burials but also from social and political policy. Its consequences went beyond opening the pores or windpipes of individuals, making them more susceptible to plague. Benedetti recounted that at the beginning of July in Venice, policies that brought fear to everyone increased in number; the princes of Italy passed bans against Venice, prohibiting even messengers to enter the city, and almost all foreigners began to leave along with noblemen, while other wealthy citizens retreated to their villas. Cloth merchants, who employed two-thirds of the city's work force, ceased operation. Judges, notaries, and other officials left, leaving only the poor ('miserabile') behind.[48]

Lorenzo Condivi, a doctor at the Sorbonne and librarian of the court of Henry III, wrote a plague tract in Italian which circulated in Italian cities and which was entirely focused on fear in plague time. In addition to seeing fear of plague as a cause of death, he attributed the problem to the state—an infinity of officers and ministers of the plague, not to speak of the health board, the sight of so many grave-diggers in the streets with their horrible faces, bizarre manners and fearsome voices:

if you pass any corner, you see the porters and boatmen ('Caronti'), carrying away the plague-stricken and healthy indifferently, both abducted and tied to the carts destined for the lazaretti, which meant to the slaughter house ('beccaria'), where above its portal stands: 'Leave all hope behind, Ye who enter', without any consolation, without any access to your own things or to speak with any living being or to say goodbye to a family

---

[46] Canobbio, *Il successo*, 2r–3v. [47] Ciappi, *Regola da preseruarsi*, 464r–v (BAV copy).
[48] Benedetti, *Raguaglio*, 482r–v.

member . . . a desperate death in terrible agony . . . without the offices of Christian piety, without funerary rites, to die like a dog and worse.[49]

Condivi, however, did not end on this desperate note or with Fioravanti's laissez-faire. He saw hope first by brushing aside fear and melancholy with banquets, singing, playing musical instruments, dancing, and after returning home and locking all the windows and doors, having a good drink.[50] Moreover, he went beyond the individual and placed hope also with the state: through its systems of financial support and provisioning of the inflected, plague could be remedied.[51]

Finally, fear itself had direct economic consequences, which plague writers in 1575–8 addressed. In addition to a breakdown in contacts within the city, 'with friends and family refusing to assist one another',[52] the prohibitions on trade and the closing of shops, fear of contagion also frightened those from the countryside coming to the city and provisioning it with food. Canobbio noted in April (even before the summer escalation of deaths) that those from villages and walled towns, near and far, even subjects of the Venetian dominion, had abandoned the capital. If they had any dealings with the city, it was with utmost fear and suspicion.[53] In the poetic praises of Verona's podestà, one of the hydra-headed challenges to Barbarigo's rule was the problem of Verona's peasants, who 'abandoned the city, refusing to bring it the things it needed to survive', and 'on the pretext of fear of plague', became stubborn, even rebels ('rubelli') against public authority, breaking every sort of law to attend to their own health'. Immediately, it caused great desperation among the *popoli* and especially for the infinite numbers who lacked all means of survival.[54]

Others were less descriptive and more analytical on the causes and consequences of mass fear during the plague. Fioravanti and Raimondo were not the only doctors to point to strategies of sequestering, locked houses, quarantine, and the lazaretti as terrorizing the poor, worsening defences against plague. Donzellini attempted to understand why the poor ('la vil plebe & gente povera') harboured the disease more than other classes and why it spread mostly in their neighbourhoods. While he admitted that there were many reasons, he seized on one: they vigorously tried to conceal the disease. Behind this problem for doctors and the community at large, he alleged, lay fear and systematic problems with the structure of health politics during plague.[55] Donzellini stressed three reasons why commoners concealed their affliction. One is borne of avarice and fear that their property, while of little value, will be burnt. The second is fear of being refused assistance by doctors and relatives. And third is the fear of being carted to the lazaretti, where most die.

---

[49] Condivi, *Medicina filosofica contra la peste*, 7v. On Condivi also see Hipp, 'Poussin's The Plague at Ashdod', 207.

[50] Condivi, *Medicina filosofica contra la peste*, 210v–11r.   [51] Ibid., 195v.

[52] Canobbio, *Il successo*, 9r.   [53] Ibid., 9r.   [54] *Raccolta delli componimenti*, 3r.

[55] Ibid., 311v–12r.

For these, Donzellini offered three recommendations—'remedies', as he called them—not for the individual but for the body politic, for the health system of Venice and, by implication, of other Italian cities. Unlike Fioravanti, he did not call for dismantling health policy but for more of it: (1) the goods of the infected and suspected should not be burnt immediately but, if possible, cleaned by water, perfume, or buried under ground or in sand; (2) to combat fear of abandonment by doctors and relatives, the city should pass an ordinance arranging for the plague-stricken to be taken from the city to a house for the afflicted, where their clothes and goods would be immediately purified, where doctors would visit them at their doors and treat them with the best remedies. The third source of fear was the lazaretti.[56] Already Baravalle's poem during the previous plague of 1555–6, had identified this fear as one of the Hydra monster's seven heads.[57] Donzellini's 1576 account went further and offered specific recommendations. First, he advised the city to appoint trustworthy servants to be stationed at the lazaretti and that those caught stealing from the poor and afflicted should be hanged.[58] In addition, 'medical physicians and intelligent surgeons' must be employed there 'and not charlatans ('ceretani'), empirics ('empirici'), vagabonds, or butchers of Christians as usually is the case'. These doctors should supply simple and compound medicines, which are good and solid ('reali') and not sophisticated or advanced drugs. The lazaretti need to be kept clean and tidy and not left with dead bodies locked inside. Rubbish and filth must be regularly and immediately removed and the rooms perfumed daily or 'even more than once a day'. He then discussed in detail the types of perfumes and how to dispense them in the lazaretti. Finally, like Ingrassia, he discussed the architectural organization and construction of lazaretti, the need for different rooms to treat different types of patients. By Donzellini's plan, they were to be divided into four *appartamenti*: one for the infected, another for the suspected, a third for those recovering but still under quarantine, and a fourth for those who have just emerged from the first section but had yet to complete their quarantine.[59]

A year later (1577), the Veronese druggist Giovan' Andrea Bellicocchi, who, unlike his compatriot Donzellini, remained in Verona, wrote a plague tract addressed to the health board of his city. Without citing Donzellini, this tract echoed almost verbatim Donzellini's complaints and 'remedies' for reforming public health, his notions of the spread of plague principally among the poor, and

---

[56] On the lazaretti of Venice and elsewhere, see Palmer, 'The Control of Plague', ch. 7; and Stevens, 'The *lazaretti* of Venice, Verona and Padua', Ph.D. thesis, Cambridge, 2008, which I read only when the book was in production.

[57] Baravalle, *L'Historia della peste di Padoa*, 513v.

[58] This appears to have been the policy of Milan's lazaretto under the draconian rule of Bellintani, who recommended capital punishment for robbing the poor in plague time; *Dialogo della peste*, 141–3 and 147–8.

[59] Donzellini, *Discorso nobilissimo*, 311v. Such recommendations were similar to Ingrassia's and went beyond current arrangements of pesthouses present anywhere in northern cities.

his ideas about the plebs' fears and how to assuage them.[60] Perhaps influenced by the Jewish doctor de Pomi and others, Bellicocchi saw the plague as a disease of poor neighbourhoods and bad housing and proposed to avoid the horrors of the lazaretti and problems of locked houses by providing the poor and plague-stricken with new and uncontaminated temporary housing within the city ('allogiamento sincero'). The health board would then clean and purify their infected homes along with all their possessions left inside. Bellicocchi added to Donzellini's resolutions: doctors were to be divided by the gates of the city charged with treating the plague-stricken in their districts; 'to the best of their abilities', they were to employ the full range of their remedies, and these must be administered in the new housing set aside for the plague-stricken. In this way, Bellicocchi maintained, 'the poor would not be abandoned by friends and kin'. Finally, in the druggist's scheme lazaretti would not disappear; they would, however, accommodate only the plague-stricken left without friends or family. Further, the lazaretti needed reforming; here he copied Donzellini's plans closely: regular and frequent visitation by proper physicians and surgeons; quarters to undergo thorough and daily cleaning; plague corpses removed immediately and rooms purged with heavy-duty 'perfumes' ('acuto et vigore'). Showing his professional expertise, the druggist provided far greater detail here than the doctor. His list of drugs included compounds with arsenic acid, sulphur, pitch, resin, liquid storax, turpentine, sandarac, antimony, incense, and myrrh; the best vinegar for washing rooms; grains from wormwood to be burnt to purify the air; and the list goes on. He then returned to Donzellini's plan of the lazaretti divided into four parts, (still without giving him credit),[61] but perhaps, because he was not a doctor, the druggist did not consider nearly so carefully as Donzellini the problems of contagion and spread of the disease back to the community.

Criticisms of the state and those employed to assist the plague-stricken did not end with the plague of 1575–8 . These later doctors, however, did not dismiss the intervention and support of the state as Fioravanti had before 1575. The proposals of the physician Arellano at the end of the century turned in exactly the opposite direction. Like Fioravanti, Arellano began with remedies and liquors of his own invention and a diatribe not against the policies of a particular city but against the behaviour of states in general and the Church. However, he attributed the cruelty of fathers abandoning children, husbands abandoning wives, and the destruction wrought by the 'horrible monster' plague to states' failure to act—their 'silence'—asserting that, when plague came, magistrates, princes, and city governors (*signori*) fled or refused to place impositions on trade and commerce from fear of losing business. But what astounded him more was that, 'because of fear of this Hydra', governors failed to care for the infected; priests refused to come to their aid, and heaps of plague dead were left unadmitted to their graves. 'With such infinite disorder, the fright of counsellors, the sequestering of men,

---

[60] Bellicocchi, *Avvertimenti*, 411v–12r.   [61] Ibid., 412r–13r.

the locking of houses, and the inexperience of doctors, all vanished into a whisper and into ruin.' Arellano's tract then pleaded to governments and 'those whose job it was to pass the necessary laws and ordinances to act and to become bold'.[62]

In his chapter on the causes of plague, fear along with many other factors accounted for the plague's spread. Once again, he poured scorn on the weakness and incompetence of governments. There were 'internal' reasons for the plague's dissemination, which involved putrefaction of the air and the body's condition to receive the contagion. But Arellano then went beyond these Galenic doctrines and concentrated on the external reasons, listing six causes. These centred on government and mass fear. First, he charged that the paucity of ordinances passed by governors, their inadequate provisioning of necessary things, and doctors' lack of experience were responsible 'for the great fear of the people that led to flight and spread of the disease'. Secondly, he pointed to the failure of the governors ('Superiori') to purge the streets, clean sewers, remove filth from alleyways and houses in the city and countryside or to supply medications and medical treatment especially to the poor. Thirdly, he saw fear leading to the 'extreme sadness of the soul', contributing further to the plague's death counts. Fourthly, fear, which led to flight, caused problems beyond merely fanning contagion; it also provoked hatred among communities and resistance to outsiders. He cited recent examples from his own region. During the current plague, gate-guards at the Piedmont town of Rivoli had added to the plague's death tolls by murdering those attempting to enter the town and those trying to escape it. Fifthly, he charged that governments' inadequate provisioning led to deaths from famine and thirst. Finally, doctors' lack of training increased mortality and fear. According to Arellano, every time such unprepared doctors discovered a glandular swelling or a *carbuculo*, they diagnosed it as plague, reported it to the health board, and ordered the house to be sequestered, which caused many deaths, 'when it is clear from many places and the most expert opinion that the simple appearance of these signs alone did not mean that the case was one of plague'.[63] As we have seen, by the last quarter of the sixteenth century, politics had now become a normal part of the doctor's terrain. Whether they praised or chided their states, they saw their expertise and grounded their remedies in political action as much as in pharmacology or theorizing about the mutation of air. With Arellano, criticism and evaluation of the political now concentrated as much on alleviating the psychological ramifications of plague as its medical pathology.

SPIRITUAL AND PSYCHOLOGICAL RENEWAL

Despite the protests, swaggers, mismanagement, and corruption, plague writers after Fioravanti to the end of the century backed governments' long-standing

---

[62] Arellano, *Trattato di peste*, 2–3.   [63] Ibid., 28–9.

structures of sequestration, quarantine, and lazaretti as necessary and efficacious. As Canobbio had concluded for the plague in 1576–7, '[t]he most
effective remedy' ('Il piú gagliardo rimedio') had been to send the infected and their goods to the lazaretti and the suspected from the city to stay
in the wooden huts ('caselle di legno').[64] The outrage of those from inside
and outside the medical profession against Mercuriale and the Paduan academy had not turned on disputed terms in Galen but on observations. They
had seen the consequences of the academicians' recommendations that loos-
ened trade restrictions and ended sequestration; mortality in Venice suddenly
reversed during the summer of 1576, soaring above that of any other major city
in Italy.

Furthermore, writers of this plague were astonished at and proud of the sums
which their states had mobilized to alleviate the pain and suffering of the plague-
afflicted, the great majority of whom, as one doctor after another noted, were
the poor. According to Canobbio, Padua spent 50,000 *scudi* in its fight against
plague. Besta estimated the Milanese expenditure on food alone to feed the poor
during the plague at 70,000 *scudi*.[65] The chronicler Bugati marvelled at the expert
and innovative administration initiated by the Milanese senate during the plague,
establishing laundries and places to purge infected goods throughout the city
and creating depots for food distribution and other necessities at every gate,
parish, and neighbourhood. The generosity of the daily rations clearly impressed
him—24 ounces of bread a day per person (10 ounces from white flour and 14
from rye), along with a half *mettà* of white rice, an ounce of salt, and various
quantities of wine, cheese, meat, fowl, mutton, game, fruit, vegetables, vinegar,
wood, and small pieces of charcoal ('carbonina') per head every ten days. Over
800 barrels (*brente*) of wine and 900 capons were doled out daily, all costing the
state many thousands of *scudi*.[66] In his poem of liberation, the Florentine exile
Borgaruccio boasted that the Venetian government constructed over 500 houses
of wood and delivered the best of care for those sent to the Lazaretto nuovo,
where over 10,000 ducats were well spent: 'the prince had spared no expense
[*ogni cosa piú cara*] helping his people'.[67] The bleak picture of life for the poor
and the horrid conditions of lazaretti described by some such as Raimondo is
here given another slant:

> Brodi, Stillati, Capponi, e Galline,
> Pollastri, e carne di Manzo, o vitello,
> Non mancan lor, né vin nelle cantine.[68]

---

[64] Canobbio, *Il successo*, 34r.   [65] Besta, *Vera narratione*, 18r.

[66] Bugati, *L'aggiunta*, 157. According to a Milanese ordinance of 3 December 1576, over 100,000
scudi was set aside to feed the poor 'who were infinite in number in this city'. The funds were taken from
part of the *dacio*, a sales tax on wine (*Gride diverse*, no. 81).

[67] Borgarucci, *L'afflition di Vinetia*, 10–11.

[68] Ibid., 10. In addition, see the generous rations stipulated in Bellintani, *Dialogo della peste*, 139.

[Broths, drippings, capons, and hens
Young fowl, beefsteak, or veal
They are wanting for nothing, including wine from the cellar.]

The Milanese gate-guard Besta went into greater detail, specifying the varying amounts of bread and *minestra di riso* allocated to men, women, and children.[69] Towards the end of his account he reflected on his own experiences as an officer of one of the poorest parishes in Milan, San Lorenzo,[70] in charge of inspecting housing, registering families, reporting their state of health, and issuing plague passports: 'I could never have believed that so large a number of poor people could have been fed so well for such a long time, with the regular provision of six *quattrini* of bread a day and small portions of other food.' For Besta, this mass provisioning depended not only on the government but also on the charity of its citizens.[71]

Furthermore, Besta and others lauded the monies raised for individual works and charities, such as the 600 *scudi* solicited by Borromeo from the populace ('fu fatta una general elemosina') for the new plague hospital outside Milan called Vittoria.[72] In gratitude for the decline of plague deaths in 1577, the Venetian government's initial payment to begin construction of 'the temple' in honour of Jesus Christ, the Redeemer, on the island of Giudecca—il Redentore—amounted to 1,500 *scudi*.[73] The bill to clean a single quarter of the city of Palermo over seven days during the height of the 1576 plague cost 1,000 *scudi*.[74] At the new lazaretto of Palermo (la Cubba), the state spent no less than 5,000 *scudi* in a single month for new clothing alone for the infected. For these and other expenses including the salaries for the construction of the lazaretto and other charities for the ill, Palermo spent more than 60,000 *scudi* in only five months and yet this was a city which in comparison with northern ones such as Trent, Mantua, Padua, Milan, and especially Venice, was largely spared the full brunt of the plague.[75] Bugati gave the largest figure for plague charities of the 1575–8 plague, one million gold *scudi*, counting contributions from the city, the nobility, and King Philip II for Milan.[76] As Carlo Cipolla has shown for seventeenth-century Italy, such enormous expenditures in plague years could cripple economies and lead to bankruptcies and future hardship across social classes that would last for decades.[77] With the seventeenth-century plagues, a more sorrowful gloss

[69] Besta, *Vera narratione*, 20v–21r.
[70] On San Lorenzo, see Saba, 'Una parrocchia milanese'; and D'Amico, *Le contrade e la città*, 34, 37, and 54.
[71] Besta, *Vera narratione*, 36v.   [72] Ibid., 16r.   [73] Benedetti, *Raguaglio*, 490r.
[74] Ingrassia, *Parte quinta*, 36–7.   [75] Ingrassia, *Informatione*, 235.
[76] Bugati, *L'aggiunta*, 170.
[77] Cipolla, *Cristofano and the Plague*, esp. 109–17. Also, see his *Faith, Reason, and the Plague*, p. 81, and the sorrowful report of Father Dragoni, head of Montelupo's health board, on 25 August 1630, two weeks after the last plague death: 'A large part [of the people] are dead, the rest are ruined or quarantined. There are plenty of debts. No one is to be found who will make loans or give credit . . . he who can pay [taxes] makes more trouble than the poor man.' In the secondary literature on the Italian plague of

was often placed on these expenditures and their consequences. By contrast, the raising and deployment of these vast sums in 1575–8 sparked civic pride, prompting plague writers such as Besta, Canobbio, Benedetti, and others to proclaim their cities' triumph over plague.

Plague literature of 1575–8 illustrates not only a celebratory relief with the plague's cessation but a new sense of triumph that swept across Italy. With earlier plagues, even major ones as in 1523–4 or 1528–30, the termination of affliction passed almost without notice, at least in publications about plague: no poems of congratulation or praise of local magistrates and functionaries as epic heroes ranging from a soon-to-be canonized saint to choir masters and bell-ringers. There may have been processions thanking God or a city's patron saint but no optimistic self-reflections embodied in artistic displays, floats, and other events mounted by secular and ecclesiastical authorities as described in verse and prose in 1576 to 1578. Only one exception emerges in the Italian plague literature as far as I find, Cristoforo Baravalle's poem celebrating Padua's liberation in 1556.[78]

For the 1575–8 plague, however, the change in mentality from fear and angst to celebration and triumph overflowed in the plague literature and not just in poems and pamphlets entitled liberation. For instance, in Milan, May 1576, with signs of the plague's decline but with the city's women and children still locked in their homes and permitted to participate only from windows, the Milanese Jesuit Bisciola described Carlo Borromeo's procession of the Holy Nail, three times around the city: 'This time there was not the same mood as the previous time', when the Holy Nail had been processed in October. Then, the cardinal had called for three days of fasting and went barefoot round the city, dressed for sadness with a large cord around his neck, a hood over his head, dragging his cloak along the ground, and accompanied by a thousand flagellants dressed the same beating themselves continually. 'But what moved the lower classes ('l'inferior del popolo') the most' was that great black cross with the Holy Nail coming from it and blood dripping from the feet of the Holy Cardinal.[79] In contrast to that morose baroque spectacle—what we might expect from plague and mass death during the Counter-Reformation—by May, Bisciola's descriptions illustrate a populace radically transformed, 'there was magnificent happiness and a sense of triumph'.[80]

The Milanese officer Besta described the same transition in the city's ceremonial life between October 1576 and February—the cardinal dressed as described

1629–33 I have found no evidence of commentators boasting about how much their governments spent to contain the plague as indicative of civic pride.

[78] Baravalle, *L'historia della peste di Padoa*, 518v, see Chapter 5 above.

[79] Bisciola, *Relatione verissima del progresso della peste*, 4r.

[80] Ibid., 5v. As shown earlier, women and children were excluded because they were believed to be more contagious and susceptible to plague. Indeed, in urban places such as Milan, they died in significantly greater numbers.

above, followed by the governor of Milan, senators and magistrates, the *popolo* and the religious orders 'filled with tears, sobbing, frightful, lachrymose cries for mercy, beseeching the Lord to pardon them for their sins and the horror of their errors, which had moved God with justified rage to punish them with the plague'.[81] In February the atmosphere changed from these dark hues to confident self-praise: the heads of families processed with their guild flags, representing the entire city. In celebration of men like himself—the ordinary officer in Milan's battle against plague—Besta concluded: 'the diligence of the inspectors and guards of the gates' have won the city's liberation and would ensure that 'Milan would never again fall into the same misery and affliction'.[82]

In Venice, the celebrations appear to have been even more elaborate and costly. We have seen that Lumina's *La Liberatione di Vinegia* described in detail the triumphal floats, governmentally led processions, and ornate works of art constructed above streets and on church portals throughout the city. Despite earlier controversies and the highest mortality of any city in Italy during that or any sixteenth-century plague, Venice's transformation in Lumina's pages was total. Even the earlier discredited government, swayed by the Paduan 'dotti', emerged triumphant: 'under their happy rule and decrees, having wiped the city clean of the contagion, they [the Doge and Senate] wished to display this happiness, which they felt might be achieved by works of art'. Written the day after the city's liberation, Lumina concluded his observations: 'Lord I confess, that had I not witnessed the plague in Venice, I would have thought not only that none had died but that the Venetian population had doubled. Such a throng of people not only filled the spacious *campo* of San Marco but all the balconies and sun terraces so that the entire Grand Canal was cloaked in people. Such was this liberation no one could get enough of it.'[83]

According to Benedetti, the celebrations and radical transformation in spirit began earlier; 1 January 1577 marked the first day since the plague's arrival without a single plague death registered. A procession 'open to all' filled the streets of Venice; 'incredible joy opened hearts that had been closed by so many tribulations; now everyone rejoiced together'.[84] Publications of short pieces celebrating cities' liberations from plague continued after 1575–8 . In a similar vein to Lumina and others in 1576–7, a short publication by Antonio Cornuto, a canon of Turin and almoner of the duke of Savoy, described in detail the elaborate floats and processions including 'great numbers of little virgins dressed in white to demonstrate the city's gratitude and happiness' upon its liberation

---

[81] Besta, *Vera narratione*, 16r.   [82] Ibid., 50r.

[83] Lumina, *La liberatione di Vinegia*, 477v and 478v. Similar amazement over throngs of people suddenly filling the banks of Grand Canal during this celebration can also be seen from archival sources; see Laughran, 'The Body, Public Health and Social Control', 263.

[84] Benedetti, *Raguaglio*, 490v. Along with other commentators of 1575–8 he emphasized the significance of processions for popular morale. On the secular role of religious processions in plague time, also see Horden, 'Ritual and Public Health', 24.

282

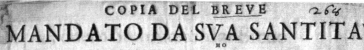

COPIA DEL BREVE

MANDATO DA SVA SANTITA'

ALL'ILLVSTRISS. DOMINIO
CON INDVLGENTIE CONCESSE
à tutti gl'Infermi di Mal Contagioso:

ET A' QVELLI CHE SERVENO ALLI PREDETTI:
& che negotiano per la liberatione di tal male, così nella città di Venetia,
come in tutti gli altri luoghi di esso Illustrissimo Dominio.

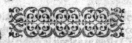

49.

GREGORIO PAPA DECIMOTERZO.

A Tvtti & cadaun Fedel di Christo de l'un'e l'altro sesso, nella Città di
Venetia, ouero luoghi ad essa soggetti, ammalati di mal contagioso; & à
quelli che per qual si uoglia modo li serueno, Salute, & Apostolica benedittio-
ne. Desiderando per il nostro Pastoral officio, & carità (quanto possiamo con
Dio) proueder opportunamente alla salute dell'anime uostre, à uoi, & à cadaun
di uoi, confessi & contriti in articolo di morte; ouero, se non ui potrete confes-
sare per causa ragioneuole, ui dolerete di uostri peccati; & con cuore almeno
(se non potrete dir con bocca) inuocareti il nome di Giesv. Indulgentia plenaria, & remission de tutti li uostri peccati, à uoi ueramente, che fareti qualche
opera de carità & pietà, uerso tali Infermi, cioè uisitandoli, seruendoli, medi-
candoli, ò ueramente facendoli qualche altra cosa necessaria, se sarete ò Laici ò
Ecclesiastici, ouero Regolari. Ancora à tutti uoi predetti, che pregareti Iddio
con mente, ouer con uoce, per liberatione della Peste, quante uolte farete alcu-
na delle cose predette, tante uolte cento anni, & tante quarantene dell'ingion-
te à uoi, & à chi si uuol di uoi; ouer per qual si uoglia modo debite penitentie.
Similmente à uoi, & ciaschedun di uoi, che reciterà deuotamente ad efferto pre-
detto, la corona, conseguite, & ciaschedun di noi consequisca le medesime Indulgentie, & remision di peccati, quali conseguiscono, ò conseguir posson
quel giorno che direte essa Corona, quelli, che uisitano le Chiese de l'alma Ci-
tà nostra, & fuori di suoi muri; confidatici della Misericordia dell'Onnipotente
Iddio, & dell'auttorità de' Beati suoi Apostoli Pietro & Paulo, misericordiosa-
mente nel Signore per le presenti, concedemo, relassemo, & donemo, non ostā-
te cadauna cosa che faccia in contrario.

Data in Roma, app... Sa... ro, sotto l'Anel del Pescatore. Adi vij Luglio.
M. D. LXXV. A... Quinto del nostro Pontificato.

Cesare Glorierio.

42.

Francesco Vianello Secretario Ducale.

Illustration 13. Pope Gregory XIII, *Mandato da sua santità all'illustriss. Dominio con indulgentie concesse a tutti gl'infermi di Mal Contagioso*, 8 July 1575.

from the plague in 1599.[85] Even in reporting the number killed by the plague in Milan that he estimated at 10,000 in the plague of 1576–7, Bugati saw success and praised the accomplishment of the Milanese people: without their diligence, humility, and prayers, 100,000 would have perished.[86]

CHURCH AND STATE

Such sentiments and praise of local administrators as Hercules triumphing over plague do not square with usual interpretations of the effects of devastating epidemics and mass mortality on mentalities. The men and women who survived the 1575–8 plague—Italy's worst of the sixteenth century and perhaps its worst since 1400—do not appear as broken, desperate figures retreating from bold secular ideals, turning to otherworldly transcendental religions, as William McNeill and others have depicted as a general trend in the world history of epidemics and mass catastrophe.[87] Far from a rejection of political power and the ideals of a strong state, the Church itself emerged as a more vigorous leader, not only of spiritual ideals, but especially in its civic organization and administration of charity, law, and health enforcement. As we have seen, the ecclesiastical statutes for Milan, Bologna, and Mantua during 1575–8 exhorted citizens to act collectively for the benefit of the poor, to obey the laws of secular magistrates and health boards, and to endure harsh measures of quarantine and other forms of sequestration. Cardinals and bishops marshalled their own troops to man dangerous positions attending the plague-stricken in huts, locked houses, and lazaretti. Even the spiritual measures consciously addressed needs that were not solely religious: by processions, the use of relics and new symbols such as Borromeo's Holy Nail, they sought to enliven, entertain, and encourage the faithful through the darkest days of contagion.[88]

Bugati presents a glowing image of the success of these spiritual practices during the general and repeated quarantines of Milan before the plague began to lift:

All the people together, in their houses, at their windows, from their balconies, or at their doors, celebrated the seven canonical hours, seven times, responding in litanies,

---

[85] Cornuato, *Breve relatione della processione solenne fatta in Torino*.

[86] Bugati, *L'aggiunta*, 164. Similar boasting of the low numbers killed in the 1575–8 plague is seen for Palermo and Verona.

[87] McNeill, *Plagues and Peoples*; Thorndike, 'The Blight of Pestilence': 'Like a cancer the fell disease [the plague] ate at the vitals of European civilization. Like an incubus it weighed upon the human imagination and spirit' (455).

[88] Jones, 'Plague and Its Metaphors', 106–14, divides the plague tract into three 'corporate' groups of writers, 'each with very different concerns and preoccupations': 'namely, medical practitioners, with their concern for health; churchmen, with their preoccupation with morality and spiritual welfare; and the representatives of secular authority, or magistrates, with their concern with community welfare and the workings of authority' (106). Such sharp divisions fail to ring true in 1575–8: a text such as Ingrassia's *Informatione* embodied all three voices simultaneously.

psalms, or prayers, responding to certain deputies [of Carlo Borromeo] placed in every *contrada*, singing in chorus to one another [*choro a choro*], men, women, and children, such that this great city appeared as a grand church in paradise, all praising and invoking the Lord.[89]

In the face of the gravest moments of the plague, with death tolls reaching ninety a day at Padua, the notary Canobbio, so sceptical of Galenic theories of corrupt air, constellations, and the like, took solace along with his citizens in prayers, devotions, and processions of Padua's most sacred image of the Virgin organized by the Church, even if controversies arose over the removal of the image from its original lunette.[90] The last hopes in those dark hours were, as Canobbio shows, in the building of new oratories and churches: in Padua these were constructed in part by the wretched themselves.[91] He fully believed in the powers of sacred paintings and Christian rituals in the fight against the plague.[92] The *Commentariolus*, whether its author was the head of Verona's health board or the city's bishop, shows complete cooperation between Church and State in their mutual effort to combat plague. If the magistrate Chiocco was its author, the centre of attention and praise was placed squarely on the city's bishop, Valier. If the bishop was the author, then the work shows collaboration between the city's highest-ranking prelate and its highest health officer, who signed this work's dedication addressed to the Veronesi.[93]

By the next transregional plague in Italy, that of 1629–31, the interaction and cooperation between Church and State appears not to have continued so seamlessly, at least in some places in Italy. Carlo Cipolla has highlighted the tensions between 'faith and reason' that erupted during the plagues in Tuscany, 1629–33, the conflict between the spiritual arm, which saw mass processions as necessary to placate God's ire—as the first remedy for curing plague—and secular health boards, which saw the assembling of crowds as the best means for spreading the contagion.[94] Already in 1348, doctors had seen plague as a disease of explosive contagion that distinguished it from all other diseases.[95] Nor had doctors in the sixteenth century lost sight of this essential characteristic; they too advised their patients and readers not to assemble in times of plague. Because of plague, the Venetian government had prohibited public preaching in 1497, 1509, 1510, and 1511; processions in 1512 and 1530; and in 1509 and 1529 feast days had been postponed.[96] It is easy to assume that tensions between the medical corps and churchmen would have grown early on in plague time and all the more during the Counter-Reformation

89 Bugati, *L'aggiunta*, 156.   90 Canobbio, *Il successo*, 25v.   91 Ibid., 26r.
92 Ibid., 28v: 'Voglio dare per la spesa che occorrerà in servigio di questa santa imagine'.
93 See the discussion in Chapter 4, 131–3.
94 Cipolla, *Faith, Reason, and the Plague*; and idem, *Fighting the Plague*, 56.
95 See Cohn, *The Black Death Transformed*, 208–9.
96 Palmer, 'The Control of Plague', 300; and idem, 'The Church, Leprosy and Plague', 96.

with powerful Church leaders such as Borromeo, Paleotti, Gonzaga, and Pope Gregory XIII in 1575–8 . As far as plague writings go, this was not, however, the case.[97]

As we have seen, this plague was not without its critics and complaints about sequestration, theories of academic doctors, the evil of grave-diggers and plague cleaners, the ingratitude of the poor masses, the disobedience and turbulence of workers and artisans, the supposed selfishness of peasants, the incompetence of doctors, and the mismanagement and negligence of the state. Plague writers criticized friars and priests who from fear shirked their spiritual obligations—Holy Communion, confession, and the celebration of last rites. But, surprisingly, in the midst of the suffering and fault finding, even writers such as Panizzone Sacco did not criticize the Church hierarchy for organizing processions and jubilees that assembled churchmen and laity in these contagious times. Instead, lay authors praised Church leaders for initiating collective religious rites, because these lifted the spirits of the poor and others who remained in plague-stricken cities.[98] In addition, ascetic strictures and notions about contagion could be mutually supportive, as the parish guard Besta observed in Milan during the height of the plague in 1576: 'And a new mode of dressing came about, because judges and senators dressed in short and light ('succinti') suits and these were seen to spread the contagion less than the various types of pompous and ornate dress, previously sported throughout the city.'[99]

[97] Hanlon, *Early Modern Italy*, 227, for instance, claims that three 'great' processions of October 'dismayed the health officers' of Milan but shows no evidence for it. As we shall see, Borromeo limited these processions to a select group and threatened others who joined with severe penalties (288–9 below). Pacagnini, 'Introduction' to Bellintani, *Dialogo della peste*, 18, maintains that conflicts between Borromeo and the civil authorities over processions were usual, but also fails to supply any evidence for it. Palmer, 'The Control of Plague', 320, comes to the same conclusion for the late sixteenth and seventeenth centuries, not only for Venice, but for Counter-Reformation culture in northern Italy in general, manifested in a conflict between the pragmatism of health boards and theology. Also see idem, 'The Church, Leprosy and Plague', 94–7, where he argues that such conflict characterized plagues from the fourteenth to the seventeenth century but intensified in the sixteenth. Horden, 'Ritual and Public Health', 38, argues that these conflicts evolved slowly from the rise of city-states in thirteenth-century Italy to the eighteenth century. His evidence comes, however, exclusively from Cipolla. On the other hand, according to Bamji, 'Religion and Disease in Venice', this was not the case even with the 1630–1 plague in Venice. Church and State 'worked together to promote the spiritual, as well as the physical health of the city' (132). However, for the fifteenth and sixteenth centuries she cites examples of conflict between Church and State during plague, such as in Venice in 1485, when church services were banned and in Geneva in the sixteenth century, when those infected with plague were excluded from church service. In retaliation, churchmen refused to cooperate with the city authorities and to provide plague hospitals with a chaplain. Finally, Bowers, 'Plague, Politics', 13, also finds cooperation and mutual respect between municipal leaders and the Church in their struggle against late sixteenth-century plagues in Seville (1581–2 and 1599–1600).

[98] See for instance Besta, *Vera narratione*, 29r–v.

[99] Ibid., 24r–v. However, as Pacagnini, 'Introduction', 30–1, argues, the severity of controls and punishments imposed by the Capuchin authority in charge of Milan's Lazaretto left lasting bitterness in the oral tradition that surfaced with the next big plague in 1630 as seen in the commentary of Giuseppe Ripamonti.

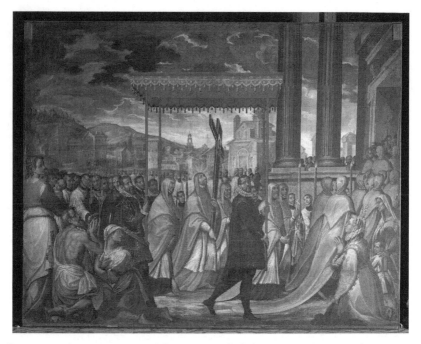

Illustration 14. Gian Battista della Rovere, called Il Fiammenighino, *Carlo Borromeo's procession of the Holy Nail, 1600.* Tempera on Canvas.

In Milan, the laity and churchmen praised their 'Good Pastor' Carlo Borromeo along with the state for their mutually supportive laws combating plague. The Jesuit Bisciola began his tract by placing Borromeo, the king of Spain's lieutenant in Milan, the Milanese Senate, and deputies of the health board all on the same high pedestal: future generations could learn from their laws and provisions during times of pestilence: Borromeo was 'the perfect pastor, who loved his flock'; the Prince and his magistrates showed how to govern in such trying times. Perhaps such praise of the cardinal is not surprising coming from a cleric. But the eulogies were not limited to the clergy. On the eve of the city's liberation from plague, Besta was as gushing:

One could only speak of him in saintly terms and this in a great city at a time when she was stripped of all sweetness [*delicie*] like a bride stripped of all signs of beauty. Oh, how the city was broken, made into a mirror of misery. But the city and its citizens were taken into his lap and now made every effort to show their gratitude toward his so loving and courteous deeds.[100]

<hr/>

[100] Besta, *Vera narratione*, 38r.

Besta saw Borromeo's processions 'as being the principal remedy of the city's liberation, lifting the sin that had so moved the wrath of God against them'.[101] The diary of the carpenter Giambattista Casale poured further devotion on the 'Illustrious Cardinal', concentrating on his deeds even more than had the Jesuit Bisciola. The carpenter saw the city's imposition of its first general quarantine as bringing great results ('uno grandissimo profitto'), but then he reflected that the improvement hinged 'not so much on the quarantine' as on acts of the Illustrious Cardinal, in particular, his barefoot processions with the Holy Nail and wearing the cord round his neck.[102]

Lay praise also flowed from the pen of the outsider Panizzone Sacco, who in the depths of despair had fired a barrage of complaints against various targets. In those days of Milan's impending fate as 'Sodom and Gomorrah', only three individuals in Panizzone Sacco's opinion were above sin, petty crime, and cowardice and worthy of praise—first, 'il mio cittadino & Pastor Carlo Borromeo', then the temporal ruler, Don Antonio de Guzman marchese d'Aimonte 'Governator mio', and later in his tract Milan's chief magistrate, Gabrio Serbelloni.[103] Even during the height of the plague, the Cardinal's fame and example had spread to other cities and was exalted by lay writers such as Canobbio, who reported that the 'Holy Pastor of Milan was always on the front-line in this horrible struggle, armed only with charity'. The notary continued by praising clerics in his own city, listing numerous religious orders of men and women who had played their part and had died as a result. His plague chronicle ended with a list of commemoration praising those men and women who faithfully stayed at their posts despite the terror of contagion. These were not only the city's highest leaders but included the choir master at the cathedral of Padua, the organist, singers, custodians, chaplains, *zaghi* (masters of ceremonies within the Venetian church), messengers, and even a cathedral bell-ringer.[104]

The plague tracts leave no trace of any strident conflict between Church and State during this plague.[105] Perhaps future archival research may reflect another face. However, against historians' assumptions that the flourishing of Church power with Counter-Reformation culture brought Church and State into conflict with drastically different notions on how to combat plague, plague writing in 1575–8 plots another story: Church and State bound together in mutual support

---

[101] Ibid., 30r.

[102] *Il diario di Giambattista Casale*, 301. Also, see Bellintani, *Dialogo della peste*, 105–6, 108–9, 112–13 and elsewhere, on Carlo Borromeo as the model of pastoral care, charity, and leadership during plague.

[103] Panizzone Sacco, *Pianto della città di Milano*, 1r, 4v, and 12v.

[104] Canobbio, *Il successo*, 14v.

[105] See Martin, *Plague?*, 199–200, on Jesuit faith in the medical profession and its enthusiasm for doctors' preservatives and remedies.

against a common enemy.[106] Such cooperation and mutual sympathy is present in plague legislation promulgated by health boards and city governments,[107] as they joined in partnership with the Church and figures such as Carlo Borromeo to plan and control religious festivals, and not only after the plague had declined or disappeared altogether. For instance, with the plague's first Christmas in Milan, 1576, the health board eased their conditions of quarantine, partially because plague mortalities had declined with the coming of winter but also so that feasts for the Nativity could be enjoyed. From 20 December to 7 January heads of households—but they alone—were permitted to join Christmas processions and festivities.[108] Doctors, such as the community physician of Udine in 1576–7, supported the practice of his health board and counselled a public procession on the second day of Pentecost as the first public measure to protect the city from the plague.[109]

This cooperation must be attributed in large part to the clergy's fear and understanding of the plague as highly contagious and its willingness to take seriously plague's 'inferior' or natural as opposed to divine causes. Ecclesiastical ordinances enacted by those at the pinnacle of the Church's hierarchy—Borromeo

---

[106] Pullan, 'Plague and Perceptions of the Poor ', 105, maintains that tensions over contagion and processions between Church and clergy, on the one hand, and the state and doctors, on the other, were present or latent during plagues in general. However, he supplies no examples. Nutton, 'Medicine in Medieval Western Europe', maintains that increasingly from the fifteenth century onwards, strong differences emerged between secular and religious approaches to plague . . . This conflict of ideas also reflects a conflict in authority . . . in opposition to the Church' (196). More emphatically, Palmer, 'The Control of Plague', 280, charges that officers of the health board and those of the Church operated according to two conflicting approaches and theories about plague, that from the late fifteenth century on 'the growing conviction that plague could be controlled by practical techniques, which was expressed in the foundation of the Health Offices, opened a division between religious and civil notions of how plague should be dealt with' (297–8). 'In northern Italy the occurrence in the 1570s, at the height of Counter-Reformation, of the most severe epidemic since the Black Death, gave new vigour to the concept of plague as a punishment for sin.' According to Palmer, this otherworldly view clashed with 'the contagionist philosophy of the Health Office'—'a wholly secular account of plague and its causes' (302). He argues for the same chronological divide in 'The Church, Leprosy and Plague', 97: in the plague of the 1570s 'in town after town the civic authorities turned ultimately to sacred remedies'. However, he cites little evidence for it; only that governments turned to sacred remedies such as the Redentore in Venice, implying that they also turned against secular ones. Yet, despite this supposed ideological conflict between the Church, on the one hand, and the health board and the medical profession on the other ('The Control of Plague', 308), he acknowledges that the two could sometimes agree and collaborate: 'At the same time, the church orders took note of the danger of contagion, and urged the clergy to cooperate fully with the Health Offices' (308). In addition, Davi, *Bernardino Tomitano*, 44, charges that the 'psychological influence of the Counter-Reformation' propelled the recovery of plague as divine retribution and the refutation of the medical realism of the previous plague in 1555–6, but produces no evidence for this.

[107] See for instance the plague ordinance in Milan (*Gride diverse*, no. 31), which alerted houses to receive benediction from Carlo Borromeo and the Church but excluded those who had been excommunicated or were prostitutes, usurers, loan-sharks ('barratarie'), ran prohibited games, or practised other criminal behaviour.

[108] *Gride diverse*, no. 87, 1576.xii.19. On 27 December the health board found that confusion and corruption had arisen in the granting of licences for heads of households to circulate through the city and that the intermingling was threatening the 'good work' of the health board; ibid., no. 88, 1576.xii.27.

[109] Daciano, *Trattato della peste*, 42.

and the Capuchin Bellintani in Milan, Gonzaga in Verona, Paleotti in Bologna, and Razzi in Florence—to protect the lives of their own clerics, who administered to the plague-stricken attests to their awareness of plague's dangers of virulent contagion.[110] At the end of the century, Rutilo Benzoni, bishop of Loreto and Recanati went further. Not only were some clerics given permission to flee the plague, they had an obligation to protect themselves against contagion and were advised to avoid any contact with the infected when administering the sacraments. In addition, they were ordered to buy and use antidotes, preservatives, and other medicines prepared by pharmacists to avoid infection and further spread of the disease.[111]

Until secular governments had officially declared their cities 'liberated' from plague, the religious leaders themselves limited religious processions to select groups of religious orders and magistrates. As Borromeo's calls for processions make clear, the uninvited were severely punished if they left their homes, regardless of their piety or religious motivation. Furthermore, he also granted licences to clergy not to participate, if they so desired.[112] Governments made accommodations for these measures by allowing processions yet passing plague ordinances to regulate them with strict limits to small minorities.[113] The health board of Milan and Carlo Borromeo even promulgated plague laws together.[114] In addition, Church leaders invented other forms of religious devotion to create a sense of religious community without risk of physical intermingling. Realizing that plague casualties were mounting in July 1576, Padua's Church leader ('Il molto Reverendo Monsignor Vicario') persuaded his flock to perform 'extra' prayers twice daily at a specified time in mid-morning and evening in their own homes. He ordered all the parish priests to ring their church bells as the signal for these prayers; 'thus all the families and all the city together at the same moment prayed to God for the liberation of Padua and Venice'.[115] In Milan, according to the carpenter Casale, even before the government imposed a general quarantine, every evening the population engaged in prayer from their windows and doorways so that the city 'appeared as one united church'.[116] And when the general quarantine was imposed in October 1576, 'every day, seven times a day', the population locked in their homes chanted the litany with 'other beautiful prayers, Pater Nostri and Ave Marie contained in a *libretto* distributed by the government'. 'Each at the window, the neighbourhood in unison' responded in these acts of devotion. The carpenter describes the means by which Church

---

110 For Bellintani, see *Dialogo della peste*, 105–6. For the others, see Chapter 8.
111 Benzoni, *Tractatus de Fuga*, 4v–5r, 8r–v, 11v–12r, and 12v–13v.
112 Borromeo, *Ordini d'orationi*, 1r–2v.
113 See the Milanese ordinance passed on 18 January 1577 for a day-long procession to the church of Saint Sebastian. On that day, the health board ruled that no one could leave their house except the few invited to participate, which, as far as the laity was concerned, seems to have included only the syndic of each parish; *Gride diverse*, nos 43, 50, 51, 52.
114 Ibid., no. 140, 1577.iv.2.   115 Canobbio, *Il successo*, 11r.
116 *Il diario di Giambattista Casale*, 292.

fathers heard confessions at doorways, carrying long white canes to measure how far they should stand from the threshold.[117] On clerics' attention to matters of contagion, physical health, and preservation of life, the plague chronicle of the canon Jacopo Strazzolini, who officiated over confessions and made daily rounds of Cividale's four lazaretti in 1598, is perhaps the most remarkable: his chronicle ends with fourteen points of advice ('Avvertimenti') 'on how best to save oneself during the plague'. Not a single one mentioned sin, God, or prayer. They instead concerned matters of quarantine, cordoning off streets, cleaning various items, carrying balls of scented herbs, and the like, and how to recognize the disease.[118]

The 1575–8 plague had not spread under the shadow of a Counter-Reformation return to apocalyptic visions of plague as divine punishment, as historians have generally assumed. Medical thinking during Counter-Reformation Italy did not then reject 'the realism' of mid-sixteenth-century medical accomplishments in Italy—Fracastoro's theories of contagion, Vesalius's breakthroughs in anatomy, supposedly new clinical teaching,[119] and the spread of botanical gardens for teaching and experimentation.[120] Evidence from plague writing shows another pathway in medical history. Doctors such as Ingrassia, who began their tracts 'in honour and glory of God' and put God as the first cause as well as the remedy of pestilence, also argued strenuously for enforced separation of the healthy from the infected.[121] Later in his text, he confronted the problem of placating God while 'extinguishing or lessening the spread of the contagion'. His chapter 14 (part four of his first plague tract of 1576–7) began with three remedies and three difficulties. The first was the divine one, involving processions carrying the Holy Sacrament, which he maintained could be 'well shown with many reasons and examples' to have been effective in fighting disease. Such measures, he contended, 'have gained God's help and have gone beyond what was humanly possible'. Processions such as a recent one in Palermo carrying the chest of the relics of Saint Christina and statues of Saints Roch, Sebastian, Cosmos and Damian could be shown to have been efficacious: the number of

---

[117] *Il diario di Giambattista Casale*, 302–3.   [118] Strazzolini, *La peste a Cividale nel 1598*, 46–7.

[119] The legend of Giovan Battista Da Monte's initiation of bedside teaching at the hospital of San Francesco goes back to 1808. Instead, the first evidence of clinical teaching there comes at the end of the plague in 1577–8, when Marco degli Oddi (1526–91), a professor of Medicine at Padua, was employed by the hospital and when it became a formal requirement of the curriculum; see Ongaro and Forin, 'Girolamo Mercuriale e lo studio di Padova', 35; and Wear, 'Medicine in Early Modern Europe', 257. Also, see Henderson, *The Renaissance Hospital*, 225–6, for earlier uses of hospitals for clinical teaching.

[120] The position is stated most dramatically by Davi, *Bernardino Tomitano*, 44; Palmer, 'The Control of Plague', 120ff; and others have also seen the mid-sixteenth century, especially at the University of Padua, as the high watermark of early modern Italian medicine and its decline coinciding with the Counter-Reformation's progress in the following decades; see n. 106. Bylebyl, 'The School of Padua', highlights the mid-sixteenth-century achievements at Padua but argues that its medical prestige did not decline until the seventeenth century.

[121] Ingrassia, *Informatione*, 2 and 10; similarly, many less famous doctors in 1575–8, such as Giovanni Battista Amiconi from Sartirana Lomellina in the territory of Pavia, did much the same: 'Deo optimo maximo', Somenzi, *De morbis*, 20r–v.

plague cases suddenly declined, and those who perished 'were not worthy of such grace anyhow'. He also held that 'one could see clearly from experience' that devotional fasting by the populace, eating bread and drinking water only, were effective in the communal fight against the contagious disease.[122]

Nonetheless, a niggling contradiction remained for the former inquisitor Ingrassia: such religious intermingling and fasting could conflict with basic medical concepts seen throughout his plague tracts. Following his first remedy, he presented two others: (1) the incarceration or 'barregiatura' of the suspected and the infected, their separation from one another and the separation of both from the healthy, and (2) the need to reduce sharply the intermingling of people ('se fusse bene levar la gran conversatione della gente') and especially women and children. For Ingrassia, 'the true cause of the spread of the *contagio*' was the intermingling of the infected with the healthy. He further emphasized the importance of keeping the poor well fed in plague time to increase their resistance to the disease: many had died because of the lack of bread, help, and hope. However, he did not fully endorse these principles when he momentarily considered the Church's recommendations for fasting. Ingrassia engaged in a convoluted discussion with himself, raising the problems of processions and intermingling of the multitudes, concluding momentarily that such processions should be prohibited. He, however, caught himself and ended by questioning how he could presume to be so condescending as to deny faithful Christians their necessary devotion, 'their wishes to cry and pray for God's grace'. His shadow boxing unresolved, he left the question to others 'wiser than himself, especially in the affairs of Sacred Theology'. Ingrassia then returned to firmer and more familiar ground—remedies and problems of sequestration, state expenses, the wickedness of the plebs, and recommendations for the full force of the law, especially against thieves of infected goods, who spread the contagion.[123]

Part Five of his *Informatione*, written just after the plague ended, hints at a slight change in stance: he appeared cautious, even critical of Pope Gregory XIII's desire for a jubilee in Sicily. Without condemning it directly, Ingrassia insisted on emphasizing the prohibition of excessive intermingling. He added: 'for this, it is advisable to publish again bans prohibiting visiting one another in their houses, and not only women, but also men visiting the sick; that every feast and festival be prohibited, along with weddings, or any other gathering for joy or sadness.'[124]

During Italy's next significant plague, that of 1585, centred in Piedmont, a tract by the physician Alessandri was less equivocal and may point to future troubles between Church and State arising in the seventeenth century. He advised prohibiting any gathering that was not absolutely necessary, including schools,

---

[122] Ingrassia, *Informatione*, 269–73.
[123] Ibid., 269–73. He clearly felt better about processions and fasting once plague had declined, 270.
[124] Ingrassia, *Parte Quinta*, 43.

universities ('studij'), markets, dances, banquets, and church attendance. 'Nor were processions so secure, even if being devout was a good idea. In these times of pestilence, it would be much better if everyday at the seventh ringing of the bells, all within their homes regardless of age would genuflect, recite the psalms of David, or pray to the Lord, responding to the litany from one street to the next.'[125] But no conflict between Church and State emerged from this plague, at least noted even marginally in the plague literature, medical or otherwise.

The interaction between clerics and the laity in 1575–8 appears to have differed from that during the Black Death of 1348, when the laity accused clerics of abandoning their flocks to save their own skins, spawning the creation of anti-clerical classics such as *The Decameron*, *Piers the Plowman*, and *The Canterbury Tales*. For the 1575–8 plague, laymen such as the notaries Besta in Milan and Canobbio in Padua saw the clergy—regular and secular—courageously shouldering the burdens imposed by plague, serving the spiritual as well as the physical needs of their parishioners and of the poor in locked houses, plague huts, and lazaretti.[126] Many clerics died, but others had learnt how to administer more safely these tasks in the face of rabid contagion, as the advice of Carlo Borromeo and other clerics to their ranks suggests. Their collaboration in deeds and published advice contrasts with seventeenth-century clerics such as the Jesuit Étienne Binet, whose plague tract of 1628, translated into Italian and published in Rome during its plague of 1656–7, praised the otherworldly benefits of plague massacre and highlighted the impotence of medicine, arguing that faith and purification of the soul were the only valid means for curing plague.[127]

***

This collusion between Church and State, the pious reverence of doctors such as Ingrassia, the confidence in Church leaders by even the most discouraged such as Panizzone Sacco, and the rallying of popular enthusiasm, obedience, and hope behind the Church in its organized processions may suggest a change in mentality towards the otherworldliness and spirituality of the Church, the triumph of a Counter-Reformation culture. Such a triumph in fact did take place, especially in Italy, and evidence such as last wills and testaments suggests that the period immediately after 1575 was the watershed in the organization of new forms of piety and the laity's acceptance of them, from merchant elites to peasants.[128] Not only did the Counter-Reformation give 'an impetus and a direction to the care of the sick and healthy poor' as Ole Peter Grell and Andrew Cunningham

---

[125] Alessandri, *Trattato della peste*, 30r.

[126] Canobbio, *Il successo*, 14v, lists numerous nunneries, monasteries, friaries, and other church groups that assisted the afflicted during the plague and the numbers each order lost as a consequence. Some may have been critical of the Jesuits for taking a less heroic stance during the 1576–7 plague in Milan than the Capuchins, who manned the most dangerous positions in the plague huts and the lazaretto, but this criticism does not surface in the published plague tracts. See Martin, *Plague?*, 175–8.

[127] Conforti, 'Peste e stampa', 150–1.   [128] Cohn, *Death and Property in Siena*, chs 9–10.

have recently argued;[129] disease and in particular the plague threat of 1575–8 strengthened its hold on states, at least in Italy. But did this religious triumph then weaken the resolve of vigorous secular states, driving sentiment from the secular to the otherworldly, marking the end of Renaissance worldly freedom and creativity? [130]

Evidence from the sixteenth-century plague tracts weighs strongly against such conclusions. Instead, the vibrancy and creativity seen in these works reflect confidence in and praise of both secular and religious rulers and their organizations, which combined forces to combat the double-pronged Italian pandemic of 1575–8 . To this end, the perceived triumph over plague achieved through charity, new laws, and stringent penalties bequeathed to the new Counter-Reformation Church and absolutist states (in places one and the same) a mandate for demanding increased obedience and respect from their subjects throughout Italy.[131] To be sure, Borromeo's fame and innovations were already on the rise by the early 1570s. But would his fame and example have been so pervasive without the plague, which first through Italy and then across Europe fuelled his legendary acts of plague heroism, winning him sanctity? In cooperation, Church and State emerged from 1575–8 triumphant and as a consequence more absolutist. The plague had strengthened the secular powers of both and their future success depended on the changed psychology wrought by the 1575–8 plague. As the plague poetry and liberation pamphlets attest, the survivors saw their fate deeply indebted to both these powers on the rise.

---

[129] Grell and Cunningham 'The Counter-Reformation', 16.

[130] Bouwsma, *The Waning of the Renaissance*, viii. For such an interpretation of the intellectual and cultural history of Europe from the Black Death to the eighteenth century, see Delumeau's trilogy on the mentality of late medieval and early modern Europe (Introduction, n. 12).

[131] In turn, according to Pomata, *Contracting a Cure*, 138 and 141, the Counter-Reformation invested physicians with powers they had not possessed in 'the egalitarian relationship between patient and healer' during the Middle Ages to the mid-sixteenth century; by the end of the sixteenth century, 'disobeying one's physician' had become a sin. For the interaction between plague writing, defence against contagion, and development of absolutism in France during the latter half of the seventeenth century, see Jones, 'Plague and Its Metaphors', 110–17.

Epilogue

Neither plague nor the ideas it stimulated were static over five centuries of western civilization as historians and scientists often assume. Just as this disease evolved in its pathology, modes of transmission, and the social characteristics of its victims, so did medical thought about it. Neither physicians nor laymen were fixed in a timeless Galenic vacuum, ever blinded by antique *scientia* until Thomas Sydenham's empiricism at the end of the seventeenth century or, even later, with the laboratory revolution of the nineteenth century. As the tracts studied in this volume illustrate, the century's most feared and devastating plague that threatened Italy top to toe from 1575 to 1578 hardly killed off creativity. Instead, it unleashed a wave of plague writing that transformed the traditional plague tract and in so doing expanded the boundaries of medical thinking and advice. Half the published plague writing of the sixteenth century appeared in two years alone, 1576–7, when the plague was at its height. Suddenly the authorship of these publications fantailed from a near monopoly of physicians to include surgeons, druggists, gentlemen magistrates, merchants, notaries, lawyers, judges, petty procurators, gate-officers, clerics from parish priests to the pope, and even artisans. From erudite books of definitions, causes, cures, and remedies, encrusted in citations from Hippocrates, Aristotle, Galen, Avicenna, and other classical, Arabic, and medieval authorities, plague tracts now appeared overwhelmingly in the vernacular and branched out in new directions. Supported by parish and health board statistics and dramatized with eyewitness descriptions of bizarre happenings, human misery, and suffering, they tracked the human spread of disease to and through their cities. The plague of 1575–8 gave rise to an explosion in plague poetry, which before 1575 had been rare, and spurred on debates over issues such as the role of drinking water and the pollution of wells in the rise of pestilence. This changed literature did not, however, represent a split between physicians and those outside the medical profession. Instead, academically trained physicians challenged old Galenic models, constellations of stars, mutation of air, seasonal changes, and even the role of God for understanding disease. Trusting their own observations and reports gathered by health boards, a new nominalism infused the plague writing of 1575–8 along with a search for new correlations pertaining to the social geography of cities.

The classical physician's plague tract, still principally the terrain of the university-trained, added new sections and assumed new dimensions that pulled the doctor from the patient's bedside to address community-wide medicine, administration, society, and politics. 'Wondrous secrets', syrups, potions, plasters, and surgical procedures continued to fill some plague tracts, but others, first in Italy and soon afterwards across the Alps, turned to what doctors now considered their most 'valiant' remedies: these were lodged within the public domain and were dependent on state power. Their publications now advised princes and city magistrates on a wide variety of practical and political measures. They engaged in social engineering with dictates on the structure of new political organizations, the election of officials, and decrees for keeping streets clean, clearing public latrines, ensuring clean water, maintaining harbours purged of mud, waste, excrement, and dead animals. Their theories turned on new ideas about relations between bad plumbing and plague-ridden neighbourhoods, and proposed fundamental economic programmes for ending dire poverty now seen as the plague's true cause.

Were these innovations and shifts in mentality a momentary aberration or did they mark a more profound watershed in the investigation and understanding of plague? As we have seen, simple statistics such as the proportion of vernacular to Latin tracts show the last twenty-two years of the sixteenth century easing back towards ratios witnessed before 1575–8. Some texts returned to pedantic exercises in antique erudition. Others, even ones written in the vernacular for a larger public, were hardly distinguishable in their notions of the causes and cures of plague from treatises written a hundred years or more before. For instance, two short treatises by the physician Antonio Carrarino from Orvieto published in 1591 presented the origins, spread, and contagion of plague as dependent on air, first in the atmosphere, then within our bodies.[1] The signs for predicting a bad or pestilential year revived old clichés with new twists such as the sudden appearance of many small toads with scales on their backs. 'The evil effects of the summer' could also auger the coming of plague. Recommendations on behaviour harkened back to old generalizations based on Galen's 'six non-naturals' that had filled plague tracts since 1348, such as not to exercise too vigorously. And throughout, Carrarino emphasized prayer as the best remedy for ending plague.[2] His second tract, *On pestilences and prodigies*, reported much the same: God sent signs and prodigies as a warning before any great human calamity, and these could be read from characteristics of the air, water, and seasons such as unusually warm summers and rainy autumns, or from an extraordinary appearance of toads, fish, locust, and other small animals. According to Carrarino, the conjunction of Saturn and Mars

---

[1] *Breve discorso*; and *Delle pestilenze et prodigii*. Edit 16 provides no information on this doctor. In the first tract he says he received his education in Siena.

[2] *Breve discorso*, 1r–4v.

foretold the plagues of 1348 and 1479. For the plague of 1523 it was the flooding of the Tiber, for 1575 it was a comet from the south.[3] Except for historical references to early modern plagues, his tracts could have been penned in the fourteenth century. He made no comments about public health, bad plumbing, overflowing excrement, water supplies, or poverty as plague's underlying causes; nor did he make recommendations to city magistrates or the prince.

For those wishing to draw an unbending line from plague tracts such as the *Compendium* of the Medical Faculty of Paris in October 1348 to medical writings at the end of the seventeenth century or beyond, Carrarino's works provide valuable evidence (even if both survive only in single copies in a single library). For the last decades of the sixteenth century, such texts, at least in Italy, were not, however, the rule. To my knowledge, no doctor in the sixteenth century or later cited them. Instead, the plague writings that were cited, later republished (especially during the seventeenth-century plagues of 1629–33 and 1656–7), and translated or plagiarized by physicians across the Alps, were those that had broken the standard mould of plague writing—works by Ingrassia, Donzellini, Daciano, Centorio Degli Ortensi, Canobbio, Besta, Benedetti, Valier, and others frequently referred to in this book.[4]

To be sure, late sixteenth-century Italian authors such as the Torinese Alessandri continued to cite remote causes and signs of future plagues and even added others equally far-fetched. These included 'when Holy Virgins or saints announced plague by means of some aspect of their sacred image'; if children perform the office of the dead, without being moved by any apparent intelligence; if bread hot out of the oven is hung up overnight and fed to dogs or chickens the next morning and they either refuse to eat it or die from it; if fruit has little taste. Alessandri's list goes on with further signs such as the fleeing of crawfish, swans, and other water fowl, dead fish floating on water turning yellow, fish stinking immediately after being caught and tasting insipid.[5] He reports that such notions

---

[3] *Delle pestilenze et prodigii*, 10r–12r. According to Alessandri, *Trattato della peste*, 35v, this comet appeared instead after most cities had been liberated from the plague in 1577.

[4] For instance, during the next big plague in Italy, that of 1629–33, a number of plague tracks from 1575–7 were republished, such as works by Lucio Boerio, Paolo Filippo Castagni, Asciano Centorio degli Ortensi, and Ascanio Oliveri. By the plague of 1656–7, Ingrassi's *Informatione*, had become a classic and was discussed in the Papal Camera for lessons on the transmission of the disease; see Rocciolo, 'Cum suspicione morbi contagiosi obierunt', 116. After the crisis of 1575–7 to 1600, however, there was some slippage back to the traditional physicians' plague tracts. About a quarter of them (eleven of forty-one) either presented secret cures and recipes or were theoretical tracts beginning with definitions and universal causes, Galenic notions of air and corruption, and were without new sections on political or public health issues; nor did they concentrate on how to recognize the detailed clinical aspects of plague. See for instance Trevisio, *De caussis*, which instructed on seasons, winds, stars, air and other superior causes of pestilential fevers; also see Frangipane, *De peste coelitus;* Gallo, *De febribus pestilentibus;* and one of the Jesuit de Loarti, *Antidoto spirituale contra la peste*. These were in Latin, and except for one, existing in only three copies, are known by a sole surviving copy.

[5] Alessandri, *Trattato della peste*, 34r–6r: 'Segni che stia per venire la peste'. Such future signs of plague, especially as regards unnatural events in the animal world, were common through the sixteenth century, at least before 1575. The sorts of animals that the plague writers observed for signs expanded

continued to be prevalent among the learned and commoners in Turin during the last decades of the sixteenth century. But like many other physicians across Italy of the post-1575 generation, he expressed a new scepticism toward such reputed premonitions and concluded his list with Occam's razor: 'All of these signs cannot possibly point to the same sad outcome. When a great mortality of large animals or men rages like a fire through dry wood, this is enough of a sign to prepare for plague whether or not any of these previous signs have been observed.'[6]

***

Yet these conclusions suggest no simple binary progression from a supposed pre-modern to modern medical thought. Instead, the intellectual trajectory over the five centuries of the Black Death's repeated returns was anything but linear. For instance, the the almost 400-page Latin plague tract of Lodovico Settala, Milan's most renowned physician of the seventeenth century, called 'the Hippocrates of our time' by contemporary doctors, returned to many of preoccupations of academic treatises before 1575.[7] Its first book is a discussion, extensive as any found from the previous century, of definitions of plague, epidemic, common, and vulgar. Parts of its second and third books engaged in lengthy discussions of air and the remote causes of plague—conjunctions of stars and planets and other prognostics of plagues—studded with frequent and numerous citations to Greek, Latin, and Arabic authorities. Further sections discussed pharmacology and treatment with strong purgatives and instructed on bloodletting both as cures and prevention of plague; other sections dwelled on the importance of Galen's six non-naturals.[8] As Nutton, Bylebyl, Wear, Israel, Maclean, and many others have shown, Galenic teaching remained vibrant in medical discourse and

from the clichés of the late Middle Ages, principally about reptiles and small animals coming out of holes and occasionally the flight of birds. For the physician Biondo, *Di preseruatione di pestilentia*, plague was signalled by the multiplication of strange and unusual animals, such as worms of various sorts: 'mossoni, cenzale, cavalette, rospi, et ranocchi, filocchi, ostri, lebecci, curine' as well as 'nuvoli pieni di pioggio senza piova', 6r. Prospero Borgarucci, *De peste perbrevis tractatus*, 27, in addition to strange behaviour of birds, serpents, worms, frogs, and 'various visions' as future signs of plague, also observed peculiarities of the eggs of chickens and wolves surrounding cities as warnings. The physician of Bergamo condemned to death by the Inquisition and practising in Basel, Gratarolo, *Pestis descriptio*, 4v–5r (in BAV, but not in Edit 16) also saw wolves and mad dogs entering and molesting towns, multitudes of frogs and moths coming out of walls, and serpents, worms, and moles as signs of plague, all brought about by increased humidity of the air.

6 Alessandri, *Trattato della peste*, 36v.

7 On Settala's medical conservatism (and on plague during 1630–1), see Cosmacini, *Storia della medicina*, 116–8. In addition, Gastaldi's *Tractatus avertenda et profliganda peste Politico-legalis* (compiled during Rome's last plague of 1656 but published in 1684) returned to astrological determinants of plague and other medieval and Renaissance notions lodged in the superior causes of contagion and disease, despite attention to details of quarantine, cleansing suspected goods, the importance of politics and public health; see for instance chs 249, 251, 256, and 257 on the influences of corrupt airs, meteorites, stars, comets, eclipses, earthquakes, and signs of predictors of future plagues.

8 Settala, *De Peste*. Book one on definitions is 71 pages; for strong purgatives and bloodletting, 162–5, 239–43, 247, and 292–304.

the bedrock of medical curricula throughout Europe until the seventeenth,[9] and in some cases even until the nineteenth century.[10]

Nor was the plague of 1575–8 the first or only time that Galenic and 'universal' principles had been questioned.[11] Yet the lesser-known late sixteenth-century authors of plague tracts—priests, notaries, gentlemen officials, druggists, and physicians—whose publications this book has described, show that the questioning, even toppling of Galen, was not solely a product of the seventeenth-century Protestant–Paracelsian alliance or of early Enlightenment thought.[12] The crisis of 1575–8 jolted entrenched physician-philosophers of the medical academies as well as the laity from complacent reliance on the old rules of medical intervention. In place of theoretical remote causes, physicians and lay authors turned to trace the spread of plague, by detailing the chronological links between people and goods. Plague tracts of successive pandemics in the seventeenth and eighteenth centuries would repeat this new approach to understanding plague.

In addition, the 1575–8 crisis planted the seeds of another transition in the history of medicine, this time thought to be solidly lodged in the politics of German bicameralism and the ideology of the last stages of the Enlightenment. The Italian crisis prised doctors from patients' bedsides to discover that their most effective remedies against plague lay in politics and community action. This change also had long-reaching ramifications for plague writing and thought into the next century, even in erudite traditional treatises such as Settala's. In one fundamental respect, his tract differed from those before 1575. Two chapters, one on quarantine, the other 'on preserving a people once plague had entered the city', concerned public health ranging from the details of the number of physicians, surgeons, nurses, gravediggers and others to be employed in plague time to the special duties and obligations of the duke of Milan. On obstetrics and nursing of infants during plague, this tract in fact went beyond any I know

---

[9] Wear, *Knowledge and Practice in English Medicine*, 275–6 and 432–3; idem, 'Medicine in Early Modern Europe', 320; Israel, 'Counter-Reformation', 44; Brockliss and Jones, *The Medical World of Early Modern France*, 1, and 99–119; Maclean, *Logic, Signs and Nature*, ch. 1, is unclear when the Galenic model lost its grip over medical science, but it was certainly after 1630.

[10] Gentilcore, *Healers and Healing*, 6; Lindemann, *Medicine and Society*, 69–70; and Nutton, 'The Fortunes of Galen', 355 and 362.

[11] For earlier attacks such as those of Alexander of Tralles (*c*.560), see Nutton, 'The Fortunes of Galen', 365; see Maclean, *Logic, Signs and Nature*, 21–3 and 32 on Giovanni Argenterio's critique delivered in the 1550s in his published lectures at the University of Pisa. For the historiographical emphasis on the middle years of the sixteenth century as innovative, especially anatomy, with the last quarter of the century falling into the clutches of the Counter-Reformation intolerance with repression on the rise and Renaissance creativity in retreat; see Palmer, 'The Control of Plague', Bouwsma, *The Waning of the Renaissance*; Davi, *Bernardino Tomitano*; and others, and my comments above.

[12] For the early seventeenth-century alliance between Calvinism and Paracelsian medicine and the intolerance of the sixteenth-century Counter-Reformation and Galenic medicine, see Trevor-Roper, *Europe's Physician*, ch. 1; and Webster, *The Great Instauration*, esp. 273–88, 'on the sudden surge of Paracelsian medicine' and attacks on Galenism after the English Civil War. For the early Enlightenment assault on Galen, see Wear, *Knowledge and Practice in English Medicine*.

from the previous century.[13] Clearly, Settala's recommendations relied on the Milanese experience of 1575–6; Centorio Degli Ortensi was here his principal source.[14]

The concern for political remedies and solutions to plague would continue as a prime concern of Italian plague tracts and other medical treatises written by physicians and those outside the profession to the end of the early modern period as seen in tracts such as Rutilo Benzoni's *Tractatus de Fuga*, written in Loreto in 1595; Paolo Zacchia's *Quaestiones medico-legales*, Rome, 1621–35; Marco Antonio Alaymo's *Consigli politico-Medici*, written in Palermo in 1652 to guard Sicily against plague that then threatened from other parts of Europe[15]; the Capuchin Mauritio da Tolone's *Trattato politico da pratticarsi ne' tempi di peste* written just after Genova's disastrous plague of 1655–7;[16] Girolamo Gastaldi's *Tractatus avertenda et profliganda peste Politico-legalis*, reflections on the 1656–7 plague at Rome and its 245 decrees promulgated to contain it, which Gastaldi as head of Rome's lazaretti ('commissario generale dei lazaretti') had in fact been instrumental in passing;[17] and finally Lodovico Muratori's, *Del Governo della peste*. As with so many of the 1575–8 tracts that took on the challenges of public health, Muratori's underlying metaphor was war.[18] As with war, plague defences were matters of state. With both plague and war, the prince was responsible for mobilizing resources, organizing a hierarchy of command, and promulgating just and effective laws to prepare the state to defeat the enemy.[19] As with thinking in 1575–8, management of the poor and marginals remained of utmost importance in Muratori's political thinking about plague in 1743. This shift in ideas and

---

[13] Settala, *De peste*, 140–48.

[14] Ibid., 148. In addition, Settala added the reforms of the Milanese health board passed under the aegis of Duke Francesco Sforza in 1534, 322–41. Moreover, he went on to write a book purely on politics; see Chapter 8, nn. 79–81.

[15] Alaymo, *Consigli politico-Medici*.

[16] Da Tolone, *Trattato politico da pratticarsi ne' tempi di peste*. On da Tolone's preventative measures, see Sansa, 'Strategie di prevenzione a confronto l'igiene urbana', 96–8. On the ground swell in the medical reasoning applied to political thought at the end of the sixteenth century, see D'Alessio, 'Per una nuova scienza'; and Chapter 8, p. 262.

[17] See Sonnino, 'Cronache della peste a Roma', 56. Donato, 'La peste dopo la peste', describes a continuing tradition of these medical-administrative tracts of plague prevention published to 1720 (such as one by the Ferrarese Ippolito Bentivoglio in 1680) in praise of the Roman model of 'buon governo della peste' developed in 1656–7.

[18] Sontag, *Illness as Metaphor*, 67, maintains that the 'military metaphor in medicine first came into wide use in the 1880s, with the identification of bacteria as agents of disease' when (supposedly) verbs such as 'to invade' were first associated with the spread of disease. (Also, see her later, more nuanced statement of the same, 95–7.) The near-ubiquitous four horsemen of the Apocalypse and the arrows of the Black Death show a much earlier presence of military analogies. Moreover, poetry and medical tracts of 1575–8 suddenly expanded military metaphors for disease; more importantly, military tactics now went beyond metaphors to guide political action against the 'invasion' of plague with specific instructions on border guards, supply lines and provisioning, military intelligence and spies to warn cities and regions of plague outbreaks.

[19] Muratori, *Del governo della peste*, esp., 16ff. Also, see the chapter on the prince's obligations towards medicine and medical education in one of his last works, *Della pubblica felicità*.

writing about plague and disease was by now no longer confined to the Italian peninsula. In translations of Italian works, especially those penned in 1575–8, these ideas had crossed the Alps, anticipating the public health doctrines of 'medical police' envisioned by Wolfgang Thomas Rau (1721–72), Franz Anton Mai (1772–1814), and especially Johann Peter Frank (1748–1821) at the end of the eighteenth and into the early nineteenth century.[20]

Finally, the crisis of 1575–8 did not move populations against robust state formations towards otherworldly transcendence and pessimism as is often envisioned as the consequences of large epidemics in world history. Instead, its effects were the opposite: the triumph over plague was a victory of rulers and civil servants. From podestà to bell-ringers they emerged in literary celebrations as Hercules overcoming the Hydra-headed monster. This plague spurred on new confidence in the combined roles of Church and State in preserving social order and the application of administrative skill and political force to remedy plague. By addressing the underlying social realities, in particular the plague's root cause—poverty—plague writers envisioned not only that a city could be liberated from a present epidemic; plague could be eradicated once and for all.

Two intellectual strands in the history of medicine arose with the plague crisis of 1575–8: (1) physicians' sudden redefinition of their craft from one centred on the patient to new notions of public health directives, and (2) the efforts of plague writers across a wide spectrum of backgrounds to understand disease by tracking its contagion and progress, anticipating developments in epidemiology of the nineteenth century. In tracing these, this book sketches a new narrative in the history of medicine and has sought to add another dimension to our understanding of Counter-Reformation culture. The questioning of antique authority with assaults on the Renaissance and Galenic medicine neither depended on breakthroughs in anatomy of the 1540s nor awaited the mid-seventeenth-century Protestant–Paracelsian alliance in northern Europe. Instead, in the heartland of Counter-Reformation Italy, the pandemic of 1575–8 unleashed creative forces that sowed seeds of doubt and unveiled new concerns and ideas within that supposedly most conservative form of medical writing, the plague tract.

---

[20] The historiography of public health continues to hold that systematic ideas and advice to governments on 'policing health' developed during the late eighteenth century and primarily in Germany; see Rosen's classic, *A History of Public Health*, 161–83; Porter, 'The Eighteenth Century', 466–8; Rosen, 'Cameralism and the Concept of Medical Police'; Risse, 'Medicine in the Age of Enlightenment'; Bourdelais, 'Per una nuova storia sociale delle epidemie', 10; and Harrison, *Disease and the Modern World*, 58–61. The one place to mention the Italian experience in the development of public health is Rosen, 'The Fate of the Concept of Medical Police', 150–1, where he devotes a paragraph to two seventeenth-century Italian doctors and to Muratori as anticipating the German cameralists.

Bibliography*

ARCHIVES

Archivio di Stato, Firenze
   Ufficiali di Sanità
Archivio di Stato, Milano
   Fondo popolazione, parte antica
   Miscellanea Storica
Archivio di Stato, Verona
   Archivio di Comune
   Archivio dell'Ufficio di Sanità di Verona, Parte antica [Sanità]

MANUSCRIPTS

Biblioteca Apostolica Vaticana
Canzone di M. Girolamo Verota veronese nella gran Pestilentia et guerra della patria seduto nella gardesana, al Lago. [R.IV. 1551, no. 26]
Sonetto sopra tutti gli rimedii che si usano contra la peste, R.I. IV. 1551 (six sonetti, nos. 98a–f).

Biblioteca Braidense, Milan
Gride diverse della sanità per la peste del 1576–1577. AO.I.14:

Biblioteca Comunale, Palermo
Carretto, Federico, *De pestilentia cohorta Agrigenti anno 1526* [*Opusculum* 2 Qq H 29].

Wellcome Library
Atti dell'officio della sanità di Monza, la peste negli anni 1576 e 1577.

PRINTED PRIMARY SOURCES

Agricola, Georg, *De peste libri tres* (Basel: per Hier. Frobenium, 1554).
Ajello, Sebastiano, *Breue discorso sopra l'imminente peste. Nel Regno di Napoli l'anno 1575, 76 et 77* . . . (Naples: appresso Horatio Saluiani, 1577).
Albert the Great, *Man and the Beasts*, trans. J. Scanlan (Binghampton, NY: 1987).
Alcuni sonetti al clarissimo sig. Nicolò Michiele dignissimo capitanio di Vicenza, l'anno 1577 (Vicenza: appresso Giorgio Angelieri, 1578).
Alessandri, Francesco, *Trattato della peste et febri pestilenti, tradotto di latino in volgare* (Turin: per Antonio de' Bianchi, 1586).
Alfani, Francesco, *Opus, de peste, Febre Pestilentiali & febre maligna. Necnon de variolis & morbillis, qutenus nondum pestilentes sunt* (Naples: apud Horatium Salvianum, 1577).

---

* Publishers' names have been included only for titles published before 1800. The absence of places, names, or dates of publication means that such information has not been indicated.

Al-Razi, *Libellus de peste de Graeco in latinum sermonem versus per Nicolaum Macchellum, Medicum Mutinensem* (Venice: apud Andream Arriuabenum ad signum Putei, 1556).

Alaymo, Marco Antonio. *Consigli politico-Medici*, ed. Corrado Dollo in *Filosofia e Scienze nella Sicilia dei Secoli XVI e XVII*, vol. II (Catania?, 1996).

Amiconi, Giovanni Battista, *De morbis, qui per finitimos populus adhuc grassantur: Et nun illi ad pestilentes referendi sint, post prima responsa Mantua allata, brevis disputatio* (Cremona: apud Christophorum Draconium, 1576).

Andrew of Wyntoun's Orygnale Cronykil of Scotland, The Historians of Scotland, ed. David Laing. 9 vols (Edinburgh, 1872–9).

The Anonimalle Chronicle 1333 to 1381, ed. V. H. Galbraith, Historical Series, XLV (Manchester, 1927).

Arellano Pietro Francesco, *Trattato di peste nel quale si contengono i più scielti & approvati rimedij, con alcuni Liquori di sua inventione, sì per curarsi come preservarsi* (Asti: appresso Virgilio Giangrandi, 1598).

Argenterio, Giacomo, *Porta tecum rimedii piu veri, et approuati, tanto preseruatiui, quanto curatiui, contra la peste* (Turin: per Aluiggi Pizzamiglio, 1598)

[Arluni, Giovanni Pietro], *La peste*, ed. and trans. Francesco di Ciaccia (Milan, 1999).

Augenio, Orazio, *Del modo di preservarsi dalla peste: Libri tre, Scritti volgarmente per beneficio commune* (Fermo: appresso Astolfo de Grandi, 1577).

Baccei, Michele, *Della peste e suoi rimedii: Discorso Accademico* (Bracciano, 1631).

Bacci, Andrea, *Delle acque de' fonti et fiumi del Mondo Libri tre* (Venice: Aldo Manuzio il giovane, 1576).

Bacon, Francis, 'Of Seditious and Troubles', in Bacon, *The Essays*, ed. John Pitcher (London, 1985), 101–07.

Bairo, Pietro, *Nouum ac perutile opusculum de pestilentia et de curatione eiusdem per utrunque regimen preseruatiuum .s et curatiuum* (Turin: per magistrum Franciscum Siluam, 1507).

Baldini, Bernardino, *In pestilentiam libellus* (Milan: apud Pacificum Pontium, 1577).

Civelli, Francesco, *Carmina, quibus ob acerbam pestem Mediolanensium status deploratur* (Milan: apud Io. Baptistam Pontium, 1577).

Bandi & Constitut. diverse di Bologna (Bologna : per Alessandro Benacci, 1576).

Bando dell'illustrissimi, et ecc. S. il S. Duca di Firenze, et di Siena . . . sopra la tere, e provincie infette dalla peste (Florence: appresso i Giunti, 1564).

Bando et ordinationi fatte per l'illustri & molto spettabili signroi offitiali della felice città di Palermo conchiuse e terminate nel la Deputatione della Sanità sopra il morbo contagioso che corre nella detta città (Palermo: Giovan Mattheo Mayda, 1575).

Baravalle, Cristoforo, *L'historia della peste di Padoa dell'anno MDLV* (Padua: Grazioso Percacino, not before 1555).

—— *Praticam medicinam profitentis de peste* (Monte Regali: ex officina Leonardi Torrentini, 1565).

Barrelli, Giovanni, *Thesoro inestimabile che insegna molti dignissimi secreti contra la peste* (Venice: nella stamperia de' Rampazetti, 1579).

Bartolomeo da San Zeno, *Sorano so chi poeti desgirlande* (1576?).

Bassino, Giovanni, *Modo e ordine securo da preservarse e curarse dal pestifero morbo: novamente aggregato* (Pavia, 1501).

Baviera, Baverio, *Trattato mirabile contra peste* (Bologna: per Hieronymo di Beneditti, 1523).

Bellintani, Paolo, *Dialogo della peste*, ed. Ermanno Pacagnini (Milan, 2001).

Bellicocchi, Giovanni Andrea, *Avvertimenti di tutto ciò che in publico da Signori & in Privato da ciascuno, si debbe far nel tempo della peste* (Verona: appresso Sebastiano dalle Donne, 1577).

Benedetti, Rocco, *Noui auisi di Venetia, ne quali si contengono tutti i casi miserabili, che in quella, al tempo della peste sono occorsi* ... (Urbino: appresso Battista de Bartoli Vinitiano, 1577) and (Bologna: per Alessandro Benacci, 1577).

_____ *Raguaglio: Minutissimo del successo della peste di Venetia: Con gli casi occorsi, provissioni fatte & altri particolari, Infino alla liberatione di essa* (Tivoli: appresso Domenico Piolato, 1577).

Benzi, Ugo, 'Trattato', ed. Arturo Castiglioni, in 'Ugo Benzi da Siena ed il "Trattato utilissimo circa la conservazione della sanitate" ', *Rivista di Storia Critica delle Scienze Mediche e Naturali*, 12 (1921): 75–105.

Benzoni, Rutilo, *Tractatus de Fuga* ... (Venice: apud Societatem Minimam, 1595).

Beroaldo 'il vecchio', Filippo, *Opusculum de Terraemotu et pestilentia cum Annotamentis Galeni* [1505] (Venice: per Bernardinum Venetum de Vitalibus, 1508).

Besta, Giacomo Filippo, *Vera narratione del successo della peste, che afflisse l'inclita città di Milano, l'anno 1576 & di tutte le provisioni fatte a salute di essa città* (Milano: per Paolo Gottardo & Pacifico Pontij fratelli, 1578).

Betholio, Bernardo, *Carmen super eventu pestis in urbe Mediolani* (Milan: Maria Metius, 1577).

Biondo, Michelangelo, *Di preseruatione di pestilentia, et di la perfetissima cura dell'appestato* (Venezia: dalla casuppula del Biondo, 1555).

Bisciola, Paolo, *Relatione verissima del progresso della peste di Milano* (Ancona and reissued in Bologna, Alessandro Benacci, 1577.

Bocca, Bernardino, *Diuini fioretti preseruatiui, & medicatiui contra peste* (Venice: per Giovannantonio e fratelli da Sabbio, 1528).

Boccaccio, Giovanni. *Decameron*, ed. Vittore Branca (Milan, 1976).

Boccalini, Giovanni Francisco, *De causis pestilentiae urbem Venetam opprimentis anno MDLVI. In Marsilii Ficini Consilium annotatiunculae* (Venice: apud Gabrielem Iolitum de Ferrariis, 1556).

Boerio, Luchino, *Trattato delli buboni, e carboni pestilenti con le loro cause, segni, e curationi* (Genoa: Giuseppe Pavoni 1630) [Genoa, 1579].

Bonagente, Vittorio, *Decem problemata de peste* (Venice, ex officina Erasmiana, 1556).

Bononia Manifesta: Catalogo dei bandi, editti, costituzioni e provvedimenti diversi, stampati nel XVI secolo per Bologna e il suo territorio, ed. Zita Zanardi, Biblioteca di Bibliografia italiana, CXLII (Florence, 1996).

Borgarucci, Borgaruccio, *L'afflition di Vinetia: nella quale si ragiona di tutti gli accidenti occorsi in Vinetia, l'Anno 1576 per cagion di Peste* (Florence: ad istantia di Antonio Padovani, 1578).

Borgarucci, Prospero, *De peste perbrevis tractatus* (Venice: ex officina Marci de Maria Salernitani, 1565).

Borromeo, Carlo, *Avisi comuni a tutto il Clero Secolare & Regolare della Città di Milano* (Milan, 1576).

_____ *Cause, et rimedi della peste . . . Con alcuni auisi dell'illustriss. e rev. Cardinal Borromeo* ... (Macerata: appresso Sebastiano Martellini, 1577).

Borromeo, Carlo, *Constitutiones, et decreta sex prouincialium Synodorum Mediolanensium* (Venice: apud Franciscum de Franciscis Senensem, 1595).

–––– *Ordini d'orationi da continarsi per i pericoli di peste, dati da Mons. Ill. Et Rev. Cardinale di Santa Prassede. Arcivescovo di Milano* (Milano: appresso Pacifico Pontio, 1576).

–––– *Pratica per i curati, et altri sacerdoti intorno alla cura dell'infermi & sospetti di peste dell'illustriss. e Rev. Monsignore Cardinale si S. Prassede Arcivescovo di Milano* (Milano: appresso Paicifico Pontio, 1576).

Borromeo, Federico *La peste di Milano*, ed. A. Torni (1987).

Branchi, Girolamo, *Oratione . . . fatta per la liberatione della sua Patria dalla Peste. L'anno MDLXXVI* (Palermo, 1577?).

'Brevis tractatus contra pestem eines Magistrus Primus de Gorllicio', *Archiv für Geschichte der Medizin* [hereafter *Sudhoff*], 17 (1925): 77–92.

Briganti, Annibale, *Avvisi e avvertimenti intorno al governo di preservarsi di pestilenza . . .* (Napoli: presso Giuseppe Cacchio, 1577).

Bucci, Agostino, *Modo di conoscere et distinguere gli influssi pestilenti* (Turin: appresso l'herede del Beuilacqua, 1585).

–––– *Reggimento preservativo degli huomini, luoghi et città dall'influsso della peste . . .* (Turin: appresso Martino Crauoto, 1564).

Bucelleni, Faustino, *Faustino Bucelleni all'eccell. m. Annibal Raimondo, sopra il discorso da lui fatto, in materia del presente male, pestifero, & contagioso* (Venice, 1576).

Bugati, Gasparo. *L'aggiunta dell'Historia universale, et delle cose di Milano . . . dal 1566 fin'al 1581* (Milan: per Francesco & heredi di Simon Tini, 1587).

–––– *I fatti di Milano al contrasto della peste, over pestifero contagio: Dal primo d'Agosto 1576 fin a l'ultimo dell'anno 1577 . . .* (Milano: ad instantia di Pietr'Antonio Leveno, 1578).

–––– *Historia universale nella . . . dal principio del mondo fino all'anno MDLXIX* (Ferrara, 1571).

Buonagrazia, Girolamo, *De provisione et cura morborum pesilentium Hieronimi de Bonagratiis Physici Florentini* (1522?).

Burlacchini, Burlacchino, *Ragionamento sopra la Peste dell'anno MDLXXVI* (Florence: appresso Bartolomeo Sermartelli, 1577).

Calori, Giovanni, *Regimento como lhomo si debbe gubernare et perseuerare nel tempo della pestilentia* (Bologna: per Iustiniano da Rubiera, 1522).

Calzaveglia, Vincenzio, *De theriacae abusu in febribus pestilentibus* (Brescia: apud Vicentium Sabiensem, 1570).

Camerarius, Joachim, *Synopsis quorundam brevium sed perutilium commentariorum de peste . . .* (Nuremberg: Edita studio Joachimi Camerarii, 1583).

–––– *De recta et necessaria ratione praeservandi a pestis contagio*, in *Synopsis*.

Campana, Cesare, *Alcune compositioni volgari et latine, nelle quali chiedendo aiuto dalla divina pietà, si ricordano le misere conditioni della mortal pestilenza, successa in Vinegia l'anno M.D. LXXVI* (Vicenza: appresso Giorgio Angelieri, Vicentino, 1576).

Canobbio, Alessandro, *Il successo della peste occorsa in Padoua l'anno MDLXXVI* (Venice: appresso Paolo Megietti libraro in Padova, 1577).

Canzone alla gloriossima Vergine del reverendo padre M. Remigio fiorentino, dell'Ordine de' Predicatori [Remigio Nannini] (Venice: appresso Gabriel Giolito de' Ferrari, 1577).

Canzone di fileremo per la patria del Clariss. Sig. Nicolò Barbarigo, Podestà di Verona meritissimo (1576 or 1577).

Canzone sopra la città di Venetia liberata da la peste (Verona: appresso S. dalle Donne, 1577).

Cappelletti, Antonio, *Apologia Marci Antonii Capelletti aduersus Bartholomeum Traffichettum Britonorien. medicum Arimini degentem, in qua quamplurima cum de laterali morbo, tum pestilenti de febri, exacta ratione disseruntur* (Pesaro: apud Hieronymum Concordiam, 1569).

Capra, Marcello. *De morbo epidemico, qui miserrime Siciliam depopulabatur anno chistianae salutis 1591, itidemque 1592, causis, syntomatibus, et curatione* (Messina: apud haeredes Fausti Bufalini, 1593).

Carcano, Archileo, *De Peste Opusculum* (Milan: Jo. Maria Metius, 1577.

____ *Trattato di peste vtilissimo* (Pavia: appresso Girolamo Bartoli, 1577).

Carmen. De urbe veneta pestilential liberate. Anno M. D. LXVII (1577?)

Carrarino, Antonio, *Breve discorso sopra l'andamento delle quattro stagioni dell'anno . . .* (Orvieto: per Antonio Coladi, 1591).

____ *Delle pestilenze et prodigii che sono stati in Italia avanti N.S. è dopo. Incominciando dall'anno del Mondo 4465. fino a quest'anno di nostra salute 1591 . . .* (Orvieto: per Antonio Coladi, 1591).

Cassal, Jean. *Traicté de la peste; avec une méthode servant pour la cognoissance d'icelle ensemble une exhortation pour consoler ceux qui seront detenus de quelques grandes maladies & principalement de la contagion* (Lyon: Par Benoist Rigaud, 1589).

Cause et rimedii della peste et d'altre infermita nelle quali oltre a diverse historie . . . Con vn sermone del venerabile Bernardino Busti (Florence: appresso i Giunti, 1577).

'Causae, signa et remedia contra pestilentiam edita per Magistrum Henricum (de Bremis oder de Ribbenicz)', in *Sudhoff*, 7 (1913): 81–9.

Cavagnino, Giovanni Battista, *Compilatione delli veri et fideli rimedii da preservarsi et curarsi dalla peste, con la cura delli antraci, carboni & giandusse* (Brescia: appresso Vincenzo Sabbio, 1576).

Centorio Degli Ortensi, Ascanio, *I cinque libri degl'avvertimenti ordini, gride, et editti* (Venice: appresso Giovanni e Gio. Paolo Gioliti de'Ferrari, 1579).

Cermisone, Antonio, *Remedii verissimi . . . esperimentati per lo eccl. M. Antonio Cermisone Medico Padovano aggionti novamente* (1555).

____ *Questo sono recepte facte quasi tutte da magistro Antonio Cermisono contro la pestilentia* (Milan: per Ludovicium de Bebulco, 1512).

Ceruti, Federico, *Prosopopeia amphitheatri Veronsensis ad Nicolaum Barbadicum praetorem* (Verona: apud Sebastianum et Ioannem à Donnis fratres, 1575).

Chronique des Pays-Bas, de France, d'Angleterre et de Tournai, in Corpus Chronicorum Flandriae, III, ed. J.-J. de Smet. (Brussels, 1837–65).

Chronique et annales de Gilles le Muisit, ed. H. Lemaître. Société d'histoire de France, vol. CCCXXIII (Paris, 1906).

Ciappi, Marcantonio, *Regola da preseruarsi in sanita in tempi de suspetto di peste . . .* (Perugia, Pietroiacomo Petrucci, 1577).

Cieco, Francesco, *Barceletta sopra il lamento di Venetia, del mal contagioso* (Brescia, 1576?).

Cittadoni da Cassia, Dionisio, *Regole per conseruar l'huomo dalla peste* (Camerino: Antonio Gioioso?, 1564?)

Civelli, Francesco, *Carmina, quibus ob acerbam pestem Mediolanensium status deploratur* (Milan: apud Io. Baptistam Pontium, 1577).

Col nome del Spirito Santo. De mandato del Serenissimo Principe, & . . . & Proveditori alla Sanità . . . publicar & propalar il presente rimedio (Venice, 1576).

Col nome d'Iddio modi, et ordini che s'hanno da tener in sborar ogni sorte di robbe infette, et suspette facilmente et sicuramente, 1576, ix novembre (Venice: Domenico de Ferri, 1576).

Columba, Gerardo, *Disputationum de febris pestilentis cognitione & curatione* (Messina: apud Petrum Bream, 1596).

'Ein Compendium epidemiae, aufbewahrt in Danzig' (beginning of the fifteenth century), *Sudhoff*, XI (1919): 165–76.

Compendium de Epidemia per collegium Facultatis Medicorum Parisius Ordinatum. ed. H. Emile Rébouis, in *Étude historique et critique sur la peste* (Paris, 1888), 70–145.

Complani, Bassiano, *Pestilentis morbi praecautione ex communi illustrium medicorum consensu . . .* (Brescia: ex Calcographia Vincentii Sabii, 1577).

Condivi [Condio], Lorenzo, *Medicina filosofica contra la peste* (Lyon: Alessandro Marsilij, 1581).

Conseil des medecins de Lyon, assemblez pour ordonner les remedes plus necessaires & plus aisez à preparer en la faueur du pauure peuple affligé de peste. . . (Lyon: Par Iean Phillehotte, 1581).

Consigli contro la peste (da un manoscritto della Braidense), ed. B. Ferrari-S. Balossi (Pisa, 1966).

Contardi, Giovanni Agostino. *Il modo di preservarsi e curarsi dalla peste* (Genoa: appresso Marc'Antonio Bellone, 1576).

Cornuato, Antonio, *Breve relatione della processione solenne fatta in Torino la prima Domenica di Quaresima con assistenza di Sua Altezza Serenissima, per la preservatione e liberatione d'essa città dalla Peste* (Torino: appresso Antonio de' Bianchi, 1599).

Corvi, Guglielmo, *De febribus tractatus optimus. De peste. De consilio observando tempore pestilentiali ac etiam de cura pestis tractatus perspicuus eiusdem . . .* (Venice: per Bonetum Locatellum, 1508).

Cronaca senese di Donato di Neri e di suo figlio Neri [aa. 1352–1381] in *Cronache senesi*, ed. Alessandro Lisini and Fabio Iacometti, *Rerum Italicarum Scriptores* [hereafter RIS], XV/6 (Bologna, 1900–).

Crotto, Leone, *Memoriale delle provisioni generali, Che a' Prencipi s'aspetta di fare in tempi di peste* (1576).

Curationes ad praevisionem pestis, ex rogatu procerum politiocum . . . (Paris: Chez Thomas Perier, 1581).

Daciano, Gioseffo, *Trattato della peste et delle petecchie* (Venice: appresso Chrisoforo Zanetti, 1576).

da Marostica, Giuliano, *Copia d' vna lettera dello eccellente . . . Giuliano da Marostica treuisano in materia di medicar la peste, & le petecchie, & di preservar dall' uno, & l' altro male* (Venice: n.p, 1556).

Darezia, Anibal, *Auisi Dongaria del'assedio de Strigonia . . . con lintrada del turcho in peste* (Mantua, 1566?).

da Tolone, Mauritio, *Trattato politico da pratticarsi ne' tempi di peste, circa gl'ordini communi, e particolari dell'infermarie, prugationi e quarantine . . .* (Genoa: Per Pietro Giovanni Calenzani, 1661).

Da Vigo, Giovanni, *Secreti mirabilissimi contra peste dell'eccellentissimo Messer Giovanni di Vigo il quale fu Medico di Papa Giulio Secondo, con alcuni conisgli circa questa materia d'altri ecclentissimi Medici* (1556).

de Courselles, Françoys, *Traité de la peste clair et très utile* (Paris: Chez Guillaume Auuray. . . , 1596).

De foeda pestis rabie in Venetam ciuitatem saevius. Diutiusque furente assiduis ad eum precibus, sollemnique voto penitus extinguenda oraculum (Venice? not before 1576).

Defoe, Daniel, *A Journal of the Plague Year* (London, E. Nutt . . . , 1722).

De Forte, Angelo, *Il trattato de la peste, dove si fa conoscere* . . . (Venice: Giovanni Griffio, 1556).

Della Croce [Crucetii], Lodovico Annibale, *Ad Deum Opt. Max. Precatio* (Milan: Ex Typographia Io. Baptistae Pontii, 1576).

Del regimento della vita. Ordine e modo di vivere a tempo de pestilentia . . . (Venice: eredi di Giovanni Padovano, 155?).

De mandato del Serenissimo Principe, & . . . *Proveditori alla Sanità. Fanno publicamente a beneficio universale, publicar & propalar il presente rimedio preservativo dal mal Contagioso* . . . *dell'Ecc M. Ascanio Oliveri Medico al Lazaretto Vecchio* (Venice: Domenico de Ferri, 1576).

De Pomi, David, *Brevi discorsi et efficacissimi ricordi; per liberare ogni città oppressa dal Mal contagioso; proposti in diversi tempi* . . . (Venice: appresso Gratioso Perchacino, 1577).

de Rubys, Claude, *Discours sur la contagion de peste qui a esté ceste presente année en la ville de Lyon, contenant les causes d'icelle, moyen et police tenue pour en purger, nettoyer et delivrer la ville* (Lyon: par Jean d'Ogerolles, 1577).

Una devota supplicatione della citta di Venetia al Signore Iddio . . . *con farci liberi del presente contagio* (1576).

'Di alcuni versi inediti sulla peste del 1575', ed. Antonio Pilot, in *Ateneo Veneto* 26 (1903): 350–9.

Il diario di Giambattista Casale (1554–1598), ed. Carlo Marcora, in *Memorie Storiche della Diocesi di Milano*, 12 (1965): 209–437.

I Diarii di Girolamo Priuli, 1494–1512, ed. Roberto Cessi, RIS 24/3 (Città di Castello, 1912).

Dominici, Ser Luca, *Cronache di Ser Luca Dominici*, ed. Giovan Carlo Gigliotti, I: *Cronaca della venuta dei Bianchi e della Moria 1399–1400* (Pistoia, 1933).

Donzellini, Girolamo, *Discorso nobilissimo e dottissimo preservativo et curativo della pesta* (Venice: appresso Horatio dei Gobi da Salò, 1576).

_____ *De natura, causis, et legitima curatione febris pestilentis* (Venice: apud Camillum & Ruttilinum Borgominerios, 1570).

_____ *Eudoxi Philalethis Adversus calumnias et sophismata cuiusdam personati, qui se euandrophilacten nominavit. Apologia* (Verona: apud Sebastianum a Donnis, 1573).

Dubois, Jacques, *De febribus commentarius ex libris aliquot Hippocratis & Galeni, parte plurima selectus* . . . (Venice: apud Andream Arriuabenum ad signum Putei, 1555).

Durante, Giulio, *Trattato della peste, et febre pestilentiale* (Venice: presso Gio. Battista Ciotti, 1600).

Emanuele, Bartolomeo, *Opus utilissimum contra pestilentiam* (Rome: per Antonium Bladum de Asula, 1525).

Ephemerides Urbevetanae dal Cod. Vaticano Urbinate 1745, (*Discorso Historico*), ed. Luigi Fumi, RIS, XV/5 (Città di Castello, 1902–20).

Essendo stato proposto alli Clarissimi Sig. Sopraproveditori & Proveditori alla Sanità (Venice, 1576).

[Eustachio, Celebrino] Giovani Pacalono, *Regimento mirabile et verissimo a conservar la Sanita in tempo di peste, co li remedii necessarii, da piu valenti Medici esperimentari . . .* (n.p., 1555).

Ewich, Johann von, *Of the Duetie of a Faithful and Wise Magistrate . . .* (London, 1583).

'Ex libro vetusto Dionysii Secundi Colle', in Heinrich Haeser, *Geschichte der epidemischen Krankheiten im Lehrbuch der Geschichte der Medizin und der epidemischen Krankheiten*, 3 vols (Jena, 1875–82), II, 169–70.

Ferro, Saladino, *Trattato della peste, et sua preservatione & cura, scritto da Saladino Ferro & tradotto da Salustio Viscanti Veletrano* (Foligno: per Agostino Colaldi appresso a Vincentio Cantagallo, 1565).

Ficino, Marsilio, *Il consiglio di .m. Marsilio Ficino fiorentino contro la pestilentia con altre cose aggiunte appropriate alla medesima malattia* (Florence: per gli heredi di Filippo di Giunta, 1522).

Fioravanti, Leonardo, *Il Reggimento della peste . . .* (Venice, appresso gli Heredi di Melchior Sessa, 1571).

Flandino, Ambrogio, *De animorum immortalitate a reuerendo sacre theologie doctore magistro Ambrosio Neapolitano . . .* (Mantua, 1519).

Follerio, Pietro, *Ad instructiones urbanas et regias pro custodia pestis brevis apparatus praefectis sanitatis non inutilis* (Rome: eredi di Antonio Blado, 1577).

Fracastoro, Girolamo, *De contagione et contagiosis morbis et eorum curatione, Libri III* [1546], ed. and trans. W. C. Wright (New York, 1930).

———— *De sympathia et antipathia rerum, Liber I*, ed. Concetta Pennuto (Rome, 2008).

Frangipane, Claudio Cornelio, *De peste coelitus illapsa anno M.D.LXXV* (Venice: Domenico Farri, 1576).

Frigimelega, Francesco, *Consiglio sopra la pestilentia qui in Padoa dell'Anno MDLV. . . .fatto a richiesta di questi illustrissimi Signori, e di questa alma città* (Padua: per Gratioso Perchacino, 1555).

Fumanelli, Antonio, *De compositione medicamentorum generis cuiuscunque ad morbos diversos, eiudem de Pestis curatione* (Venice: apud Hieronymum Scotum, 1548).

Gabrielli, Andreas, *De Peste, opus perutile ac praesidio locupletissimorum auctorum roboratum* (Bologna: apud Peregrinum Bonardum, 1577?).

Gallo, Andrea, *Fascis de peste, Peripneumonia pestilentiali cum sputo sanguinis, febre pestilentiali ac de quibusdam symptomatibus, in quinque dasciolos digestus* (Brescia: ex officina Io. Baptistae Bozolae, 1566); reprinted as *Fascis Aureus, De peste ac febre pestilentiali* (Frankfurt: Ex officina typographica Ioannis Saurii, 1606).

Gallo, Carlo, *De febribus pestilentibus, ac malignis, tractatus bipartitus . . .* (Ferrara: apud Victorium Baldinum, 1600).

Gastaldi, Girolamo, *Tractatus de avertenda et profliganda peste politico-legalis* (Bologna: Ex camerali typographia Manolessiana, 1684).

Giudici, Giovanni Battista, *Il trattato della peste diviso in tre libri* (Lucca: appresso Vincenzo Busdraghi, 1577).

Glisenti, Antonio, *Oratione divotissima per ringratiare il nostro Signore Iddio, nella liberatione del Male Contagioso di Venetia* (n.p., not before 1576).

_____ *Il summario delle cause che dispongono i corpi de gli huomini a patire la corrottione pestilente del presente anno MDLXXVI* (Venice: Rutilio e Camillo Borgominieri, 1576).

_____ *Trattato del Regimento del vivere et delle altre cose che deveno usare gli uomini per preservarsi nelli tempi Pestilenti* (Venice: appresso Rutilio e Camillo Borgominerij, 1576?).

Goselini, Giuliano, *Componimenti Christiani in materia de la peste* (Milan: per Gio. Battista Pontio, 1577).

Gratarolo, Guglielmo, *Pestis descriptio, causae, signa omnigena & praeservatio* (Basel: Ludovicus Lucius, 1554).

Grassi, Girolamo, *Diario empirico dell'eccellente M. Girolamo Crasso . . . Nel quale si dimostra il modo di curare ogni sorta di ferita nel corpo humano. Aggiuntoui vn breue trattato in materia della peste* (Venice: appresso gli heredi di Francesco Rampazetto, 1577).

Gratiolo di Salò, Andrea, *Discorso di peste: nel quale si contengono utilissime speculationi intorno alla natura, cagioni, e curatione della peste, con un catalogo di tutte le pesti più notabili de' tempi passati* (Venice: appresso Girolamo Polo, 1576).

Gregorii PP. XIII Iubileum ad avertenda pestis pericula Venetiis (Venice: apud Danielem Zanettum, 1576).

Gregorii PP. XIII [S.D.N.D.] Iubileum ad avertenda pestis pericula (Rome: apud haeredes Antonij Bladij Impressores Camerales, 1576).

[Gregorii PP] *Il sommario del Giubileo del.S .S. N. S. Gregorio papa XIII per rimover i pericoli della Peste* (Venice: appresso Daniel Zanetti, 1576).

Guinther of Andernach, Johann [Johann Winter], *De Pestilentia Commentarius: In quatuor dialogus distinctus* (Strasbourg: Mylius, 1565).

Guy de Chauliac (Guigonis de Caulhiaco), *Inventarium sive chirurgia magna*, vol. I. *Text*, ed. Michael R. McVaugh (Leiden, 1997).

_____ *Chiurgia*, Tract. II, cap. 5, in Haeser, *Geschichte der epidemischen Krankheiten*, 175–6.

Horrox, Rosemary, ed. and trans. *The Black Death*, Manchester Medieval Sources series (Manchester, 1994).

'Die Identität des Regimen contra pestilentiam des Kanutus Episcopus Arusiensis (1461–2) . . . mit der Pestschrift des Johannes Jacobi', *Sudhoff*, V (1911): 56–8.

Ingrassia, Giovanni Filippo, *Avertimenti contra la peste raccolti dalli scritti di Gio. Filippo Ingarsia [sic], Protomedico di Sicilia* (Genoa: 1579).

_____ *Informatione del pestifero et contagioso morbo . . .* (Palermo: Giovan Mattheo Mayda, 1576; reprinted with introduction and notes by Luigi Ingaliso (Milan, 2005).

_____ *Parte quinta di Giouan Filippo Ingrassia del pestifero, & contagioso morbo . . .* (Palermo: Giovan Mattheo Mayda, 1577).

_____ *Trattato assai bello et utile di doi mostri nati in Palermo in diversi tempi . . . Agiontovi un ragionamento, fatto in presenza del Magistrato sopra le infermita epidemiali e popolari successe nell'anno 1558 in detta Città . . .* (Palermo: Giovan Matthei Mayda, 1560).

Ionni, Donato, *Carmen. De urbe Veneta pestilentia liberata, Anno M.D. LXXVII* (1576).

Iordan, Thomas, *Pestis phaenomena seu de iis quae circa febrem pestilentiem apparent, exercitatio* (Frankfurt: apud Andream Wechelum, 1576).

Johanns de Tornamira, 'Praeservatio et cura apostematum antrosum pestilentialium' (around 1360), *Sudhoff*, V (1911): 46–53.

Johannes Jacobi, 'Tractatus de peste ad honorem sancte et individue Trinitatis', *Sudhoff*, XVII (1925): 16–32.

'Ein Kölner Pestinkunabel kurz vor 1500', *Sudhoff*, XVI (1925): 152–3.

Lamento della città di Vicenza, L'anno M. D. LXXVII, Aggiuntovi alcuni sonetti in Lode del Signor Gieronimo Schio (Vicenza: appresso Giorgio Angelieri, 1578).

Landi, Bassiano, *De Origine et causa pestis Patavinae, Anni MDLV* (Venice: Ioan. Gryphius excudebat, 1555).

La Legislazione medicea sull'ambiente. I. I Bandi (1485–1619), ed. Giovanni Cascio Pratilli and Luigi Zangheri (Florence, 1994).

Legislazione Toscana, ed. Lorenzo Cantini, 31 vols (Florence, 1800–1808).

Le lagrime di Palermo. Canzone per la peste di Palermo nell'anno 1575 (Palermo?, 1575?).

Le Paulmier, Julien, *Bref discours de la preservation et curation de la peste* (Angers: par Anthoine Hernault, 1584).

Lettera pastorale di Monsig. Ill Card. Paleotti, Vescovo di Bologna, al Popolo suo nel pericolo della Peste (Bologna: per Alessandro Benaccio, 1576).

'Leve Consilium de pestilentia a Francischino de Collignano Florentiae (1382)', *Sudhoff*, V (1912), 365–84.

Leveroni, Giovenale, *Due discorsi volgari in materia di Medicina consecrati al SS. N. S. Papa Sisto V* (Turin: Antonio de' Bianchi, 1590).

Lini da Correggio, Giovanni Antonio. *Trattato contra peste novamente e succuntamente composto all'utilità publica dal Magnifico et ingeniosissimo . . .* (Bologna, 1576).

Loarti, Gaspar de, *Antidoto spirituale contra la peste* (Genoa: per Marc' Antonio Bellone, 1577).

Locati, Umberto, *Italia trauagliata novamente posta in luce, nellaqual si contengono tutte le Guerre, Seditioni, Pestilentie & altri Travagli* (Venice: appresso Daniel Zanetti, & compagni, 1576).

Lumina, Muzio, *La liberatione di Vinegia, insieme con il voto fatto dalli Signori di vna Chiesa dedicata al Sommo Nostro Redentore. . .* (Bologna: per Alessandro Benacci, 1577).

Machiavelli, Niccolò, *Opere di Niccolò Machiavelli cittadino e segretario fiorentino*, 5 vols (1813).

Madrigali spirituali nel tempo della peste nella città di Vicenza, l'anno, M. D. LXXVII (Vicenza: appresso Giorgio Angelieri, 1578).

Maganza, Giovanni Battista, *Canzone di Gio. Battista Maganza, nel calamitoso stato di Venetia, l'anno M.D.LXXVI* (Vicenza, 1576).

Mainardi, Pietro, *De preservatione hominum a pestiphero morbo* (Venice, c.1523).

Marinelli, Giovanni, *De peste, ac de pestilenti contagio liber: in quo disputatur, quantum inter se distent pestis, & pestilens contagium: & quae contagioni pestilenti, quales sunt bubones pestiferi . . .* (Venice: apud Gratiosum Perchacinum, 1577).

Massa, Niccolò, *De essentia causis et cura pestilentiae Venetiis grassantis anno 1556*, published as Letter 35 in his *Epistolarum medicinalium tomus primus* (Venice: Stellae Iordini Zilleti, 1558).

—— *Liber de febre pestilentiali, ac de pestichiis, morbillis, variolis & apostematibus pestilentialibus . . .* (Venice: apud Andream Arrivabenum ad signum Putei, 1556).

—— *Ragionamento dello eccellentiss.M. Nicolo Massa sopra le infermità, che vengono dall'aere pestilentiale del presente Anno 1555* (Venice: all'insegna della Stella, 1556).

Massaria, Alessandro, *De abusu medicamentorum vesicantium et theriacae in febribus pestilentibus disputatio* (Padua: apud Paulum Meiettum, 1591).

_____ *De peste: Libri duo* (Venice: apud Altobellum Salicatium, 1579).

Massucci, Marino, *La preseruatione dalla pestilenza* . . . (Macerata: appresso Sebastiano Martellini, 1577).

Mead, Richard, *A Discourse on the Plague*, 9th edn (London, 1744).

Il Memoriale di Iacopo di Coluccino Bonavia medico Lucchese (1373–1416), ed. Pia Pittino Calamari in *Studi di Filologia Italiana*, 24 (Florence, 1966).

'Le "Memorie" di Giovan Ambrogio Popolano', 9–15, in Filippo Maria Ferro, *La Peste nella cultura Lombarda* (Venice, 1975), first published as 'Diario di un popolano milanese la peste del 1576, *Archivio Storico Lombardo* (1877): 124–40.

Mercuriale, Girolamo, *De pestilentia* . . . *in quibus de peste in universum, praesertim vero de Veneta & Patavina* (Venice: apud Paulum Meietum, 1577).

Mignoto, Giovanni Maria, *Mignotydea de peste* . . . (Milan: Gotardus Ponticus, 1535).

Minutoli, Antonio, *Avvertimenti sopra la preservatione dalla peste* (Lucca: appresso Vincenzo Busdraghi, 1576).

Mocca, Cesare, *Discorsi preservativi e curativi per la peste, co'l modo di purgare le case & robbe appestate* (Venice: Ghirardo Imberti, 1630).

_____ *Trattrato della peste* (Carmagnola: appresso Marc'Antonio Bellone, 1599).

Montecchio, Sebastiano, *Carmen epicum super hoc lethifero anno MDLXXVI* (Padua: Laurentius Pasq., 1576).

Morea, Vitangelo, *Storia della peste di Noja* (Naples: A. Trani, 1817).

Morosini, Andrea, *Degl'istorici delle cose veneziane i quali hanno scritto per pubblico decreto*, 7 vols (Venice: appresso il Lovisa, 1718–9).

Moulton, Thomas, *Myrour or glasse of healthe: Necessary & nedefull for euery person to loke in, that wyll kepe their bodye from the syckenesse of the pestilence* (London: Robert Toye, c.1546).

Mugino, Giuseppe, *Trattato breve sopra la preservatione & cura della Peste* (Milan: per Iacomo Maria Meda, 1577; reprinted, Gio.Battista Bidelli, 1630).

Muratori, Lodovico, *Del governo della peste, e delle maniere di guardarsene* . . . *divio in Politico, Medico, ed Ecclesiastico* . . . (Rome: per Girolamo Mainardi, 1743).

_____ *Della pubblica felicità, oggetto de' buoni prìncipi* in *La letteratura italiana: storia e testi*, 44, 1, ed. Giorgio Falco and Fiorenzo Forti (Milan, 1964), ch. 11, 1566–72.

Mutinelli, Fabio. *Storia arcana ed aneddotica d'Italia raccontata dai veneti Ambasciatori*, 4 vols (Venice, 1855–8).

Napolitano, Giovanni Battista, *Opera et trattato che insegna molti dignissimi secreti contra la peste, con li quali subito si guarisce Composto per il Venerabile frate Giovanni Battista Napolitano governatore sopra li amorbati in Napoli de Reame* (Venice: per Bernardinum de Vitalibus, 1527).

_____ *Opera et trattato che insegna* (Venice, 1556).

_____ *Trattato di mirabili secreti contro la peste* (Brescia,: appresso Giacome & Policreto de Turlini fratelli, 1576).

Nevizzano, Giovanni. *Summarium decretorum Sabaudiae* . . . *M.ccccxxij* (1522).

'Notizen zur Pestkur von Antonius de Salomonibus, Canonicus bei Sanct Petronio zu Bologna vom Jahre 1464', *Sudhoff*, XVI (1925): 124–5.

Oddi, Oddo degli, *De pestis & pestiferorum omnium affectuum causis, signis, Praecautione & Curatione, Libri IIII* (Venice: apud Paulum & Antonium Meietos Fratres, 1570).

'Opuscule relatif à la peste de 1348 composé par un contemporain', ed. E. Littré. *Bibliotèque d'École des chartes*, 2 (1841): 201–43.

Oratione devoto da dirsi ogni giorno da tutti li fideli Christiani massime in questi tempi calamitosi, per placar l'ira del N.S. Iddio (c.1576).

Oratione al Signore Iddio per la liberatione del male contagioso (c. 1576).

Oratione alla Vergine Maria contra la peste (c.1576).

Orationi devotissime contra la peste (c.1576).

'Gli Ordinamenti sanitari del Comune di Pistoia contra la pestilenza del 1348', ed. A. Chiappelli, *Archivio Storico Italiano*, ser. 4, 20 (1887): 8–22.

Ordine et modo tenuto da monsig. Antonio Giannotto, vescouo di Forli, in celebrare il Giubileo dell'Anno Santo, et quello della peste. Raccolto da vn pio sacerdote, con alcune altre cose, degne di notizia (Cesena: appresso Bartolomeo Raverij, 1578).

Ordonnances contre la peste et autres ordonnances concernant la salubrité publique dans la ville de Rouen rendues par la cour de l'échiquier . . . , ed. Charles Lormier (Rouen, 1863).

Ordonnance de la police de la ville & faulxbourgs de Paris, pour obvier au dangier de la peste. . . 16 sept 1533. . . (Paris, 1553).

Les ordonnances faictes et publiees a son de trompe par les carresfours de ceste ville de Paris. Pour eviter la dangier de peste (1512).

Orsini, Giovanni [Jean Ursin], *Elegiae de peste de eaque medicinae parte quae in victus ratione consistit . . .* (Alessandria: Francesco e Simone Moschini, 1549).

Ottimi remedi per mantenersi sani nel tempo della peste (1576).

'Ein Paduaner Pestkonsilium von Dr. Stephanus de Doctoribus', *Sudhoff*, VI (1913): 355–61.

Paleotti, Gabriele, *Sommario delle cose ordinate da Mons. Ill. Card Parleotti Vescovo di Bologna nella Congregatione de Pievani & Visitatori, sopra i sospetti della Pestilentia & altri bisogni delle loro Chiese, alli 2. d'Ottobre 1576* (Bologna : per Alessandro Benacci, 1576).

——— *Lettera pastorale di . . . Paleotti* [within Razzi, Cause, 113–35].

Panebianco, Domenico, ' "De preservatione a pestilencia" di Cardone de Spanzotis de Mediolano, del 1360', *Archivio Storico Lombardo*, 102 (1977): 347–54.

Panizzone Sacco, Olivero, *Giubilo della citta di Milano per la gratia ricevuta dalla Maestà Divina, della liberatione della contagiosa infermità pestilentiale* (Alessandria: apresso Hercole Quinciano, 1578).

——— *Pianto della città di Milano per la pestilenza dell'anno 1576 & 1577* (Alessandria: appresso Hercole Quincino, 1578).

Parisi, Pietro, *Auuertimenti sopra la peste, e febre pestifera, con la somma delle loro prencipali cagioni* (Palermo: per Gio. Antonio de Franceschi, 1593).

——— *Trattato della peste et febre pestifera* (Palermo: per Gio. Antonio de Franceschi, 1593).

Pasini, Lodovico, *De pestilentia Patavina anno 1555* (Padua: apud Gratiosum Perchacinum, 1556).

Pastarino, *Preparamento del Pastarino per medicarsi in questi sospetosi tempi di peste* (Bologna: per. Gio. Rossi, 1577).

'Eine Pestbeulenkur unter dem Namen des Kardinals Philipp von Alenzolo', *Sudhoff*, VI (1913): 342–4.

'Die Pestschrift des "Blasius Brascinensis" (Barcelonensis)', *Sudhoff*, XVII (1925): 103–19.

'Die Pestschriften des Johann von Burgund und Johann von Bordeaux', *Sudhoff*, V (1911): 58–75.

'Pestilence', in *Galar y Beirdd: Marwnadau Plant/ Poets' Grief: Medieval Welsh Elegies for Children*, ed. Dafydd Johnston (Cardiff, 1993), 50–8.

'Der Pesttraktat des Pietro di Tussignano (1398)', *Sudhoff*, V (1912): 390–5.

'Ein Pesttraktat eines Magister Berchtoldus', *Sudhoff*, XVI (1925): 77–95.

'Das Pestwerkchen des Raymundus Chalin de Vinario', *Sudhoff*, XVII (1925): 35–9.

Petrarca, Francesco, *Opere*, ed. E. Bigi (Milan, 1963).

——— *Francesco Petrarca Poesia Latine*, ed. Guido Martellotti and Enrico Bianchi (Turin, 1976).

Il pianto della sconsolata città di Vicenza, l'anno M. D. LXXVII, dove lei determinate d'emendarsi de' suoi peccati, conseguisse gratia da Dio per sua salute (Vicenza: appresso Giorgio Angelieri, 1577).

Picegaton di memorosi Beretaro de la contra di San Lazaro al clarissimo podestà (1577?).

Pisanelli, Baldassare, *Discorso di M. Baldassarre Pisanelli bolognese medico di S. Spirito sopra la peste diuiso in due parti* (Rome: per gli eredi di Antonio Blado, stampatori camerali, 1577).

Podiani, Luca Alberto, *Preservatio a peste nuper compilata numquam ante impressa* (Perugia: arte & impensa Cosimi Ver. Blanchini, 1523).

Politi, Lancellotto, *Rimedio a la pestilente dottrina de frate Bernardino Ochino* (Rome: ne la contrada del Pellegrino, 1544).

Politici e moralisti del Seicento: Strada, Zuccolo, Settala, Accetto, Brignole Sale, Malvezzi, ed. Benedetto Croce and Santino Caramella (Bari, 1930).

Porto, Antonio, *De peste libri tres: De morbillis liber vnus. Recenter recogniti et copiosius aucti* (Roma: apud Dominicum Basam, 1589).

Preghi al Signore Iddio per la liberatione del popolo di Vinegia dalla pestilenza (Venice, 1576).

Previdelli, Girolamo, *Tractatus legalis de peste, In quo continetur quid de iure fieri debeat, et possit tam circa ea, quae salubritatem civitatum respiciunt quam circa ultimas voluntates, iudicia et ceteros actus inter vivos, tempore quo peste affligimur* (Bologna: excusus a Ioanne Baptista Phaello, 1524).

Prezati, Gabriele, *Tractatus flagellum Dei intitulatus de praeservatione ac curatione pestis* (Pavia: Giacomo Pocatela, 1504).

'Prophylaxe und Kur pestilentialischer Fieber nach Nicolaus Florentinus (Niccolò Falcucci, end of the fourteenth century)', Sudhoff, VI (1913): 338–41.

Pucci, Antonio, 'Delle crudeltà della pestilenza', in *Storia letteraria d'Italia*, ed. Natalino Sapegno (Milan, 1948), p. 413.

Puccinelli, Alessandro, *Dialoghi sopra le cause della peste universale* (Lucca: appresso Vincenzo Busdraghi, 1577).

Quattrami, Frate Evangelista, *Breve trattato intorno alla preservatione, et cura della peste* (Roma: nelle stamparia de Vincentio Accolti, 1586).

Raccolta delli componimenti scritti in Lodi del Clarissimo Signor Nicolò Barbarigo Podestà di Verona (Verona: apud Sebastianum & Iannem à Donnis frates, 1576).

Raccolta di avvertimenti et raccordi per conoscer la peste: Per curarsi & preservarsi & per purgar robbe & case infette. Presentata al Magistrato eccellent.mo della Sanità di Venetia (Venice: Presto Combi & là Noù, 1630).

Raimondo, Annibale, *Apologia di Annibale Raimondo Veronese, Intorno alcuni amorevoli avisi mandateli & per la risolutione di variij & diversi Dubij* (Venice: Domenico Nicolini da Sabbio, 1576).

Raimondo, Annibale, *Discorso de Annibale Raimondo veronese nel quale chiaramente si conosce la viva et vera cagione, che ha generati le fiere infermità, che tanto hanno molestato l'anno 1575 & tanto il 76* . . . (Padua, 1576).

Razzi, Silvano, *Cause et rimedi della peste et d'altre infermità . . . Fatti raccogliere per ordine di Mons. Rev.ssmo Marco Gonzaga Vescovo di Mantova* . . . (Florence: Giunti, 1577).

—— *Modo di conservarsi sano per regola di vita* (Florence: appresso Bartolomeo Sermartelli, 1577).

Regesti di bandi, editti, notificazioni e provvedimenti diversi relative alla città di Roma ed allo Stato Pontificio: I *(anni 1234–1605)*, ed. Francesco Scaduto (Rome, 1920).

Ricordi di m. Paolo Clarante da Terni medico in Roma, Ricordi per gli Infermi (c.1576).

Righi, Alessandro, *Historia contagiosi morbi, qui Florentiam populatus fuit anno 1630* (Florence: Typis Francisci Honufrii, 1633).

Rime di diverso a gli habitani di Venetia, et a quelli che sono partiti per la peste (Venice, 1576).

Rivetti, Giorgio, *Trattato sopra il mal delle pettechie, peste è gianduissa, & il modo, che si ha da tener per curar le Febre Pestilentiali & altri simili mali raccolti da varij auttorii* (Bologna: Vittorio Benacci, 1592).

Roffredi, Filippo Maria, *Pestis, et calamitatum Taurini Subalpinae Galliae metropolis anni MDXCIX* (Turin, 1600).

Rondinelli, Francesco, *Relazione del contagio stato in Firenze l'anno 1630 e 1633. Con un breve ragguaglio della Miracolosa Immagine della Madonna dell'Impruneta* (Florence: Giovanni Battista Landini, 1634).

Royet, Antoine, *Traicté de la peste, monstrant les causes et signes dicelle* . . . (Lyon: Pour Iean Durant, 1583).

Rufini, Giacomo, *Carmen de pestilentia Venetam urbem vexante MDLVI* (Venice: dagli eredi di Lucantonio Giunta il vecchio, 1557).

Rustico, Pietro Antonio, *Qui atrocem horres pestem* . . . (1520?).

Sale, Cristoforo, *Trattato di Epidemia* (Trevigio: appresso Euangelista Dehuchino, 1599).

Sassonia, Ercole, *Disputatio de Phoenigmorum, quae vulgo Vesicantia appellantur & de Theriacae usu in febribus pestilentibus, in qua etiam de natura pestis & pestilentium febrium* (Padua: apud Paulum Meiettum, 1591).

—— *Praticam medicinam in Patavino gymnasio* (Padua: apud Paulum Meiettum 1591).

Settala, Lodovico, *De peste et pestiferis affectibus. Libri quinque* (Milan: apud Joannem Baptistam Bidellium, 1622).

Scelta de i piu belli e bizari motti che si sono veduti scritti sopra le Botteghe serrate di Venetia (c.1576).

Somenzi, Tommaso, *De morbis, qui per finitimos populus adhuc grassantur* (Cremona: apud Christoporum Draconium, 1576).

Sorboli, Girolamo, *Discorso del vero modo di preseruare gli huomini dalla peste* . . . (Bologna: per Gio. Rossi, 1577).

Sovirolius, Guillielmus, *Brevis & accurata de peste disputatio* (Paris, 1571).

Squacialupi, Marcello, *Difesa contra la peste* (Milan: appresso Francesco Moscheni, 1565).

Stabile, Francesco, *Breuis quaedam defensiocontra nonnullos asserentes pudendorum inflammationem non esse pestis signum* . . . (Venice: apud Gratiosum Perchacinum, 1576).

Sudhoff, Karl, 'Pestschriften aus den ersten 150 Jahren nach der Epidemie des "schwarzen Todes" 1348' in *Archiv für Geschichte der Medizin [Sudhoff]*, VI–XVII (1910–25).

Strazzolini, Jacopo, *La peste a Cividale nel 1598*, in Mario Brozzi, *Peste, fede e sanità in una cronaca cividalese del 1598* (Milan, 1982), 29–57.

Supplicatione divotissima sopra queste due parole, Ave Maria, in otto stanze . . . (Venice, 1576).

Susio, Giovanni Battista, *Libro secondo del conoscere la pestilenza: dove si mostra, che in Mantova non è stato male di simil sorte l'anno M.D.LXXV . . .* (Brescia: appresso Giacoma, & Policreto Turlini Frat., 1579).

Tiani [Theani], Bartolomeo, *De singulari pestilentiae magnitudine & atrocitate quae Brixianam civitatem & Agrum fere totum nuperrime invasit, ac pene diripuit* (Brescia: apud Vincentium Sabbium, 1578).

*Tempore pestis oratio (c.*1576).

Tomai [Thomaii], Camillo, *De medendis febribus humoralibus . . . commentariolus* (Venice: apud Andream Arivalbenum, 1542).

Tomitano, Bernardino, *Il consiglio sopra la peste di Vinetia l'anno 1556* (Padua: appresso Gratioso Perchacino, 1556).

Tommasi, Francesco, *Tractatus de peste. Ad Illustrem & Reuerendiss. D. Ioannem Baptistam Ruynum Hospitalis S. Spiritus in Saxia . . .* (Rome: Iacobi Tornerij & Bernardini Donangeli, 1587).

Tommaso del Garbo, *Consiglio contro a pistolenza*, ed. Pietro Ferrato, Scelta di Curiosità letterarie inedite o rare dal secolo XIII al XVII, 74 (Bologna, 1866).

Torella, Gaspar, *Qui cupit a peste non solum preservari sed & curari hoc legat consilium* (Rome, 1504).

Thomae Walsingham, quondam monachi S. Albani, Historia Anglicana, ed. Henry T. Riley, in *Rerum Britannicarum Medii Aevi Scriptores* 28/1, vol. 1, 1272–1381 (London, 1863).

'Der Tractatus pestilentialis eines Theobaldus Loneti aus Aurigny in der Diözese Besançon', *Sudhoff*, XVII (1925): 53–65.

'Tractatus de praeservationibus . . . Hinricum Rybbinis de Wartislavia', *Sudhoff*, IV (1910): 205–22.

Traffichetti, Bartolomeo, *Antidosis Bartolomaei Traffichetti Britonoriensis medici, aduersus Marcum Antonium Capellettum Calliensem medicum, in qua plurimæ soluuntur difficultates cum circa pleuritidem, tum febrem pestilentem. . .* (Venice: apud Gratiosum Perchacinum, 1572).

Tranquilli, Vincenzo, *Pestilenze che sono state in Italia da anni MMCCCXI in qua, co i prodigii osseruati inanzi all'auuenimento loro, et i remedij et prouisioni usatevi di tempo in tempo* (Perugia: per Baldo Saluiani, 1576).

Tranzi, Sebastiano, *Trattato di peste* (Rome: Per gl'Heredi di Giovanni Gigliotto, 1587).

Trevisio, Andrea, *De caussis, natura moribus ac curatione pestilentium febrium* (Milan: apud Pacificum Pontium, 1588).

Tronconi, Jacobo, *De peste et pestilenti morbo, Libri Quatuor* (Florence: in officina Georgii Marescoti, 1577).

Turini, Andrea, *De bonitate aquarum fontanae, et cisterninae* (Rome: in vico Pellegrini apud Balthasarem de Cartulariis Persusinum, 1542).

―――― *Utile consiglio preservativo & curativo delle peste, facto per generale comodita & bene del Populo de Roma* (Rome: J.Mazochius, *c.*1505–1510?).

Valdagni, Giuseppe, *De theriacae usu in febribus pestilentibus Iosephi Valdanii medici libellus* (Brescia: apud Vincentium Sabiensem, 1570).

Valier, Agostino, *Commentariolus quo explicatur qua ratione Dominus pestilentiae suspicione comminatus sit Veronae, anno sanctissimi iubilei, M.D.LXXV* (Verona, apud Sebatianum a Donnis & Ioannem fratres, 1576).

⸺ *Lettera consolatoria del reverendiss. Mons. Agostino Valerio Vescovo di Verona . . .* (Venice: appresso Pietro Farri, 1575).

Venusti, Antonio Maria, *Consilium de peste* (Milan: apud Paulum Gottardum Pontium 1577).

Il vero e santo rimedio . . . (Venice: appresso Gabriel Giolito de Ferrari, 1556).

Villani, Matteo, *Cronica con la continuazione di Filippo Villani*, ed. Giuseppe Porta, 2 vols (Parma, 1995).

Viscanio, Giuseppe, *Regimento del viver commune a' sani in tempo di peste, o di sospetto* (Venice: appresso il Griffio, 1576).

Vives, Juan Luis, *De subventione pauperum. Libri II* (Leiden: Melchioris & Gasparis Trechsel fratru, 1532).

Zacchia, Paolo, *Quaestionum medico-legalium, tomi tres*, ed. Joan Danielis Orstii (Frankfurt, 1666).

SECONDARY SOURCES

Albini, Giuliana, *Guerra, fame, peste: crisi di mortalità e sistema sanitario nella Lombardia tardomedioevale* (Bologna, 1982).

Alfani, Guido and Samuel Cohn, 'Nonantola 1630. Anatomia di una pestilenza e meccanismi del contagio (con riflessioni a partire dalle epidemie milanesi della prima Età Moderna)', *Popolazione e Storia*, (2007): 99–138.

Amelang, James S, *A Journal of the Plague Year: The Diary of the Barcelona Tanner Miquel Parets 1651* (New York, 1991).

Arcangeli, Alessandro and Vivian Nutton (eds), *Girolamo Mercuriale: Medicina e cultura nell'Europa del Cinquecento, Atti del convegno 'Girolamo Mercuriale e lo spazio scientifico e culturale del Cinquecento (Forlì, 8–11 novembre 2006)'*.

Aymard, Maurice, 'Epidémies et médecins en Sicile à l'époque moderne', *Annales cisalpines d'histoire sociale'*, série 1, no. 4 (1973): 9–37.

Bazin-Tacchella, Sylvie, 'Rupture et continuité du discours médical à travers les écrits sur la peste de 1348 . . . ', in Sylvie Bazin-Tacchella, Danielle Quéruel, and Évelyne Samama (eds), *Airs, Miasmes et contagion: Les épidémies dans l'antiquité et au Moyen Age* (Langres, 2001), 105–31.

Babinger, F, 'Barbarigo, Niccolò', *Dizionario biographico degli Italiani* [hereafter *DBI*], 6 (1964), 76–8.

Baehrel, René, 'La haine de classe en temps d'épidémie', *Annales E. S. C.* 7 (1952): 351–60.

Bailey, Gavin, Pamela Jones, Franco Mormando, and Thomas Worcester (eds), *Hope and Healing: Painting in Italy in a Time of Plague, 1500–1800* (Chicago, 2005).

Bamji, Alexandra, 'Religion and Disease in Venice, c. 1620–1700' (Cambridge, PhD thesis, 2007).

Barkai, Ron, 'Jewish Treatises on the Black Death (1350–1500): A Preliminary Study', in French, Arrizabalaga, Cunningham, and García-Ballester, *Medicine from the Black Death to the French Disease*, 6–25.

Bell, Rudolph M, *How to Do It: Guides to Good Living for Renaissance Italians* (Chicago, 1999).

Belloni, Luigi, 'Carlo Borromeo e la storia della medicina', in *San Carlo e il suo tempo: Atti del Convegno Internazionale nel IV centenario della morte (Milano, 21–26 maggio 1984*, 2 vols (Rome, 1986), I, 165–77.

Bennassar, Bartolomé, *Recherches sur les grandes épidémies dans le nord de l'Espagne à la fin du XVIe siècle: Problèmes de documentation et de méthode* (Paris, 1969).

Bergdolt, Klaus, *La Pesta Nera e la fine del Medioevo: La più spaventosa epidemia nella storia dell'Occidente stermino millioni di persone*, trans. Anna Frisan (Casale Monferrato [AL], 2002).

Besozzi, Leonida, *Le magistrature cittadine milanesi e la peste del 1576–1577*, *Biblioteca dell' 'Archivio Storico Lombardo'*, no. 2 (Bologna, 1988).

Besta, Beatrice, 'La popolazione di Milano nel periodo della dominazione spagnola', in Corrado Gini (ed.), *Atti del Congresso Internazionale per gli studi sulla popolazione* (Rome 1933), I, 593–610.

Bibliografia cronologica di leggi sanitari; *Leggi e bandi del periodo mediceo posseduti dalla Biblioteca nazionale centrale di Firenze*, I: *1534–1600*, Gustavo Bertoli (Florence, 1992).

Bibliografia cronologica di leggi sanitarie toscane dall'anno 1161 all'anno 1841 (Florence, 1856).

Biraben, Jean-Noël. *Les hommes et la peste en France et dans les pays européens et méditerranéens*. Civilisations et Sociétés 35–6, 2 vols (Paris, 1976).

Bisgaard, Lars and Leif Søndergaard (eds), *Living with The Black Death* (Odense, 2009).

Black, Christopher, *Early Modern Italy: A Social History* (London, 2001).

Blockmans, W. P., 'The Social and Economic Effects of Plague in the Low Countries 1349–1500', *Revue belge de philologie et d'histoire*, 58 (1980): 833–63.

Bottero, Aldo, 'La peste in Milano nel 1399–1400 e l'opera di Gian Galeazzo Visconti', *Atti e Memorie dell'Accademia di Storia dell'Arte. Sanitaria La Rassegna di Clinica, Terapia e Scienze Affini*, 41, fasc. 6 (1942): 17–28.

Bourdelais, Patrice, 'Per una nuova storia sociale delle epidemie', *Epidemie e società nel Mediterraneo di età moderna*, ed. Giuseppe Restifo (Messina, 2001), 9–14.

Bouwsma, William J., *The Waning of the Renaissance 1550–1640* (New Haven, 2000).

Bowers, Kirsty Wilson. 'Plague, Politics and Municipal Relations in Sixteenth-Century Seville' (University of Indiana, PhD thesis, 2001).

Bowsky, William, 'The Medieval Commune and Internal Violence: Police, Power, and Public Safety in Siena, 1287–1355', *American Historical Review* 73 (1967): 1–17.

Brockliss, Lawrence and Colin Jones, *The Medical World of Early Modern France* (Oxford, 1997).

Bulst, Neithard and Robert Delort (eds), *Maladies et société (XIIe –XVIIIe siècles): Actes du colloque de Bielefeld novembre 1986* (Paris, 1989).

Burnet, Sir Macfarlane. *Natural History of Infectious Disease*, 3rd edn (Cambridge, 1962).

Bylebyl, Jerome J., 'The School of Padua: Humanistic Medicine in the Sixteenth Century', in Charles Webster (ed.), *Health, Medicine and Mortality in the Sixteenth Century* (Cambridge, 1979), 335–70.

Calvi, Giulia, 'L'oro, il fuoco, le forche: la peste napoletana del 1656', *Archivio Storico Italiano*, 507 (1981): 405–58.

———, *Histories of a Plague Year: The Social and the Imaginary in Baroque Florence*, trans. Dario Biocca and Bryant T. Ragan, Jr. (Berkeley, 1989).

Cantor, Norman, *In the Wake of the Plague: The Black Death and the World it Made* (New York, 2001).

Capasso, Gaetano, 'L'Officio della Sanità di Monza la peste degli anni 1576–7', *Archivio Storico Lombardo* 33 (1906): 299–330.

Carabellese, Francesco, *La peste del 1348 e le condizioni della sanità pubblica in Toscana* (Rocca S. Casciano, 1897).

Carmichael, Ann, *Plague and the Poor in Renaissance Florence* (Cambridge, 1986).

——— 'Contagion Theory and Contagion Practice in Fifteenth-Century Milan', *Renaissance Quarterly*, 44 (1991): 213–56.

——— 'History of Public Health and Sanitation in the West before 1700', in Kenneth F. Kiple (ed.), *The Cambridge World History of Human Disease* (Cambridge, 1993), 192–9.

——— 'Epidemics and State Medicine in Fifteenth-Century Milan', in French, Arrizabalaga, Cunningham, and García-Ballester, *Medicine from the Black Death to the French Disease*, 221–47.

——— 'The Last Past Plague: The Uses of Memory in Renaissance Epidemics', *Journal of the History of Medicine and Allied Sciences*, 53 (1998): 132–60.

——— 'Universal and Particular: The Language of Plague, 1348–1500', in Nutton, *Pestilential Complexities*, 43–51.

Carniel, Elisabeth, 'Plague Today', in Nutton, *Pestilential Complexities*, 115–22.

Carpentier, Elisabeth, *Une ville devant la peste: Orvieto et la peste noire de 1348* (Paris, 1962).

——— 'Famines et épidémies dans l'histoire du XIVe siècle', *Annales: E.S.C.*, 17 (1962), 1062–92.

Carreras Panchón, *Antono, La peste y los médicos en la España del Renacimiento* (Salamanca, 1976)

Cartwright, Frederick F, *A Social History of Medicine* (London, 1977).

Castiglioni, Arturo, 'Ugo Benzi da Siena ed il "Trattato utilissimo circa la conservazione della sanitate" ', *Rivista di Storia Critica delle Scienze Mediche e Naturali*, 12 (1921): 75–105.

——— 'I libri italiani della pestilenza', in Castiglioni, ed., *Il Volto di Ippocrate: Istorie di Medici e Medicine d'altri tempi* (Milano, 1925), 147–69.

——— *A History of Medicine*, trans. E. B. Krumbhaar, 2nd edn (New York, 1947).

Cavini, Giovanni., *L'influenza epidemica attraverso i secoli* (Rome, 1959).

Choksy, N. H., 'The Various Types of Plague and their Clinical Manifestations', *American Journal of Medical Sciences*, 138 (1909): 351–66.

Christensen, Peter, 'Appearance and Disappearance of the Plague: Still a Puzzle?' in Bisgaard and Søndergaard (eds), *Living with The Black Death*, 11–22.

Chun, J. W. H., 'Clinical Features', in Wu Lien-Teh, Chun, Pollitzer, and C. Y. Wu, (eds), *Plague: A Manual for Medical and Public Health Workers* (Shanghai Station, 1936), 309–33.

Cipolla, Carlo, *Cristofano and the Plague: A Study in the History of Public Health in the Age of Galileo* (London, 1973).

_____ 'Origine e sviluppo degli Uffici di Sanità in Italia', *Annales Cisalpines d'histoire sociale*, 1 (1973): 83–101.

_____ *Public Health and the Medical Profession in the Renaissance* (Cambridge, 1976).

_____ *Faith, Reason, and the Plague: A Tuscan Story of the Seventeenth Century*, trans. Muriel Kittel (Brighton, 1977).

_____ 'A Plague Doctor', in Harry A. Miskimin, David Herlihy, and A. L. Udovitch (eds), *The Medieval City* (New Haven, 1977), 64–72.

_____ *Fighting the Plague in Seventeenth-Century Italy* (Madison, WI, 1981).

_____ and Dante E. Zanetti, 'Peste et mortalité différentielle', *Annales de démographie historique* (1972): 197–202.

Cohn, Samuel, *Death and Property in Siena: Strategies for the Afterlife* (Baltimore, 1988).

_____ *The Black Death Transformed: Disease and Culture in Early Renaissance Europe* (London, 2002).

_____ *Lust for Liberty: The Politics of Social Revolt in Medieval Europe, 1200–1425* (Cambridge, MA, 2006).

_____ 'The Black Death and the Burning of Jews', *Past & Present*, 196 (2007): 3–36.

_____ and Guido Alfani, 'Households and Plague in Early Modern Italy', *Journal of Interdisciplinary History*, 38/2 (2007):177–205.

_____ 'Epidemiology of the Black Death and Successive Waves of Plague', in Nutton, *Pestilential Complexities*, 74–100.

Coleman, William, *Death Is A Social Disease: Public Health and Political Economy* in Early Industrial France (Madison, WI, 1982).

_____ *Yellow Fever in the North: The Methods of Early Epidemiology* (Madison, WI, 1987).

Conforti, Maria. 'Peste e stampa: Trattati, relazioni e cronache a Roma nel 1656', in Fosi, *La Peste a Roma*, 35–58.

Conrad, Lawrence I., Michael Neve, Nutton, Roy Porter, and Andrew Wear (eds), *The Western Medical Tradition 800 B.C. to A D 1800* (Cambridge, 1995).

Cook, Raymond A., 'The Influence of the Black Death on Medieval Literature and Language', *Kentucky Foreign Language Quarterly*, 11/1 (1964): 5–13.

Corradi, Alfonso, *Annali delle epidemie occorse in Italia dalle prime memorie fino al 1850*, 5 vols (Bologna, 1865–92).

Cosmacini, Giorgio, *Storia della medicina e della sanità in Italia: Dalla peste europea alla guerra mondiale, 1348–1918* (Bari, 1988).

Coville, Alfred, 'Écrits contemporains sur la peste de 1348 à 1350', in *Histoire littéraire de la France*, 37 (Paris, 1938), 325–90.

Craven, Robert B., 'Plague', in Paul D. Hoeprich, M. Colin Jordan, and Allan R. Ronald (eds), *Infectious Diseases: A Treatise of Infectious Processes*, 5th edn (Philadelphia, 1994), 1302–12.

D'Alessio, Silvana, 'Per una nuova scienza. Medicina e politica nella prima età moderna', in Antonella Argenio (ed.), *Biopolitiche* (Rome, 2006), 1–27.

D'Amico, Stefano, *Le contrade e la città: Sistema produttivo e spazio urbano a Milano fra Cinque e Seicento* (Milan, 1994).

Davi, Maria Rosa, *Bernardino Tomitano: Filosofo, medico e letterato (1517–1576): Profilo biografico e critico*. Centro per la storia dell'università di Padova (Trieste, 1995).

Del Panta, Lorenzo, *Le epidemie nella storia demografica italiana: secoli XVI–XIX* (Turin, 1980).

Del Panta, and Massimo Livi Bacci, 'Chronologie, intensité et diffusion des crises de mortalité en Italie: 1600–1850', *Population*, 32 (1977): 401–46.

Delumeau, Jean. *La peur en Occident (XIVe –XVIIIe siècle: Une cité assiégée* (Paris, 1978).

—— *Le péché et la peur: la culpabilisation en Occident (XIIIe–XVIIIe siècles)* (Paris, 1983).

—— *Rassurer et protéger: le sentiment de sécurité dans l'Occident d'autrefois* (Paris, 1989).

de Vivo, Filippo, *Information and Communication in Venice: Rethinking Early Modern Politics* (Oxford, 2007).

De Witte, Sharon N. and James W. Wood, 'Selectivity of Black Death Mortality with Respect to Preexisting Health', *Proceedings of the National Academy of Sciences*, 105 (2008): 1436–41.

Di Scala, Spencer M., *Italy: From Revolution to Republic, 1700 to the Present* (Boulder, CO, 1995).

Dollo, Carrado, *Filosofia e scienza in Sicilia: Catalogo di testi inediti (1501–1700)* (Catania, 1984).

Donato, Maria Pia, 'La peste dopo la peste: Economia di un discorso romano (1656–1720)', in Fosi, *La Peste a Roma*, 159–74.

Dubois, Henri, 'La depression: XIVe et XVe siècles', in Jacques Dupâquier (ed.), *Histoire de la population française* (Paris, 1988), I, 313–66.

Durling, Richard J., *A Catalogue of Sixteenth Century Printed Books in the National Library of Medicine* (Bethesda, 1967).

—— 'A Chronological Census of Renaissance Editions and Translations of Galen', *Journal of the Warburg and Courtauld Institutes*, 24 (1961): 230–305.

Eamon, William, *Science and the Secrets of Nature: Books of Secrets in Medieval and Early Modern Culture* (Princeton, 1994).

Evans, Richard, *Death in Hamburg: Society and Politics in the Cholera Years 1830–1910* (Oxford, 1987).

Fabbri, Christiane Nockels, 'Treating Medieval Plague: The Wonderful Virtues of Theriac', *Early Science and Medicine*, 12/3 (2007): 247–83.

Falsini, Aliberto Benigno, 'Firenze dopo il 1348. Le consequenza della peste nera', *Archivio Storico Italiano*, no. 472, CXXIX (1971): 425–503.

Ferrario, G., *Statistica medico-economica di Milano dal secolo XV fino ai nostri giorni* (Milan, 1838).

Fenlon, Iain, *The Ceremonial City: History, Memory and Myth in Renaissance Venice* (New Haven, 2007).

Findlen, Paula, *Possessing Nature: Museums, Collecting, and Scientific Culture in Early Modern Italy* (Berkeley, 1994).

—— 'The Formation of a Scientific Community: Natural History in Sixteenth-Century Italy', in Grafton and Siraisi, *Natural Particulars*, 369–400.

Firpo, L. 'Borgarucci', in *DBI*, 12 (1970), 565–8.

Fosi, Irene (ed.), *La Peste a Rome (1656–1657). Roma moderna e contemporanea*, 14 (2006).

Foucault, Michel, *Madness and Civilization: A History of Insanity in the Age of Reason*, trans. Richard Howard (New York, 2001).

French, Roger, Jon Arrizabalaga, Andrew Cunningham and Luis García-Ballester, *Medicine from the Black Death to the French Disease* (Aldershot 1998).

Gani, Raymond and Steve Leach, 'Epidemiologic Determinants for Modeling Pneumonic Plague Outbreaks', *Emerging Infectious Diseases* 10/4 (2004): 608–14.

Gatacre, W. F. *Report on the Bubonic Plague in Bombay, 1896–97 with Plans* (Bombay, 1897).

Gentilcore, David, ' "All that Pertains to Medicine": Protomedici and Protomedicati in Early Modern Italy', *Medical History*, 38 (1994): 269–96.

____ *Healers and Healing in Early Modern Italy* (Manchester, 1998).

____ *Medical Charlatanism in Early Modern Italy* (Oxford, 2006).

Giordano, Davide, *Leonardo Fioravanti, Bolognese* (Bologna, 1920).

Gnudi, Martha and Jerome Webster, *The Life and Times of Gaspare Tagliacozzi, Surgeon of Bologna, 1545–1599: With a Documented Study of the Scientific and Cultural Life of Bologna in the Sixteenth Century* (New York, 1950).

Gordon, Daniel, 'The City and the Plague in the Age of Enlightenment', *Yale French Studies*, 92 (1997): 67–87.

Gottfried, Robert S, 'Plague, Public Health and Medicine in Late Medieval England', in Bulst and Delort, *Maladies et société*, 337–65.

Grande dizionario della lingua italiana, 21 vols (Milan, 1961–2002).

Grell, Ole Peter, 'Plague in Elizabethan and Stuart London: The Dutch Response', *Medical History*, 34 (1990): 424–39.

____ and Andrew Cunningham, 'The Counter-Reformation and Welfare Provision in Southern Europe', in Grell, Cunningham and Arrizabalaga, *Health Care and Poor Relief*, 1–17.

____ Andrew Cunningham with Jon Arrizabalaga (eds), *Health Care and Poor Relief in Counter-Reformation Europe* (London, 1999).

Grendler, Paul F., 'Form and Function in Italian Popular Books', *Renaissance Quarterly*, 46 (1993): 451–85.

Guenée, Bernard, *Between Church and State: The Lives of Four French Prelates in the Late Middle Ages*, trans. Arthur Goldhammer (Chicago, 1991).

Hanlon, Gregory, *Early Modern Italy, 1550–1800*, European Studies Series (London, 2000).

Harrison, Mark, *Disease and the Modern World: 1500 to the Present Day* (Cambridge, 2004).

Henderson, John, 'Epidemics in Renaissance Florence: Medical Theory and Government Response', in Bulst and Delort, *Maladies et société*, 165–86.

____ 'The Black Death in Florence: Medical and Communal Responses', in Steven Basset (ed.) *Death in Towns: Urban Response to the Dying and the Dead, 100–1600* (Leicester, 1992), 136–50.

____ *Piety and Charity in Late Medieval Florence* (Oxford, 1994).

____ 'Charity and Welfare in Early Modern Tuscany', in Grell, Cunningham, and Arrizabalaga, *Health Care and Poor Relief*, 56–86.

____ *The Renaissance Hospital: Healing the Body and Healing the Soul* (New Haven, 2006).

____ 'Public Health, Pollution and the Problem of Waste Disposal in Early Modern Tuscany', in S. Cavaciocchi (ed.), *Le interazioni fra economia e ambiente biologico nell'Europa preindustriale. Secc. XIII-XVIII*. XLI Settimana di Studi, Prato, 26–30 aprile 2009 (Florence, forthcoming, 2010).

Herlihy, David, *The Black Death and the Transformation of the West*, Cohn ed. and introd. (Cambridge, MA, 1997).

Herlihy, David, and Christiane Klapisch-Zuber, *Les Toscans et leurs familles: Une étude du Catasto de 1427* (Paris, 1978).

Hipp, Elizabeth, 'Poussin's The Plague at Ashdod: A Work of Art in Multiple Contexts', in Franco Mormando and Thomas Worcester (eds), *Piety and Plague from Byzantium to the Baroque* (Kirksville, MO, 2007), 177–224.

Hirsch, Rudolf, *Printing, Selling and Reading, 1450–1550*, 2nd edn (Wiesbaden, 1974).

Horden, Peregrine, 'Ritual and Public Health in the Early Medieval City', in Sally Sheard and Helen Power (eds), *Body and City: Histories of Urban Public Health*, (Aldershot, 2000), 17–40.

Israel, Jonathan, 'Counter-Reformation, Economic Decline, and the Delayed Impact of the Medical Revolution in Catholic Europe, 1550–1750', in Grell, Cunningham, and Arrizabalaga, *Health Care and Poor Relief*, 40–55.

Jarcho, Saul, *Italian Broadsides Concerning Public Health: Documents from Bologna and Brescia in the Mortimer and Anna Neinken Collection, New York Academy of Medicine* (Mt. Kisco, 1986).

Jones, Colin. 'Plague and Its Metaphors in Early Modern France', *Representations*, 53 (1996): 97–127.

Kinzelbach, Annemarie, 'Infection, Contagion, and Public Health in Late Medieval and Early Modern German Imperial Towns', *Journal of the History of Medicine and Allied Sciences*, 61/3 (2006): 369–89.

Kiple, Kenneth F, 'Scrofula: The King's Evil and Struma africana', in Kiple (ed.), *Plague, Pox and Pestilence* (London, 1997), 44–9.

La Cava, A. Francesco, *La peste di S. Carlo: Note storico—Mediche sulla peste del 1576* (Milan, 1945).

La Croix, E., 'Vergelijkende studie van de opvattingen omtrent oorzaken, ziektemechanismen entherapieën van pest op basis van de Pesttraktaten van de Medische Faculteit te Parijs (1348–1349), van Joannes de Vesalia (na 1454), en van Thomas Montanus (1669), *Koninklijke Academie voor Geneeskunde van België*, 61/2 (1999): 325–61.

Laforce, F. Marc, et al., 'Clinical and Epidemiological Observations on an Outbreak of Plague in Nepal', *Bulletin of WHO*, 45 (1971): 693–706.

Laughran, Michelle Anne, 'The Body, Public Health and Social Control in Sixteenth-Century Venice' (University of Connecticut, PhD thesis, 1998).

Leven, K. H., ' "At Times these Ancient Facts Seem to Lie before Me Like a Patient on a Hospital Bed"—Retrospective Diagnosis and Ancient Medical History', in H. F. J. Horstmanshoff and M. Stol (eds), *Magic and Rationality in Ancient Near Eastern and Graeco-Roman Medicine* (Leiden, 2004), 369–86.

Lindemann, Mary, *Medicine and Society in Early Modern Europe* (Cambridge, 1999).

Little, Lester, *Plague and the End of Antiquity: The Pandemic of 541–750* (Cambridge, 2007).

—— 'Life and Afterlife of the First Plague Pandemic', in idem, *Plague and the End of Antiquity*, 3–32.

Lombardi, Daniela, '1629–1631: crisi e peste a Firenze', *Archivio Storico Italiano*, no. 499 (1979): 3–50.

Lyttelton, Adrian (ed.), *Liberal and Fascist Italy* (Oxford, 2002).

Macchiavello, Atilio, 'Plague' in R. B. H. Gradwohl, Luiz Benitez Soto, and Oscar Felsenfeld (eds), *Clinical Tropical Medicine* (London, 1951), 444–76.

Maclean, Ian, *Logic, Signs, and Nature in the Renaissance: The Case of Learned Medicine* (Cambridge, 2002).

McNeill, William, *Plagues and Peoples* (New York, 1976).

Manson's Tropical Diseases, ed. Philip H. Manson-Bahr, 7th edn (London, 1921).

Manson's Tropical Diseases, ed. P. E. C. Manson-Bahr and D. R. Bell, 19th edn (London, 1987).

Manson's Tropical Diseases, ed. G C. Cook and Alimuddin Zumla, 20th edn (London, 1996).

Manson's Tropical Diseases, ed. G. C. Cook and Alimuddin I. Zumla, 22nd edn (Edinburgh, 2009).

Maragi, Mario, 'La santé publique dans les anciens status de la ville de Bologne (1245–1288)', *Histoire des sciences médicales*, 17 (1983): 81–7.

Martin, A. Lynn, *Plague? Jesuit Accounts of Epidemic Disease in the 16th Century* (Kirksville, MO, 1996).

Martinez Vinueza, Juan, 'Peste eruptiva (viruela pestosa) y angina pestosa: formas raras de la peste', *Boletin de la Officina Sanitaria Panamericana (SP)* 9 (1930): 1189–95.

Mavalankar, Dileep V., 'Indian "Plague" Epidemic: Unanswered Questions and Key Lessons', *Journal of the Royal Society of Medicine*, 98 (1995): 547–51.

Michielse, H. C. M., 'Policing the Poor: J. L. Vives and the Sixteenth-Century Origins of Modern Social Administration', *Social Service Review*, 64 (1990): 1–21.

Moote, A. Lloyd and Dorothy C. Moote, *The Great Plague: The Story of London's Most Deadly Year* (Baltimore, 2004).

Mormando, Franco and Thomas Worcester (eds), *Piety and Plague from Byzantium to the Baroque* (Kirksville, MO, 2007).

Moseng, Ole Georg, 'Climate, Ecology and Plague: The Second and Third Pandemic Reconsidered', in Bisgaard and Søndergaard, *Living with the Black Death*, 23–46.

Naso, Irma. 'Les hommes et les épidémies dans l'Italie de la fin du Moyen Age: Les réactions et les moyens de défense entre peur et méfiance', in Bulst and Delort, *Maladies et société*, 307–26.

Nicoud, Marilyn, 'Médecine et prévention de la santé à Milan à la fin du Moyen Age', in Philippe Bourdin (ed.), *Assainissement et salubrité publique en France méridionale à la fin du Moyen Age-Epoque moderne* (Clermont-Ferrand, 2001), 23–37.

_____ *Les régimes de santé au Moyen Age: Naissance et diffusion d'une écriture médicale (XIIIe-XVe siècle)*, 2 vols (Rome, 2007).

Nutton, Vivian, 'Continuity or Rediscovery? The City Physician in Classical Antiquity and Mediaeval Italy', in Andrew W. Russell (ed.), *The Town and State Physician in Europe from the Middle Ages to the Enlightenment*, Wolfenbütteler Forschungen, 17 (Wolfenbüttel, 1981), 9–46.

_____ 'Seeds of Disease: An explanation of contagion and infection from the Greeks to the Renaissance', *Medical History*, 27 (1983): 1–34.

_____ 'Humanist Surgery', in Andrew Wear, Roger French, and I. M. Lonie (eds), *The Medical Renaissance of the Sixteenth Century* (Cambridge, 1985), 75–99.

_____ 'Introduction', in his *Pestilential Complexities*, 1–16.

_____ 'The Reception of Fracastoro's Theory of Contagion: The Seed That Fell among the Thorns?', *OSIRIS*, 2nd series 6 (1990): 196–234.

_____ 'Medicine in Medieval Western Europe, 1000–1500', in Conrad et al., *The Western Medical Tradition*, 139–214.

Nutton, Vivian, 'The Changing Language of Medicine, 1450–1550', in Olga Weijers
    (ed.), *Vocabulary of Teaching and Research Between Middle Ages and Renaissance: Pro-
    ceedings of the Colloquium, London, Warburg Institute, 11-12 March 1994* (Turnhout,
    1995), 184–98.

_____ 'Medicine in the Greek World, 800–50 BC', in Conrad et al., *The Western Medical
    Tradition*, 11–38.

_____ 'Roman Medicine, 250 BC to AD 200', in Conrad et al., *The Western Medical
    Tradition*, 39–71.

_____ *Ancient Medicine* (London, 2004).

_____ 'Books, Printing and Medicine in the Renaissance', *Medicina nei Secoli, arte e
    scienza*, 17/2 (2005): 421–442.

_____ 'With Benefit of Hindsight: Girolamo Mercuriale and Simone Simoni on Plague',
    Medicina & storia: Rivisita di Storia della Medicina e della Sanità, 11 (2006):
    5–19.

_____ 'The Fortunes of Galen', in R. J. Hankinson (ed.), *The Cambridge Companion to
    Galen* (Cambridge, 2008), 355–90.

_____ (ed.), *Vocabulary of Teaching and Research between Middle Ages and Renaissance: Pro-
    ceedings of the Colloquium, London, Warburg Institute, 11–12 March 1994* (Turnhout,
    1995), 184–98.

_____ (ed.), *Pestilential Complexities: Understanding Medieval Plague* (*Medical History*,
    Supplement No. 27) (London, 2008).

Niebyl, Peter H., 'The Non-Naturals', *Bulletin of the History of Medicine*, 45 (1971):
    486–92.

Ongaro, Giuseppe and Elda Martellozzo Forin, 'Girolamo Mercuriale e lo studio di
    Padova', in Alessandro Arcangeli and Nutton (eds), *Girolamo Mercuriale: Medicina e
    cultura nell'Europa del Cinquecento, Atti del convegno "Girolamo Mercuriale e lo spazio
    scientifico e culturale del Cinquecento" (Forlì, 8–11 novembre 2006)* (Florence, 2008),
    29–50.

Palmer, Richard J., 'The Control of Plague in Venice and Northern Italy, 1348–1600'
    (University of Kent at Canterbury, PhD thesis, 1978).

_____ 'Nicolò Massa, his family and his fortune', *Medical History*, 25 (1981): 385–410.

_____ 'The Church, Leprosy and Plague in Medieval and Early Modern Europe', in
    Studies in Church History, 19 (1982): 79–99.

_____ 'Physicians and the Inquisition in Sixteenth-Century Venice', in Grell and Cun-
    ningham (eds), *Medicine and the Reformation* (London, 1993), 118–33.

_____ 'Physicians and the State in Post-Medieval Italy', in Russell, *The Town and State
    Physician*, 47–61.

_____ 'Girolamo Mercuriale and the plague of Venice', in Arcangeli and Nutton, *Girolamo
    Mercuriale*, 51–65.

Panseri, Guido, 'La nascita della polizia medica: l'organizzazione sanitaria nei vari Stati
    italiani', in Gianni Micheli (ed.), *Storia d'Italia: Annali 3: Scienza e tecnica nella cultura
    e nella società dal Rinascimento a oggi* (Turin, 1980), 155–96.

Park, Katherine, 'Natural Particulars: Medical Epistemology, Practice, and the Literature
    of Healing Springs', in Grafton and Siraisi, *Natural Particulars*, 346–67.

Pasa, Marco, 'Quadri urbani e strutture territori nel Veronese: L'epoca veneta ed i caratteri
    originari', *Storia urbana*, 95 (2001), 139–66.

Pastore, Alessandro, 'Note su criminalità e giustizia in tempo di peste: Bologna e Ginevra fra '500 e '600', in *Città italiane del '500 tra riforma e controriforma: Atti del Convegno Internazionale di Studi. Lucca, 13–15 ottobre 1983* (Lucca, 1988), 31–43.

_____, Crimine e giustizia in tempo di peste nell'Europa moderna (Bari, 1991).

Pennuto, Concetta, *Simpatia, fantasia e contagio: Il pensiero medico e il pensiero filosofico di Girolamo Fracastoro* (Rome, 2008).

Pettegree, Andrew, 'Centre and Periphery in the European Book World', *Transactions of the Royal Historical Society*, 6th ser. 18 (2008): 101–28.

Pinault, J. R., *Hippocratic Lives and Legends* (Leiden, 1992).

Pitrè, G., *Medici, barbieri e speziali antichi in Sicilia* (Rome, 1939).

Pomata, Gianna, *Contracting a Cure: Patients, Healers, and the Law in Early Modern Bologna* (Baltimore, 1998).

Porter, Roy, 'The Eighteenth Century', in Conrad et al., *The Western Medical Tradition*, 371–476.

_____ *The Greatest Benefit to Mankind: A Medical History of Humanity from Antiquity to the Present* (London, 1997).

Preti, C., 'Giovanni Filippo Ingrassia', in *DBI*, 62 (2004), 396–9.

Preto, Paolo, *Peste e società a Venezia nel 1576* (Venice, 1978).

_____ 'Catalogo: Le pesti dell'età moderna: Scheda', in *Venezia e la peste*, 127–48.

_____ 'Le grandi pesti dell'età moderna 1575–7 e 1630–1', in *Venezia e la peste*, 123–6.

_____ 'Peste e demografia: L'età moderna: le due pesti del 1575–77 e 1630–1', in *Venezia e la peste*, 97–8.

_____ 'La società veneta e le grandi pesti dell'età moderna', in *Storia della cultrua veneta* 4/II (1984) 377–406.

_____ *Epidemia, paura e politica nell'Italia moderna* (Bari, 1987).

Pullan, Brian, *Rich and Poor in Renaissance Venice* (Oxford, 1971).

_____ 'Plebi urbane e plebi rurali: da poveri a proletari', in Ruggiero Romano and Corrado Vivanti (eds), *Storia d'Italia: Annali I: Dal feudalismo al capitalismo* (Turin, 1978), 981–1047.

_____ 'Plague and Perceptions of the Poor in Early Modern Italy', in Terence Ranger and Paul Slack (eds), *Epidemics and Ideas: Essays on the Historical Perception of Pestilence* (Cambridge, 1992), 101–23.

Pullapilly, Cyriac K., 'Agostino Valier and the Conceptual Basis of the Catholic Reformation', *The Harvard Theological Review*, 85/3 (1992): 307–33.

Putnam, Robert, *Making Democracy Work: Civic Traditions in Modern Italy* (Princeton, 1992).

Pyle, Gerald F., *The Diffusion of Influenza: Patterns and Paradigms* (Totowa, NJ, 1986).

Radicchi, Rino, 'Descrizione della peste di Firenze dell'anno 1527 di Niccolò Machiavelli', *Lanternino*, 12 (1989): 11–16.

Rawcliffe, Carole, 'The Concept of Health in Late Medieval Society', in S. Cavaciocchi (ed.), *Le interazioni fra economia e ambiente biologico nell'Europa preindustriale. Secc. XIII–XVIII. XLI Settimana di Studi, Prato, 26–30 aprile 2009* (Florence, forthcoming, 2010).

Redmond, Collen Linda, 'Girolamo Donzellino, Medical Science and Protestantism in the Veneto', (Stanford University, PhD thesis, 1984).

Rees, Willaim, 'The Black Death in England and Wales, as exhibited in Manorial Documents', *Proceedings of the Royal Society of Medicine*, 16: *Section of the History of Medicine* (1922–3): 27–45.

Restifo, Giuseppe. *Le ultime piaghe: le pesti nel mediterraneo (1720–1820)* (Milan, 1994).

Rocciolo, Domenico, '*Cum suspicione morbi contagiosi obierunt*: Società, religione e peste a Roma nel 1656–1657', in Fosi, *La Peste a Roma*, 111–34.

Rinaldi, Stefania Mason (ed.), 'Catalogo: le immagini della peste', 246–86.

Risse, Guenter, 'Medicine in the Age of Enlightenment', in Andrew Wear (ed.), *Medicine in Society: Historical Essays* (Cambridge, 1992), 149–96.

Robin, Diana, *Publishing Women: Salons, the Presses, and the Counter-Reformation in Sixteenth-Century Italy* (Chicago, 2007).

Rodenwaldt, Ernst, *Pest in Venedig 1575–1577: Ein Beitrag zur Frage der Infektkette bei den Pestepidemien West-Europas* (Heidelberg 1953).

Rosen, George, *A History of Public Health* (New York, 1958).

—— 'Cameralism and the Concept of Medical Police', in Rosen, *From Medical Police to Social Medicine: Essays on the History of Health Care* (New York, 1974), 120–41.

—— 'The Fate of the Concept of Medical Police, 1780–1890', in *From Medical Police*, 142–58.

Russell, Andrew W. (ed.), *The Town and State Physician in Europe from the Middle Ages to the Enlightenment*, Wolfenbütteler Forschungen, 17 (Wolfenbüttel, 1981).

Saba, Franco, 'Una parrocchia milanese agli inizi del XVII secolo: S. Lorenzo Maggiore, Materiali per una storia demografica', *Nuova Rivista Storica*, LIX (1975): 407–57.

Sabine, Ernst L., 'Butchering in Medieval London', *Speculum*, 8 (1933): 335–53.

—— 'Latrines and Cesspools of Mediaeval London', *Speculum*, 9 (1934): 303–21.

Sallares, Robert, 'Ecology, Evolution, and Epidemiology of Plague', in *Plague and the End of Antiquity*, 231–89.

San Juan, Rose Marie, 'The Contamination of the Modern City: Marketing Print in Rome during the Plague of 1656–1657', in Fosi, *La Peste a Roma*, 205–25.

Sansa, Renato, 'Strategie di prevenzione a confronto l'igiene urbana la peste romana del 1656–1657', in Fosi, *La Peste a Roma*, 93–109.

Scott, Susan and Christopher J. Duncan, *Biology of Plagues: Evidence from Historical Populations* (Cambridge, 2001).

—— *Return of the Black Death: The World's Greatest Serial Killer* (Chichester, 2004).

Schutte, A. Jacobson, 'Donzellini, Girolamo', *DBI*, 41 (1992), 238–43.

Singer, Charles, *The Development of the Contagium Vivum* (London, 1913).

Siraisi, Nancy, 'The *Expositio Problematum Aristotelis* of Peter of Abano', *Isis* 60 (1970): 321–39.

—— *History, Medicine, and the Traditions of Renaissance Learning* (Ann Arbor, MI, 2007).

—— *Medieval and Early Renaissance Medicine: An Introduction to Knowledge and Practice* (Chicago, 1990).

Slack, Paul, 'The Disappearance of Plague: An Alternative View', *Economic History Review*, new series 33 (1981): 469–76.

—— 'Responses to Plague in Early Modern Europe: The Implications of Public Health', *Social Research*, 55 (1988), 433–53.

—— *The Impact of Plague in Tudor and Stuart England*, 2nd edn (Oxford, 1990).

Smail, Daniel Lord, 'Telling Tales in Angevin Courts', *French Historical Studies*, 20 (1997): 183–215.

Smith, Michael, 'Plague', in *Manson's Tropical Diseases*, 22nd edn, 1119–26.

_____ and N. D. Thanh, 'Plague', in *Manson's Tropical Diseases*, 20th edn, 918–24.

Sonnino, Eugenio, 'Cronache della peste a Roma: Notizie dal Ghetto e lettere di Girolamo Gastaldi (1656–1657)', in Fosi, *La Peste a Roma*, 35–74

Sontag, Susan, *Illness as Metaphor and Aids and Its Metaphors* (London, 1991).

Stevens, Jane. 'The *lazaretti* of Venice, Verona and Padua (1520–1580)' (Cambridge, PhD thesis, 2007).

Tagarelli, Sebastiano. *La peste di Noja (1815–1816)* (Noicattaro 1934).

Taschereau, J. (ed.), *Catalogie des sciences médicales* (Paris, 1857).

Temkin, Oswei, *Galenism: Rise and Decline of a Medical Philosophy* (Ithaca, 1973).

_____ 'The Scientific Approach to Disease: Specific Entity and Individual Sickness', in A. C. Crombie (ed.), *Scientific Change: Historical Studies in the Iintellectual, Social and Technical Conditions for Scientific Discovery . . .* (London, 1963), 629–47.

Testa, Antonia Pasi, 'Alle origini dell'Ufficio di Sanità nel Ducato di Milano e Principato di Pavia', *Archivio Storico Lombardo*, CII (1977), 376–86.

Thorndike, Lynn, 'The Blight of Pestilence on Early Modern Civilization', *American Historical Review*, 32 (1927): 455–74.

_____ 'A Pest Tractate before the Black Death', *Sudhoffs Archiv für Geschichte der Medizin*, 23 (1930): 346–56.

_____ 'Sanitation, Baths, and Street-Cleaning in the Middle Ages and Renaissance', *Speculum*, 3 (1928): 192–203.

Toppi, Nicolò, *Biblioteca napoletana, et apparato a gli huomini illustri in lettere di Napoli, e del Regno* (Naples, 1678).

Trevor-Roper, Hugh, *Europe's Physician: The Various Life of Sir Theodore de Mayerne* (New Haven, 2006).

Trillat, A, 'Étude historique sur l'utilisation des feux et des fumées: Comme moyen de défense contre la peste', *Annales de l'nistitut Pasteur*, 19 (1905): 734–52.

Varanini, Gian Maria, 'La peste del 1347–50 e i governi dell'Italia centro-settentrionale: un bilancio', in *La Peste Nera: Dati di una realtà ed elementi di una interpretazione. Atti del XXX Convegno storico internazionale, Todi, 10–13 ottobre 1993* (Spoleto, 1994), 285–317.

Venezia et la peste: 1348-1797 (mostra a cura del Comune di Venezia) (Venice, 1980).

Wallis, Patrick, 'Plagues, Morality and the Place of Medicine in Early Modern England', *English Historical Review*, 121 (2006): 1–24.

Walløe, Lars, 'Medieval and Modern Bubonic Plague: Some Clinical Continuities', in Nutton, *Pestilential Complexities*, 59–73.

_____ *Plague and Population: Norway 1350–1750* (Oslo, 1995).

Watson, Gilbert, *Theriac and Mithridatium: A Study in Therapeutics* (London, 1966).

Wear, Andrew, 'Medicine in Early Modern Europe, 1500–1700', in Conrad et al., *The Western Medical Tradition*, 215–361.

_____ *Knowledge and Practice in English Medicine, 1550–1680* (Cambridge, 2000).

Webster, Charles, *The Great Instauration: Science, Medicine and Reform 1626–1660* (London, 1975).

_____ 'The Historiography of Medicine', in Pietro Corsi and Paul Weindling (eds), *Information Sources in the History of Science and Medicine* (London, 1983).

Wheeler, Jo, 'Stench in Sixteenth-Century Venice', in Alexander Cowan and Jill Steward (eds), *The City and the Senses: Urban Culture Since 1500* (Aldershot, 2007), 25–38.

Wilkins, Ernest H., 'On Petrarch's *Ad Seipsum* and *I' vo pensando*', *Speculum*, 32 (1957): 84–91.

Winslow, Charles-Edward Amory, *The Conquest of Epidemic Disease* (Princeton, 1943).

Worcester, Thomas, 'Plague as Spiritual Medicine and Medicine as Spiritual Metaphor: Three Treastises by Etienne Binet, S.J. (1569–1639)', in Mormando and Worcester, *Piety and Plague from Byzantium to the Baroque*, 224–36.

Zanetti, D. E., 'La morte a Milano nei secoli XVI–XVIII: Appunti per una ricerca, *Rivista Storica Italiana*, 88 (1976): 804–52.

Zitelli, Andreina (ed.), 'Catalogo: le teorie mediche sulla peste', in *Venezia e la peste*, 29–70.

Index